Passing the
FRACP Written
Examination

QUESTIONS AND ANSWERS

This edition is also available as an e-book.
For more details, please see
www.wiley.com/buy/9781118454954
or scan this QR code:

Passing the FRACP Written Examination

QUESTIONS AND ANSWERS

Jonathan Gleadle
Professor of Medicine
Flinders University
Consultant Nephrologist
Flinders Medical Centre
Adelaide
South Australia

Tuck Yong
Senior Lecturer
Flinders University
Consultant Physician
Flinders Medical Centre
Adelaide
South Australia

Jordan Li
Senior Lecturer
Flinders University
Consultant Physician and Nephrologist
Flinders Medical Centre
Adelaide
South Australia

Surjit Tarafdar
Registrar in Nephrology and General Medicine
Flinders Medical Centre
Adelaide
South Australia

Danielle Wu
Registrar in Nephrology
Royal Adelaide Hospital
Adelaide
South Australia

WILEY Blackwell

This edition first published 2014 © 2014 by John Wiley & Sons, Ltd.

Registered office: John Wiley & Sons, Ltd, The Atrium, Southern Gate, Chichester, West Sussex, PO19 8SQ, UK

Editorial offices: 9600 Garsington Road, Oxford, OX4 2DQ, UK
The Atrium, Southern Gate, Chichester, West Sussex, PO19 8SQ, UK
111 River Street, Hoboken, NJ 07030-5774, USA

For details of our global editorial offices, for customer services and for information about how to apply for permission to reuse the copyright material in this book please see our website at www.wiley.com/wiley-blackwell

Library of Congress Cataloging-in-Publication Data

Gleadle, Jonathan, author.
  Passing the FRACP written examination : questions and answers / Jonathan Gleadle, Tuck Yong, Jordan Li, Surjit Tarafdar, Danielle Wu.
    p. ; cm.
  Passing the Fellow of the Royal Australasian College of Physicians written examination
  Includes bibliographical references and index.
  ISBN 978-1-118-45495-4 (pbk. : alk. paper) – ISBN 978-1-118-45502-9 (eMobi) – ISBN 978-1-118-45503-6 (ePdf) – ISBN 978-1-118-45504-3 (ePub)
  I. Yong, Tuck, author. II. Li, Jordan, author. III. Tarafdar, Surjit, author. IV. Wu, Danielle, author. V. Title. VI. Title: Passing the Fellow of the Royal Australasian College of Physicians written examination.
  [DNLM: 1. Medicine–Australia–Examination Questions. 2. Medicine–New Zealand–Examination Questions. WB 18.2]
  R834.5
  610.76–dc23
                                    2013017941

A catalogue record for this book is available from the British Library.

Wiley also publishes its books in a variety of electronic formats. Some content that appears in print may not be available in electronic books.

Cover image: © iStockphoto.com/Kalawin
Cover design by Sarah Dickinson

Set in 8.5/11 pt Frutiger Light by Toppan Best-set Premedia Limited
Printed and bound in Malaysia by Vivar Printing Sdn Bhd

Contents

Introduction

If you want to get out of medicine the fullest enjoyment, be students all your lives.

David Reisman (1867–1940)

Background to the examination

The Royal Australasian College of Physicians (RACP) examination consists of two parts – a written examination and a clinical examination. The written examination has two papers – Paper 1 (70 questions) and Paper 2 (100 questions), which focus on 'Basic Sciences' and 'Clinical Practice', respectively. The primary focus of this book is to help candidates prepare for the written component of the examination. The written examination is important because trainees are required to pass this before proceeding to the clinical examination and commencing advanced training in a subspecialty. Questions in the written examination are based on the curriculum and all candidates should familiarise themselves with the RACP curriculum for Basic Physician training, which is available electronically from the College website (http://www.racp.edu.au/page/curricula/adult-internal-medicine). It is vital to carefully read the most updated examination instructions (https://www.racp.edu.au/page/basic-training/written-exam), and any past questions provided by the RACP (https://www.racp.edu.au/share/page/site/pastexams/documentlibrary).

Although this book is written mainly for trainees in Australia and New Zealand, physician trainees in other programmes should still find these questions provide an opportunity for self-assessment and learning.

Questions are of two styles – multiple choice questions (MCQs) and extended matching questions (EMQs). In the MCQs, one correct answer must be selected from five possible responses to the stem. Commencing in 2013, EMQs will also be included. EMQs are organised into four parts:

1. **Theme.** There is a theme for each EMQ. This can include a symptom, investigation, diagnosis or treatment, e.g. back pain, dyspnoea, diabetes, corticosteroids.
2. **A list of possible answers, also called an option list.** This is a list of eight possible answers marked A–H.
3. **The question, also called the lead in statement.** This tells you what is being asked and clarifies the question being asked. It indicates the relationship between the clinical vignettes and the options.
4. **Clinical problems or vignettes, also called the stems.** This will usually consist of a clinical problem. There may be more than one clinical vignette for each theme.

This book has included a significant number of EMQs to help trainees familiarise themselves with this new and likely expanding format of assessment.

Question answering strategies

In Paper 1, the questions posed are commonly of the type, 'What is the likely mechanism for this disease process or treatment modality?', requiring the candidate to understand the underlying mechanism of disease pathophysiology and/or mechanism of actions for treatments that are used.

The knowledge and evidence gained from textbooks or journal articles and its application to clinical situations is one of the most challenging tasks in medicine. The retention of information, organisation of facts and recall of a myriad of data in relation to a patient is one of the crucial processes in clinical reasoning. One of the purposes of this book is to facilitate this process.

There are typically several steps in patient clinical management – making the diagnosis, assessing the severity of the disease, administering treatment according to the stage of disease and following the patient's response to treatment. Often in the MCQs or EMQs, more focused information is provided and candidates have to look for discriminating features to narrow the differential diagnosis. This is often a challenging but essential step to master as a physician. The question 'What is the next step?' is challenging because the next step may be more diagnostic evaluation, or staging, or therapy.

In general, the questions will assess knowledge of the following:
- Aetiology, epidemiology and genetics
- Anatomy, physiology, pathology and pathogenesis
- Clinical manifestations
- Diagnosis and investigations
- Treatment and prevention of disease
- Complications and outcomes
- Ethical, legal, social, economic, humanistic and historical aspects.

Candidates taking the written examination can sometimes be troubled by the wording of the questions, as when asked which features are *classical*, *characteristic* or *typical* of certain disorders, whether events are *likely*, *frequent*, *common*, *unusual* or *rare* and whether findings are expected in the *majority* or *minority* of cases or in *few* or *many* patients. For this reasons, we prefer, wherever possible, to minimise language problems with stems and responses. However it is not always possible to provide accurate numeric percentages (even approximate ones).

When answering questions and taking the examination we would emphasise the following:
- **Read the question carefully!**
- **Read the possible answers carefully!**
- **Answer all of the questions! (Make an informed guess if you are uncertain)**
- If you are uncertain about the correct response, look at which options you think are definitely incorrect. Think about why the question is being asked; what it

is 'getting at?'; what are the important 'teaching points' that are being tested? If you still are uncertain, move to the other questions and then come back to those you are not certain of.

'Hints and tips' for preparing for the FRACP examination

The best way of preparing for the physician examination, both written and clinical, is to learn from every encounter with a patient and the rest of the treating team (consultant physicians, advanced physician trainees, nurses and other health team members). Then, trainees are encouraged to use information gained from medical books (and increasingly electronic books) and journal articles to complement their education through reflection on their patient encounter. All trainees are encouraged to make the most of their learning encounters with patients; question what a symptom or sign indicates, what the most specific or sensitive diagnostic test to undertake is, what the evidence for the treatment being recommended is, how a complication can be prevented or a patient outcome improved. Even a small amount of reading or thought around a specific patient can be a very powerful learning experience.

Study effectively, do not just randomly read an article from a journal or a few pages in a textbook. Link your study to a question you could not answer or to a patient you saw last night. Cover the RACP curriculum fully, including the less obviously mainstream topics, such as statistics and psychiatry. Make sure you are studying not just reading. Make your own study notes, write down important facts, and practise relevant examination questions. Be disciplined about your study, switch off your phone, disconnect the internet and reward yourself with well-defined and enjoyable breaks.

Many trainees have found getting together as a small group to discuss and learn from each other is a useful way of preparing for this examination. Such small group dynamics are also a helpful way of supporting one another through the intense preparation.

Ensure that you have undertaken practice examinations multiple times under examination conditions and timings. **Make sure you have answered and understood all of the practice questions provided by the RACP.**

Using this book as a learning tool

This book is intended as a tool to direct basic physician trainees in their learning of core knowledge and skills in internal medicine, as well as the development of sound clinical reasoning. The content of this book sets out factual information, but also translates knowledge to clinical practice. Preparing for the physician examination is part of a lifelong process of learning, which should expand the trainee's attitude, skills and knowledge. It is this process of learning that enables a physician to cope with the ever-changing context in the practice of internal medicine. The trainee or groups of trainees can use this book in their personal studies or as part of their study group discussion. This book is not intended to cover the entire internal medicine curriculum comprehensively, but we have attempted to cover in particular topics that are rapidly evolving. For example, we have given attention to issues related to healthcare in an ageing population, disparity in indigenous health outcomes, advances in molecular science and genetics, and the complexity of care arising from multiple chronic illnesses in individual patients.

Whist we hope that many of the questions are similar to those in the actual examination, some are designed to 'teach' particularly important issues or to draw attention to contemporary topics. The commentaries explain the correct and incorrect responses. These commentaries have been prepared by the authors with input from experienced specialist physicians. For many subjects we have provided a reference, usually the best and most contemporary review we could identify at the time of writing. Reference texts are listed for further reading and as additional guides to study.

Some of the electronic or written resources on general internal medicine we recommend for use in the examination preparation are:

Up-to-date (www.uptodate.com)
New England Journal of Medicine (www.nejm.org)
Lancet (www.thelancet.com)
British Medical Journal (www.bmj.com)
Internal Medicine Journal (www.racp.edu.au/page/publications/internal-medicine-journal)
Medical Journal of Australia (www.mja.com.au)

Preparation time

In the lead-up to the examinations, it is important to maintain a healthy life of adequate sleep, exercise, food intake and socialization. Trainees are encouraged to set aside time for their clinical work, studies, family, social and recreational activities in a manner that is appropriate to each of them. It is best to study when the trainee's mind is fresh and able to concentrate on learning. As already mentioned, trainees should also make the most of their time in clinical work where experience will enhance the learning process.

Preparing for this examination should not lead to 'burn-out' for trainee-physicians. During the preparation period, the trainee should value the support received from family, peers and friends.

Disclaimer

Clinical practice and basic biomedical sciences are constantly changing and today's incontrovertible facts can quickly become outdated. Therefore, trainees are strongly encouraged to keep up-to-date with their reading and learning, and to check appropriate drug selection, dosage and route of administration. If you have any questions or suggestions, please write to us care of the publisher.

We hope that our contribution will assist you in your preparation for the examination in internal medicine. For every trainee that uses this book for their preparation, we wish you success in the RACP written examination or equivalent.

To all students of medicine who listen, look, touch and reflect;
may they hear, see, feel and comprehend.
Professor John B. Barlow in *Perspectives on the Mitral Valve*

Jonathan Gleadle
Tuck Yong
Jordan Li
Surjit Tarafdar
Danielle Wu

Acknowledgements

We would like to thank the following for their expert reviews and suggestions:
A/Professor Nicholas Antic FRACP, Consultant Respiratory and Sleep Physician
Paul Hakendorf MPH, Clinical Epidemiologist
Dr Matthew Doogue FRACP, Consultant Endocrinologist and Clinical
    Pharmacologist
Dr Ganessan Kichenadasse FRACP, Consultant Medical Oncologist
A/Professor Ann Kupa FRACP, Consultant Immunologist
Dr Stephen Lam FRACP, Intensive Care Consultant
Dr Timothy Lu FRACP, Consultant Rheumatologist
Dr Anand Rose FRACP, Consultant Respiratory and Sleep Physician
Dr Roshan Prakash, Advanced Trainee in Cardiology
Dr Su Yin Lau, Advanced Trainee in Gastroenterology and Hepatology

Basic physician trainees in the Southern Adelaide Local Health Network who
have 'tested' these questions and provided valuable feedback.

Features contained in your study aid

Question and answer sections are clearly indicated for quick reference.

Question sections:

1 Cardiology

Questions
BASIC SCIENCE

Answers can be found in the Cardiology Answers section at the end of this chapter.

1. Beta-blockers are recommended as first-line therapy for stable angina by both the American College of Cardiology/American Heart Association (ACC/AHA) and the European Society of Cardiology. Their mechanism of action in this condition is explained by:
- **A.** Plaque stabilisation
- **B.** Increased coronary blood flow
- **C.** Reduction in blood pressure
- **D.** Reduction in myocardial oxygen demand
- **E.** Reduction in systemic vasodilatation

CLINICAL

9. A 47-year-old man presents with chest pain. He reports moderately severe central chest pain of 24 h duration. The pain is worse with inspiration and is alleviated by maintaining an upright position. He also reports having had a fever recently. His medical history and physical examination are unremarkable. His ECG is shown below. What is the most likely diagnosis and the most appropriate treatment approach for this patient?

Answer sections:

16   Cardiology

Answers
BASIC SCIENCE

1. Answer D
The beneficial effects of beta-blockers in stable angina are secondary to reduction in myocardial oxygen demand. Myocardial oxygen demand varies directly according to the heart rate, contractility and left ventricular wall stress, each of which is decreased by beta-blockers.

CLINICAL

9. Answer B
The clinical diagnosis of acute pericarditis rests primarily on the findings of chest pain, pericardial friction rub and ECG changes (Imazio et al., 2010). The chest pain of acute pericarditis typically develops suddenly and is severe and constant over the anterior chest. In acute pericarditis, the pain worsens with inspiration – a response that helps to distinguish acute pericarditis from myocardial infarction.

Answers are linked to an authoritative reference to supplement your study. Scan the QR code on your mobile device to be taken directly to the reference.

 Phan, T.T., Shivu, G.N., Choudhury, A., et al. (2009). Multi-centre experience on the use of perhexiline in chronic heart failure and refractory angina: old drug, new hope. *Eur J Heart Failure* 11, 881–886.
http://eurjhf.oxfordjournals.org/content/11/9/881.long

1 Cardiology

Questions

BASIC SCIENCE

Answers can be found in the Cardiology Answers section at the end of this chapter.

1. Beta-blockers are recommended as first-line therapy for stable angina by both the American College of Cardiology/American Heart Association (ACC/AHA) and the European Society of Cardiology. Their mechanism of action in this condition is explained by:
  A. Plaque stabilisation
  B. Increased coronary blood flow
  C. Reduction in blood pressure
  D. Reduction in myocardial oxygen demand
  E. Reduction in systemic vasodilatation

2. Which one of the following compensatory mechanisms occurs in heart failure?
  A. Decreased ventricular preload
  B. Peripheral vasodilatation
  C. Increased renal sodium and water excretion
  D. Activation of the adrenergic nervous system
  E. Myocardial atrophy

3. Which is the most common origin of idiopathic ventricular tachycardia in the absence of structural heart disease?
  A. Aortic annulus
  B. Aortic sinuses
  C. Great cardiac vein
  D. Epicardium
  E. Right ventricular outflow tract

Passing the FRACP Written Examination: Questions and Answers, First Edition. Jonathan Gleadle, Tuck Yong, Jordan Li, Surjit Tarafdar, and Danielle Wu.
© 2013 John Wiley & Sons, Ltd. Published 2013 by John Wiley & Sons, Ltd.

4. Which one of the following viral infections is the commonest cause of myo-carditis in developed countries?

    A. Enterovirus

    B. Cytomegalovirus

    C. Hepatitis C virus

    D. Human immunodeficiency virus (HIV)

    E. Influenza virus

5. Which one of the following statements is correct regarding the electrical conduction and contraction of the heart?

    A. Electrical conduction is transmitted from the sino-atrial node to the bundle of His to the atrioventricular node to the Purkinje fibres to the myocardium

    B. Muscle contraction is associated with release of calcium by the sarcoplasmic reticulum

    C. Repolarisation of cardiac muscle is due to flow of potassium into the myocytes

    D. On an electrocardiogram the QRS complex corresponds to ventricular repolarisation

    E. The perfusion of the coronary arteries increases during systole

6. Perhexiline has been used in patients with chronic heart failure and refractory angina. Which one of the following statements about perhexiline is correct?

    A. It is metabolised by cytochrome P450 3A4

    B. About 7–10% of Caucasians are slow metabolisers

    C. The recommended dose for slow metabolisers is 100 mg on alternate days

    D. It can cause hyperglycaemia in diabetic patients

    E. It improves 5-year survival

Theme: Beta-blockers (for Questions 7 and 8)

    A. Propranolol

    B. Metoprolol

    C. Nebivolol

    D. Atenolol

    E. Pindolol

    F. Sotalol

    G. Bisoprolol

    H. Carvedilol

Select the drug that best fits the description in each of the following statements.

7. A non-selective beta-blocker with α_1-adrenoreceptor blocking activity.

8. A selective $\beta1$-adrenoreceptor blocker with nitric-oxide potentiating vasodilatory effect.

CLINICAL

9. A 47-year-old man presents with chest pain. He reports moderately severe central chest pain of 24 h duration. The pain is worse with inspiration and is alleviated by maintaining an upright position. He also reports having had a fever recently. His medical history and physical examination are unremarkable. His ECG is shown below. What is the most likely diagnosis and the most appropriate treatment approach for this patient?

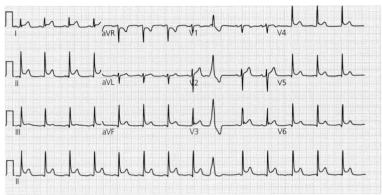

25mm/s 10mm/mV 100Hz 7.1.1 12SL 86 CID: 1   EID: 23 EDT: 12:03 29-JAN-2013 ORDER:

    A. Acute pericarditis; perform an echocardiogram in 1 week to confirm diagnosis

    B. Acute pericarditis; start a non-steroidal anti-inflammatory drug (NSAID)

    C. Acute pericarditis; start prednisolone

    D. ST elevation myocardial infarction; start thrombolytics

    E. Pericardial tamponade; requires pericardiocentesis

10. A 21-year-old Aboriginal woman presents with a sore throat for 2 days. She has fever (38°C) and coryza. On physical examination, the patient appears well but has a markedly infected posterior pharynx and exudates over her tonsils. Streptococcal pharyngitis is suspected. Which one of the following approaches to management is most appropriate?

    A. A throat swab is adequate to establish diagnosis in Aboriginal patients

    B. Intravenous benzylpenicillin 1.2 g four times a day for 10 days is the treatment of choice in eradicating Group A streptococci from the nasopharynx

    C. Treatment should be started within 9 days of the onset of symptoms to prevent acute rheumatic fever

    D. Aspirin can prevent rheumatic chorea

    E. Asymptomatic family contacts of patients with streptococcal pharyngitis should have throat swabs for streptococcal infection

11. A 50-year-old man presents with a 2-h history of severe chest pain. The pain started suddenly while eating, was constant and radiated to the back and inter-scapular region. His past medical history includes hypertension and hyperlipidae-mia. On examination, his heart rate is 120 beats/min and his blood pressure is 80/40 mmHg. Jugular venous pressure is not visualised. All peripheral pulses are present and equal. While stabilising the patient, which one of the following investigations should be undertaken?

    A. Serum lipase
    B. Computed tomography (CT) angiography of the chest
    C. D-dimer
    D. Lung ventilation–perfusion scan
    E. Upper gastrointestinal endoscopy

12. Which one of the following best describes the use of plasma brain natriuretic peptide (BNP) in the assessment of congestive heart failure (CHF)?

    A. BNP level is more useful in detecting diastolic heart failure than systolic heart failure
    B. Measurement of BNP is recommended as routine in the diagnosis of CHF
    C. BNP offers additional diagnostic information beyond that provided by echocardiogram
    D. BNP levels have been shown to predict all-cause mortality, including sudden death
    E. Plasma BNP or N-terminal pro-BNP measurement is not useful in patients presenting with new-onset breathlessness

13. A 46-year-old woman presents with a 2-week history of shortness of breath and ankle swelling. On examination her jugular venous pressure (JVP) is elevated and there are fine crackles at the bases of both lungs on auscultation. She was diagnosed with breast cancer a year ago and has been treated with surgery, doxorubicin, cyclophosphamide and radiotherapy. She has no cardiac risk factors or family history of cardiac disease. Computed tomography pulmonary angiogra-phy (CTPA) is normal and chest X-ray shows interstitial pulmonary oedema. What is the most likely cause for this presentation?

    A. Anthracycline cardiotoxicity
    B. Constrictive pericarditis
    C. Pulmonary fibrosis
    D. Radiation-induced cardiomyopathy
    E. Pulmonary embolism

14. All of the following drugs can be utilised in patients with heart failure. Which one is the most effective in improving systolic function?

    A. Spironolactone
    B. Angiotensin converting enzyme (ACE) inhibitor
    C. Digoxin

D. Frusemide

E. Hydralazine

15. A 72-year-old man describes substernal chest pressure while walking for more than 100 m and this is relieved by rest. His medical history is remarkable for hypertension and a myocardial infarction 3 years ago. His medications include aspirin 150 mg daily; metoprolol 50 mg twice daily; atorvastatin 40 mg daily; perindopril 5 mg daily; and isosorbide mononitrate 120 mg daily. He had a cardiac catheterisation 1 month ago that showed a left main coronary artery stenosis of 85%, a proximal left anterior descending artery stenosis of 70% and a 80% stenosis of the first obtuse marginal branch. His left ventricular ejection fraction (LVEF) was estimated at 45%. Which one of the following therapies would be most beneficial for this patient?

A. Addition of clopidogrel

B. Regular exercise programme

C. Percutaneous transluminal angioplasty (PCTA)

D. Coronary artery bypass grafting (CABG)

E. Transmyocardial revascularisation procedure (TMR)

16. The use of computed tomography coronary angiography (CTCA) is most appropriate in which one of the following patients?

A. An asymptomatic patient who has a strong family history of ischaemic heart disease

B. A patient with coronary stents presenting with chest pain in whom you suspect in-stent restenosis

C. A patient presenting with severe crushing chest pain and an ECG showing ST-elevation myocardial infarction (STEMI)

D. A patient presenting with chest pain and palpitations and an ECG showing rapid atrial fibrillation (heart rate: 125 beats/min)

E. A patient with chest pain with normal serial cardiac enzymes and ECGs who you think has a low-to-intermediate pre-test probability of coronary artery disease

17. An 86-year-old woman with a history of ischaemic heart disease, atrial fibrillation and type 2 diabetes presented to the emergency department with flank pain and symptomatic anaemia with haemoglobin of 69 g/L. After abdominal CT imaging, she was found to have a retroperitoneal haemorrhage. Three weeks prior to the presentation she had been changed from warfarin to dabigatran (taking a standard dose of 150 mg twice a day) for stroke prevention. Prior to this change, her INR has been within the target range for 6 years. What is the most likely explanation for the significant haemorrhagic complication in this patient after commencing dabigatran?

A. She is also taking phenytoin

B. She has impaired renal function

C. Her atrial fibrillation had reverted to sinus rhythm
D. Her INR has not been checked during the 3 weeks on the new medication
E. She is also taking digoxin

18. A 60-year-old man has had an inferior myocardial infarction 5 days ago. Today he is feeling lightheaded and his pulse rate is 40 beats/min. Blood pressure is 85/65 mmHg. An ECG is done immediately. Which one of the following findings is an indication for temporary pacing?
   A. (ECG A)
   B. (ECG B)
   C. (ECG C)
   D. (ECG D)
   E. (ECG E)

ECG A

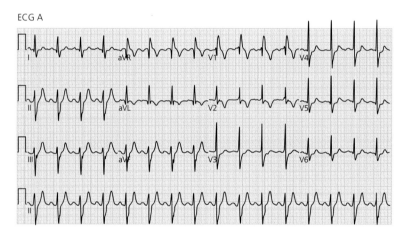

ECG B

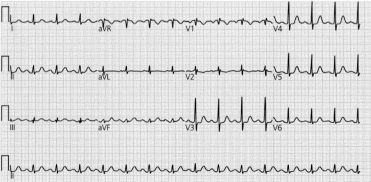

ECG C

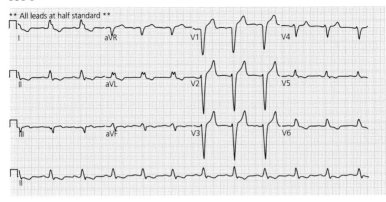

ECG D

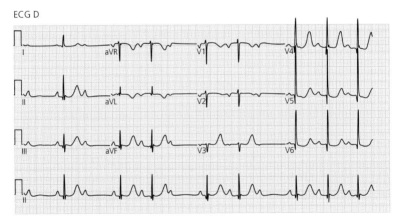

ECG E

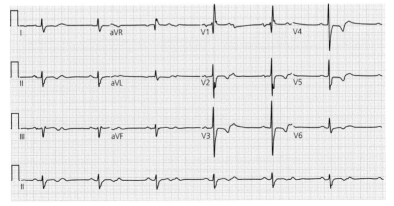

19. During pregnancy, which one of the following heart diseases is associated with the highest maternal mortality?
   A. Aortic stenosis
   B. Atrial septal defect
   C. Coarctation of aorta
   D. Eisenmenger syndrome
   E. Mitral stenosis

20. A 22-year-old man who is known to have hypertrophic cardiomyopathy undergoes physical and echocardiographic examination. Which one of the following findings is most predictive of this patient's risk of sudden cardiac death?
   A. Hypertension
   B. Double apex beat
   C. Atrial dilatation
   D. Intensity of systolic murmur
   E. Septal wall thickness of 3 cm or greater

21. Which is the commonest organism causing prosthetic valve infective endocarditis?
   A. *Staphylococcus aureus*
   B. Coagulase-negative staphylococcus
   C. *Streptococcus bovis*
   D. Candida
   E. *Streptococcus viridans*

22. A 16-year-old girl has a cardiac arrest while visiting her grandmother in hospital and has the ECG shown below. She revives after DC shock and all the subsequent ECGs show a prolonged QT interval. Blood tests rule out any metabolic derangement. Two of her first-degree relatives died suddenly at a young age. She should be treated with:

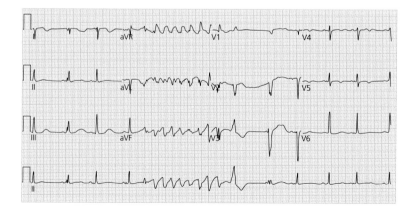

A. An implantable cardioverter–defibrillator
B. Beta-blocker
C. Quinidine
D. Sotalol
E. Verapamil

23. A 35-year-old man who is from an indigenous community in New Zealand has had mitral stenosis due to rheumatic heart disease. He has experienced some exertional dyspnoea recently. He attends a cardiology clinic with his most recent echocardiography results. Which one of the following features should prompt a referral for him to have a percutaneous balloon mitral valvuloplasty (PBMV)?
   A. Mitral orifice area of 1.2 cm^2 with minimal calcification
   B. The presence of severe mitral regurgitation
   C. Dyspnoea classified as New York Heart Association functional class I
   D. Mitral orifice area of 3 cm^2 with fusion of the subvalvular apparatus
   E. Large left atrial thrombus

24. A 68-year-old male farmer is transferred from a country hospital following a late presentation with acute myocardial infarction. He suffered severe chest pain 2 days ago but did not seek medical treatment. While you are examining the patient you hear a pericardial rub and make a diagnosis of peri-infarction pericarditis. Which one of the following statements is correct?
   A. Aspirin and heparin infusion should be stopped immediately
   B. The patient should be commenced on ibuprofen
   C. Reperfusion therapies are associated with a reduced incidence of peri-infarction pericarditis
   D. The patient should be commenced on high-dose prednisolone
   E. The echocardiogram is likely to show preserved ejection fraction

25. A 35-year-old man presents to the emergency department with a 1-h history of feeling his heart racing and slight chest discomfort. He has had two similar episodes previously following alcohol binges. An electrocardiography shows a regular narrow complex tachycardia with a rate of 180 beats/min. He otherwise feels well, his blood pressure is 98/68 mmHg and pulse oximetry on air shows oxygen saturation of 97%. What treatment should be administered?
   A. Electrical cardioversion
   B. Intravenous lignocaine
   C. Intravenous adenosine
   D. Intravenous digoxin
   E. Intravenous verapamil

26. A 45-year-man presents with a 24-h history of palpitations and chest discomfort. He had one similar episode 5 years ago. He is known to have asthma since childhood and uses a salbutamol inhaler two to three times a week. His initial examination reveals blood pressure of 110/60 mmHg, pulse rate 152 beats/min and oxygen saturation on room air of 95%. There is a scattered expiratory wheeze but no cardiac murmur. His ECG taken 5 years ago when he was admitted with an acute asthma attack is shown below (A) and his current ECG (B). His biochemistry results are unremarkable and the troponin T level is normal. Which one of the following medications should be administered to achieve rate control?

(A)

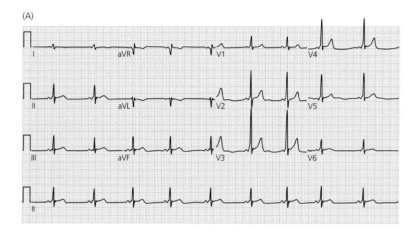

(B)

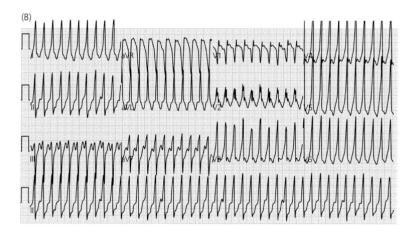

A. Intravenous adenosine
B. Intravenous atenolol
C. Intravenous loading dose of digoxin
D. Intravenous flecainide
E. Intravenous verapamil

27. A 75-year old man presents to hospital with a 2-week history of malaise and low-grade fever. He also has had chronic diarrhoea for the past 3 months and a 5-kg weight loss. On examination, his blood pressure is 100/70 mmHg, heart rate 110 beats/min and temperature of 38.4°C. A diastolic murmur (3/6) is heard at the left sternal edge. He is mildly anaemic with mean cell volume (MCV) of 76 fL (normal reference range 80–100 fL). Blood cultures grow *Streptococcus bovis* and transoesophageal echocardiography reveals vegetations on the aortic valve. What additional investigations should be undertaken?
  A. Cardiac magnetic resonance imaging
  B. Computed tomography of the abdomen
  C. Orthopantomogram (OPG)
  D. Colonoscopy
  E. White cell scan

28. Which one of the following disorders does NOT cause high-output heart failure?
  A. Hyperthyroidism
  B. Paget disease
  C. Brachio-cephalic arteriovenous fistula
  D. Cirrhosis
  E. Amyloidosis

29. A 60-year-old woman is diagnosed with *Streptococcus viridians* endocarditis involving the mitral valve. Which one of the following is a poor prognostic factor?
  A. Left ventricular ejection fraction of 50%
  B. Perivalvular extension of infection
  C. Recent dental extraction
  D. Previous adverse drug reaction to penicillin
  E. Previous abdominal aortic aneurysm repair

30. A 72-year-old man presents with a 2-day history of pain in his toes. He presented to another hospital with chest pain and received a coronary angiography 7 days ago. His other medical problems include hypertension, type 2 diabetes, chronic kidney disease with a serum creatinine of 156 μmol/L and osteoarthritis. He is taking aspirin, clopidogrel, metformin, atorvastatin and perindopril. On examination, he is afebrile, peripheral pulses are difficult to palpate and toes are painful to touch. His initial blood test results are shown below. Which one of the following diagnoses is most likely?

	Value	Reference range
Haemoglobin	82 g/L	115–155 g/L
White blood cells	13.0×10^9 cells/L	$4.0–11.0 \times 10^9$ cells/L
Platelet count	593×10^9 cells/L	$150–400 \times 10^9$ cells/L
Lactate dehydrogenase	344 U/L	110–230 U/L
Creatinine	287 μmol/L	80–120 μmol/L
Urate	0.69 μmol/L	0.21–0.48 μmol/L

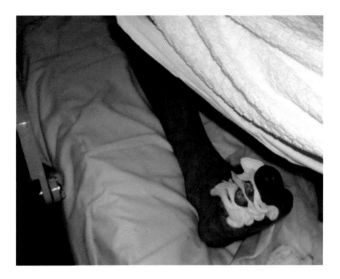

A. Contrast nephropathy
B. Renal embolus
C. Cholesterol emboli
D. Cryoglobulinaemia
E. Metformin-induced renal failure

31. A 72-year-old man who was admitted with an inferior myocardial infarction has a cardiac arrest on the way to the angiogram suite. After three cycles of cardiopulmonary resuscitation (CPR), two boluses of 1 mg epinephrine (adrenaline) and two defibrillator shocks, his electrocardiography remains unchanged and is shown below. What is the next most appropriate step?

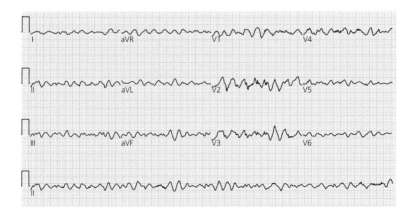

   A. 3 mg of epinephrine (adrenaline)
   B. 40 units of vasopressin
   C. 10 ml of 10% calcium chloride
   D. 10 ml of magnesium sulphate
   E. 300 mg of amiodarone

32. A 66-year-old woman is admitted for fixation of a left hip fracture. She has a history of osteoporosis and hypertension, but is otherwise in good health. She has no history of chest pain, but she says she experiences dyspnoea after walking about 400 m. She has a 30 pack-year smoking history but stopped 5 years ago. She is currently taking an angiotensin converting-enzyme inhibitor for her hypertension. What is the next most appropriate step in her assessment?
   A. Transthoracic echocardiography
   B. Dobutamine stress echocardiography
   C. Coronary angiography
   D. No further cardiac investigation
   E. Cardiac magnetic resonance imaging

33. Which one of the following is the modality of choice for diagnosing and monitoring transplant coronary artery disease after orthotopic heart transplantation?
   A. Clinical history
   B. Coronary angiography
   C. Exercise electrocardiography (ECG)
   D. Myocardial contrast echocardiography
   E. Intravascular ultrasound

34. A 53-year-old woman presents with dyspnoea and ankle oedema for 1 month. Her blood pressure is 110/80 mmHg. On examination, her jugular venous pressure rises with inspiration. She has a soft systolic murmur and a third heart sound. Electrocardiography (ECG) shows poor R-wave progression. An echocardiogram shows no pericardial effusion, increased ratio of early diastolic filling-to-atrial filling and systolic function is mildly impaired. Which one of the following is the most likely diagnosis?
   A. Restrictive cardiomyopathy
   B. Dilated cardiomyopathy
   C. Constrictive pericarditis
   D. Ischaemic cardiomyopathy
   E. Pulmonary embolus

35. A patient with acute fulminant myocarditis is most likely to present with:
   A. Dyspnoea
   B. Palpitations
   C. Hypotension
   D. Fever
   E. Chest pain

36. A 63-year-old woman is worried because her elder sister has just had a disabling stroke. Her blood pressure is 148/94 mmHg and her BMI is 30 kg/m². She wishes to reduce her blood pressure by non-pharmacological means. You should recommend which one of the following evidence-based measures?
  A. Weight reduction and a sodium intake of 5 g/day
  B. A diet reduced in sodium intake to less than 1 g/day
  C. Insist on starting an antihypertensive medication
  D. A diet reduced in potassium and sodium intake
  E. Weight reduction and the Dietary Approaches to Stop Hypertension (DASH) diet

Theme: Congenital heart disease (for Questions 37–40)
  A. Ostium secundum atrial septal defect
  B. Ventricular septal defect
  C. Patent ductus arteriosus
  D. Eisenmenger syndrome
  E. Tetralogy of Fallot
  F. Pulmonary stenosis
  G. Bicuspid aortic valve
  H. Coarctation of the aorta

For each of the following patients, select the most likely diagnosis.

37. A 32-year-old man presents to a hospital with fatigue and fever of 2 weeks' duration. He has no chest pain, dyspnoea or orthopnoea. He is known to have a 'heart murmur' since birth. On physical examination the only abnormal findings are a temperature of 38.3°C; a harsh systolic murmur is heard in the left lower sternal border; and the presence of small tender nodules are noted on two fingers. Which cardiac anomaly is most consistent with this patient's clinical presentation?

38. A 21-year-old woman is being evaluated for exertional dyspnoea. She has been having these symptoms for the past 4 months. Her medical history includes one episode of atrial fibrillation 1 month ago. Her physical examination shows fixed splitting of the second heart sound and a systolic murmur in the pulmonic area. An electrocardiogram shows slight right axis deviation and incomplete right bundle-branch block. A chest X-ray reveals an enlarged right atrium and main pulmonary artery. Which cardiac anomaly is the most likely diagnosis for this patient?

39. An 18-year-old man is being evaluated for a murmur and hypertension. He is asymptomatic. On physical examination his blood pressure is 170/100 mmHg in the right arm. The femoral pulses are diminished in amplitude compared to the radial pulses. His cardiac examination reveals a short mid-systolic murmur in the left infrascapular area. Which cardiac anomaly is the most likely diagnosis for this patient?

40. A 19-year-old woman presents with breathlessness on exertion and mild fatigue. She has no significant medical history. She does not smoke and is not on regular medication. Her cardiac examination reveals a systolic murmur at the second left intercostal space, which increases with inspiration. What is the most likely diagnosis for this patient?

Answers

BASIC SCIENCE

1. Answer D

The beneficial effects of beta-blockers in stable angina are secondary to reduction in myocardial oxygen demand. Myocardial oxygen demand varies directly according to the heart rate, contractility and left ventricular wall stress, each of which is decreased by beta-blockers.

Catecholamine activation of the beta-1 receptors, which are primarily found in the heart muscle, leads to increased heart rate, contractility and atrioventricular (AV) conduction, with a decrease in AV node refractoriness. Beta-blockers act by competitively inhibiting catecholamines from binding to these receptors.

No randomised trials have studied the effect of beta-blockers on survival in patients with angina, but survival benefits have been seen in patients with systolic heart failure and following myocardial infarction.

In the treatment of patients with angina, titrating the dose of beta-blocker to achieve a target resting heart rate of 55–60 beats/min is recommended. Adverse side effects can include bradycardia, AV node conduction problems, reduced contractility, bronchoconstriction (notably in patients who are taking a beta-2 adrenergic agonist), worsening of peripheral vascular disease, Raynaud phenomenon, fatigue, nightmares and erectile dysfunction.

2. Answer D

Compensatory mechanisms that are activated in heart failure include:
- Increased ventricular preload with ventricular dilatation and volume expansion
- Peripheral vasoconstriction, which initially maintains perfusion to vital organs
- Myocardial hypertrophy to preserve wall stress as the heart dilates
- Renal sodium and water retention to enhance ventricular preload
- Activation of the adrenergic nervous system, which increases heart rate and contractile function.

These processes are controlled mainly by activation of neurohormonal vasoconstrictor systems, including the renin–angiotensin–aldosterone system, the adrenergic nervous system, and non-osmotic release of arginine–vasopressin. These and other mechanisms contribute to the symptoms, signs and poor natural history of heart failure. In particular, an increase in wall stress along with neurohormonal activation facilitates pathological ventricular remodelling; this process has been closely linked to heart failure disease progression. Management of chronic heart failure targets these mechanisms and, in some instances, results in reverse remodelling of the failing heart (Krum and Abraham, 2009).

Krum, H. and Abraham, W.T. (2009). Heart failure. *Lancet* 373, 941–955.
http://www.ncbi.nlm.nih.gov/pubmed/19286093

3. Answer E

Ventricular tachycardia without structural heart disease is often referred to as idiopathic ventricular tachycardia (John et al., 2012). Idiopathic ventricular tachycardia in the absence of structural heart disease most often originates from the right ventricular outflow tract. Diseases such as arrhythmogenic right ventricular cardiomyopathy and sarcoidosis often need to be excluded before a diagnosis is made. Idiopathic ventricular tachycardia must be distinguished from ventricular tachycardia with structural heart disease, because the latter often warrants an implantable cardioverter defibrillator (ICD). Detection of ventricular scar on cardiac imaging can be helpful. Although idiopathic monomorphic ventricular tachycardia can cause syncope, sudden death is rare. Beta-blockers, calcium-channel blockers or catheter ablation are often effective.

Catheter ablation is a reasonable first-line therapy for many patients with symptomatic idiopathic ventricular tachycardias. Success rates approach 80–90% in experienced centres. Success rates are lower for those tachycardias arising in less common locations, such as along the aortic annulus, within the aortic sinuses, within the great cardiac vein or from the epicardium. Failure of ablation is usually due to the inability to induce the arrhythmia for precise localisation, or ventricular tachycardia origin in a location that is inaccessible or in close proximity to a coronary artery, which precludes safe ablation.

John, R.M., Tedrow, U.B., Koplan, B.A., et al. (2012). Ventricular arrhythmias and sudden cardiac death. *Lancet* 380, 1520–1529.
http://www.ncbi.nlm.nih.gov/pubmed/23101719

4. Answer A

Myocarditis is most commonly caused by a viral infection in developed countries (Magnani and Dec, 2006). Enteroviruses, including the Coxsackie virus, are the most commonly associated viral species. The Coxsackie virus has a myocardial affinity because of its easy entrance into the myocardial cell through the Coxsackie–adenoviral receptor, which triggers the host immune response.

Cytomegalovirus is commonly associated with post-transplantation myocarditis. Influenza myocarditis is often associated with haemorrhagic pulmonary oedema. HIV has been reported to cause myocarditis. However, it may be difficult to determine the exact cause of cardiac dysfunction because symptoms may be due to the inflammatory response to HIV; the HIV infection itself; or coexisting opportunistic infections, side effects of anti-retroviral treatment, or a combination of these causes.

Hepatitis C, adenovirus, parvovirus B19 and Epstein–Barr virus (EBV) have been reported to cause myocarditis.

Magnani, J.W., and Dec, G.W. (2006). Myocarditis: current trends in diagnosis and treatment. *Circulation* 113, 876–890.
http://circ.ahajournals.org/content/113/6/876.long

5. Answer B

Electrical propagation of the cardiac impulse is transmitted from the sino-atrial node to the anterior, middle, and posterior internodal tracts, to the AV node and to the bundle of His (AV bundle), and then via the right and left bundle branches to the Purkinje fibres and thence to the myocardium.

Myocytes have a negative membrane potential when at rest. Stimulation induces the opening of voltage-gated ion channels, leading to flow of cations into the cell. The positively charged ions enter the cell, causing the depolarisation characteristic of an action potential. The action potential spreads through the muscle network of T-tubules, depolarising the inner portion of the muscle fibre. The depolarisation activates L-type voltage-dependent calcium channels (dihydro-pyridine receptors) in the T-tubule membrane, which are in close proximity to calcium-release channels (ryanodine receptors) in the adjacent sarcoplasmic reticulum. Activated voltage-gated calcium channels physically interact with calcium-release channels to activate them, causing the sarcoplasmic reticulum to release calcium. Calcium release is the main trigger of muscle contraction by causing alterations in the binding of troponin and tropomyosin to actin and leading to the ATP-driven myosin–actin bonding, sliding and releasing interactions that generates contraction. Repolarisation occurs due to a flow of potassium out of the cardiac cells.

In an electrocardiogram the P wave corresponds to the depolarisation of the atria; the QRS complex to right and left ventricular depolarisation; the ST-T wave to ventricular repolarisation; the PR interval is the time from onset of atrial depolarisation (P wave) to onset of ventricular depolarisation (QRS complex); the QRS duration is duration of ventricular muscle depolarisation; and the QT interval is the duration of ventricular depolarisation and repolarisation.

During diastole the pressure within the left ventricle is lower than that in aorta, allowing blood to circulate into the heart itself through the epicardial coronary arteries.

6. Answer B

Perhexiline has been used in the treatment of congestive heart failure and refractory angina. It relieves symptoms of angina, improves exercise tolerance and increases workload needed to induce ischemia. The drug works in part by modifying myocardial substrate utilisation from fatty acids to carbohydrates, which is energetically more efficient for the heart to metabolise, thus reducing myocardial oxygen consumption. Study has demonstrated the effectiveness of perhexiline in relieving symptoms, but there is no evidence that it provides mortality benefit (Phan et al., 2009).

Its major side effects include hepatotoxicity, peripheral neuropathy and hypoglycaemia. To prevent these toxicities, perhexiline plasma levels should be closely monitored and maintained between 0.15 and 0.60 mg/L. Perhexiline is metabolised by cytochrome P450 2D6. Drug level monitoring is essential to identify patients who are slow metabolisers, which occurs in about 7–10% of Caucasians who harbour mutations in *CYP2D6*. In normal metabolisers, perhexiline's half-life is between 3 and 12 days. In slow metabolisers this half-life can be as long as 30 days. The usual loading dose is 200 mg twice a day for 3 days, then 100 mg/day. Blood is taken 3 days after commencing the drug to determine metaboliser status. If there is no metabolite peak, then the patient is a slow metaboliser, and the dose should be reduced to 100 mg weekly. If the metabolite is present, dose is continued at 100 mg daily. Plasma perhexiline trough concentrations should be monitored monthly until stable, then 3–6 monthly.

Phan, T.T., Shivu, G.N., Choudhury, A., et al. (2009). Multi-centre experience on the use of perhexiline in chronic heart failure and refractory angina: old drug, new hope. *Eur J Heart Failure* 11, 881–886.
http://eurjhf.oxfordjournals.org/content/11/9/881.long

7. Answer H

8. Answer C

Commentary for Questions 7 and 8:

Beta-adrenoreceptor blocking agents, commonly known as beta-blockers, are useful in the treatment of angina, myocardial infarction, cardiac failure, hypertension and cardiac arrhythmias. Beta-blockers given long-term have been shown to diminish mortality following acute myocardial infarction.

Some beta-blockers possess beta-agonist activity. Agents with partial agonist activity include pindolol, which causes little or no depression of resting heart rate (partial agonist effect) while blocking the increase in heart rate that occurs in response to exercise or the administration of a beta-agonist such as isoproterenol. The presence of partial agonist activity may be useful when bradycardia limits treatment in patients with slow resting heart rates. Pindolol also produces mild vasodilation. Agents with partial agonist activity cause less change in blood lipid levels than agents without agonist properties.

Non-selective beta-blockers, such as propranolol, sotalol, timolol and carvedilol, induce competitive blockade of both β_1 and β_2 receptors. Metoprolol and atenolol possess relative selectivity for the β_1 receptor. Although β_1(cardiac)-selective agents have the theoretical advantage of producing less bronchoconstriction and less peripheral vasoconstriction, a clear clinical advantage of cardioselective agents is unestablished. Bronchoconstriction may occur when β_1-selective agents are administered in therapeutic doses.

Various beta-blockers differ in their water and lipid solubility. The lipophilic agents (e.g. propranolol, metoprolol, bisoprolol and carvedilol) are readily absorbed from the gastrointestinal tract, metabolised by the liver, have large volumes of distribution and penetrate the central nervous system well. The hydrophilic agents (e.g. atenolol) are less readily absorbed, not extensively metabolised and have relatively longer plasma half-lives, resulting in their ability to be administered once per day. Hepatic impairment may prolong the plasma half-life of lipophilic agents whereas renal impairment may prolong the action of hydrophilic agents. Nebivolol is a $\beta 1$-receptor blocker with a nitric-oxide potentiating vasodilatory effect.

Carvedilol has both α_1-adrenoreceptor blockade and non-selective beta-blockade actions and is devoid of intrinsic sympathomimetic activity (Frishman, 1998). Carvedilol is indicated to slow the clinical progression of heart failure, as evidenced by reductions in hospitalisation rates and mortality. Contraindications to carvedilol therapy in patients with heart failure include severe decompensation requiring inotropic therapy, marked bradycardia, the sick sinus syndrome, and partial or complete atrioventricular block, unless a permanent pacemaker is in place.

Frishman, W.H. (1998). Carvedilol. *N Engl J Med* 339, 1759–1765.
http://www.ncbi.nlm.nih.gov/pubmed/10328713

CLINICAL

9. Answer B

The clinical diagnosis of acute pericarditis rests primarily on the findings of chest pain, pericardial friction rub and ECG changes (Imazio et al., 2010). The chest pain of acute pericarditis typically develops suddenly and is severe and constant over the anterior chest. In acute pericarditis, the pain worsens with inspiration – a response that helps to distinguish acute pericarditis from myocardial infarction. Low-grade fever and sinus tachycardia are often present. A pericardial friction rub can be detected in most patients when symptoms are acute. ECG changes are common in most patients with acute pericarditis, particularly in those with an infectious aetiology in which the associated inflammation in the superficial layer of myocardium is prominent. The characteristic change is an elevation in the ST segment in multiple leads. The diffuse distribution and the absence of reciprocal ST segment depression distinguish the characteristic pattern of acute pericarditis from acute myocardial infarction. Depression of the PR segment, which reflects superficial injury of the atrial myocardium, is as frequent and specific as ST segment elevation and is often the earliest ECG manifestation. Analgesic agents or non-steroidal anti-inflammatory drugs (NSAIDs) are often effective in reducing pericardial inflammation. Corticosteroids should be reserved for severe cases that are unresponsive to other therapy, because symptoms may recur after steroid withdrawal.

Imazio, M., Spodick, D.H., Brucato, A., Trinchero, R., and Adler, Y. (2010). Controversial issues in the management of pericardial diseases. *Circulation* 121, 916–928.
http://circ.ahajournals.org/content/121/7/916.long

10. Answer C

Acute rheumatic fever (ARF) remains common in the developing world. Indigenous populations in northern Australia have among the highest burden of ARF and rheumatic heart disease in the world, with one in 300 children developing ARF each year and up to 2% of people of all ages having rheumatic heart disease. Similar rates are seen throughout the Western Pacific region, including in Maori and Pacific Islander populations in New Zealand, where some of the most reliable data are available.

Oral penicillin V is the drug of choice in treating streptococcal pharyngitis; twice-daily dosing is as effective as four times a day dosing and may improve compliance. Group A streptococci (GAS) are isolated from throat swabs in less than 10% of ARF cases in New Zealand, and less than 5% of cases in Australian Aboriginal people. Streptococcal antibody titres are therefore crucial in confirming the diagnosis. The most commonly-used tests are the plasma anti-streptolysin O (ASO) and the anti-DNase B titres. Previous data suggest that a rise in the ASO titre occurs in 75–80% of untreated Group A streptococci pharyngeal infections, and that the addition of anti-DNase B titre increases the sensitivity of testing.

Treatment should be started within 9 days of the onset of symptoms to prevent rheumatic fever. Aspirin is recommended as the first-line treatment for arthritis or arthralgia in ARF. Sydenham chorea is self-limiting. Most cases will resolve within weeks and almost all cases within 6 months, although rare cases may last as long as 2–3 years. Because chorea is benign and self-limiting, and anti-chorea medications are potentially toxic, treatment should only be considered if the movements interfere substantially with normal activities. Aspirin does not have a significant effect on rheumatic chorea. Group A streptococci are responsible for only 5% of cases of pharyngitis in adults. Screening asymptomatic family contacts is controversial and probably unnecessary.

 RHDAustralia (ARF/RHD writing group), National Heart Foundation of Australia and the Cardiac Society of Australia and New Zealand (2012). *Australian Guideline for Prevention, Diagnosis and Management of Acute Rheumatic Fever and Rheumatic Heart Disease*, 2nd edn. National Heart Foundation of Australia. http://www.rhdaustralia.org.au/sites/default/files/guideline_0.pdf

11. Answer B

The sudden onset of chest pain radiating to the interscapular area and signs of shock suggest a diagnosis of acute aortic dissection, especially in those with risk factors such as hypertension, dyslipidaemia and peripheral vascular disease (Golledge and Eagle, 2008). Computed tomography (CT) angiography or echocardiography is usually needed in patients in whom acute aortic dissection is clinically suspected on the basis of presentation and initial investigations. A systematic review of the diagnostic accuracy of transoesophageal echocardiography, CT angiography and MRI reported a mean sensitivity and specificity of more than 95% for all three investigations. In addition to assisting in the diagnosis of aortic dissection, the results of imaging can help to plan management. Important findings include the extent of the dissection, the size of the true and false lumen, localisation of the intimal tear, the involvement of aortic branches, the presence and extent of aortic regurgitation, and the presence of periaortic haematoma, mediastinal haematoma, or effusion. Guidelines recommend the use of echocardiography or CT angiography, or both, in the initial imaging of patients suspected to have acute aortic dissection, whereas MRI is favoured for the assessment of chronic dissection. Contrast angiography is recommended in patients in whom visceral hypoperfusion is suspected or percutaneous interventions are being considered.

Patients can present with aortic dissection either in the ascending aorta (type A) or in the more distal aorta (type B). The risk factors most probably relate to a combination of inherited and acquired weakening of the aortic media and intimal disease. Marfan syndrome is an important risk factor for aortic dissection, especially in young patients. Other inherited disorders, including Ehlers–Danlos syndrome type IV and Turner syndrome, have been associated with aortic dissection.

 Golledge, J. and Eagle, K.A. (2008). Acute aortic dissection. *Lancet* 372, 55–66. http://www.ncbi.nlm.nih.gov/pubmed/18603160

12. Answer D

Brain natriuretic peptide (BNP) levels reflect the severity of congestive heart failure (CHF), the risk of hospitalisation and survival. Changes in BNP level in response to medical therapy also predict survival.

Plasma BNP or N-terminal pro-BNP measurement may be helpful in patients presenting with recent-onset dyspnoea; it has been shown to improve diagnostic accuracy with a high negative predictive value. BNP measurement has been demonstrated to be useful for differentiating dyspnoea caused by CHF from dyspnoea due to other causes, especially in the Emergency Department. A cut-off value of 100 pg/mL has a sensitivity of 90% and a specificity of 76%. However, routine use of BNP in the diagnosis of CHF is not recommended. There is no evidence that BNP provides additional diagnostic information to that provided by echocardiogram.

BNP levels appear more useful in detecting systolic heart failure than diastolic heart failure. BNP levels do not discriminate well between elderly female patients with diastolic heart failure (the most common patient group with this condition) and healthy age-matched controls.

 National Heart Foundation of Australia and the Cardiac Society of Australia and New Zealand (Chronic Heart Failure Guidelines Expert Writing Panel) (2011). *Guidelines for the Prevention, Detection and Management of Chronic Heart Failure in Australia Update 2011.* National Heart Foundation of Australia. http://www.heartfoundation.org.au/sitecollectiondocuments/chronic_heart_failure_guidelines_2011.pdf

13. Answer A

Cardiomyopathy and heart failure are well recognised complications of prolonged anthracycline treatment (Yeh and Bickford, 2009). Anthracycline cardiotoxicity can be divided into acute/sub-acute or late/chronic, with the latter being more common. In adults, chronic anthracycline-related cardiotoxicity typically presents within 1 year after finishing chemotherapy, with the peak time for the appearance of symptoms being about 3 months after the last dose. Late cardiotoxicity is characteristically seen in survivors of childhood malignancy treated with an anthracycline.

A number of risk factors for the development of chronic anthracycline cardiotoxicity have been identified. The strongest predictor is cumulative dose. Studies that have looked at the cumulative probability of doxorubicin-induced heart failure have found that it occurs in 3–5% at 400 mg/m^2, 7–26% at 550 mg/m^2 and 18–48% at 700 mg/m^2. However, intravenous administration, concomitant administration of other cardiotoxic chemotherapeutic agents (particularly paclitaxel, cyclophosphamide and trastuzumab), concurrent or prior chest irradiation, pre-existing cardiovascular disease or risk (including coronary artery disease, hypertension and diabetes mellitus) are also major risk factors.

Dexrazoxane is an EDTA-like chelator that significantly reduces the risk of chronic cardiotoxicity when used with anthracyclines. Dexrazoxane given with either doxorubicin or epirubicin significantly reduced the incidence of clinical and subclinical cardiotoxicity. It is recommended in patients who are being treated for metastatic disease and are receiving high cumulative doses of anthracyclines.

All patients should have a baseline echocardiogram and serial monitoring of myocardial function during therapy with anthracyclines. Although chest radiotherapy in the past was associated with significant cardiotoxicity, contemporary techniques with minimal exposure to the heart has lessened this complication.

Yeh, E.T. and Bickford, C.L. (2009). Cardiovascular complications of cancer therapy: incidence, pathogenesis, diagnosis, and management. *J Am Coll Cardiol* 53, 2231–2247.
http://www.ncbi.nlm.nih.gov/pubmed/19520246

14. Answer B

Pharmacological treatment of systolic heart failure consists of symptom relief with diuretics and disease modification is achieved with ACE inhibitors or angiotensin receptor blockers (ARBs), beta-blockers, spironolactone or a combination of hydralazine and isosorbide dinitrate (McMurray, 2010).

ACE inhibitors are the first-line therapy for patients with systolic heart failure; therapy should be initiated promptly and continued indefinitely. ACE inhibitors reduce ventricular size, increase the ejection fraction modestly and reduce symptoms.

The efficacy of ARBs is similar to ACE inhibitors but they are usually reserved for those who develop cough or other adverse effects with ACE inhibitors (on account of their higher cost). ARBs are sometimes prescribed for those who are symptomatic despite treatment with optimal doses of ACE inhibitors and beta-blockers.

Beta-blockers are essential first-line therapy in patients with heart failure and left ventricular systolic dysfunction. Treatment with beta-blockers improves systolic function, resulting in an increase in ejection fraction of 5–10%, and reduces symptoms. Bisoprolol, carvedilol or metoprolol CR/XL (metoprolol succinate, controlled release or extended release) can reduce the rate of hospital admissions and mortality by up to 34%.

Spironolactone is indicated in severe heart failure, that is NYHA class III or IV despite treatment with a diuretic, an ACE inhibitor (or ARB) and a beta-blocker. Digoxin when added to a diuretic and ACE inhibitor has no effect on mortality but may reduce risk of hospitalisation for heart failure.

Diuretic treatments with loop diuretics should be prescribed to minimise fluid retention and pulmonary oedema.

It is always important to also consider the underlying aetiology of the heart failure, correct this accordingly and address the possible need for anti-platelet agents, rhythm correction, implantable defibrillators, cardiac resynchronisation, coronary bypass surgery and lipid treatment. The presence of other problems such as renal insufficiency, thyroid disease and anaemia should be considered.

McMurray, J.J. (2010). Clinical practice. Systolic heart failure. *N Engl J Med* 362, 228–238.
http://www.ncbi.nlm.nih.gov/pubmed/20089973

15. Answer D

Coronary artery bypass graft (CABG) is recommended in patients with any of the following criteria: significant left main coronary artery disease, three-vessel disease [in patients with three-vessel disease, those with left ventricular ejection fraction (LVEF) <50% have the greatest survival benefit] and two-vessel disease with significant left anterior descending coronary artery involvement or abnormal LV function (i.e. LVEF <50%) (Pfisterer et al., 2010). In patients with three-vessel disease and abnormal LVEF, the survival benefit and symptom relief of CABG are superior to those of percutaneous transluminal angioplasty (PCTA) or medical therapy. In transmyocardial revascularisation procedure (TMR), a laser is used to create channels in the myocardium to relieve angina. This procedure has been shown to improve severe refractory angina in patients who could not be treated with conventional revascularisation techniques (PCTA or CABG). For the patient described here, CABG is the preferred procedure.

Pfisterer, M.E., Zellweger, M.J., and Gersh, B.J. (2010). Management of stable coronary artery disease. *Lancet* 375, 763–772.
http://www.ncbi.nlm.nih.gov/pubmed/20189028

16. Answer E

Computed tomography coronary angiography (CTCA) is a new imaging test that has been shown in meta-analyses to have excellent sensitivity (98%) and good specificity (88%) for significant coronary artery disease (stenosis >50%). Its high negative predictive value (96–100%) indicates that CTCA is an excellent test for ruling out significant disease in patients with low-to-intermediate pretest probability of coronary artery disease. Current data do not support the use of CTCA in asymptomatic patients. CTCA is not routinely recommended in patients with previous coronary stents since stents are likely to cause artefacts and make the results difficult to interpret. In patients who are likely to require invasive coronary angiograms, such as a patient with ST-elevation myocardial infarction, it is more appropriate to proceed with percutaneous coronary intervention without delay.

To avoid artefacts that may hamper interpretation of the results, the patient should be in sinus rhythm with a heart rate of less than 65 beats/min, able to hold his/her breath for 10s, able to tolerate beta-blockers and nitrates (nitrates are given to dilate the coronary arteries by most centres) and able to hold his/her arms above the head during the scan. Previous contrast allergy and renal impairment should be ruled out prior to CTCA.

Liew, G., Feneley, M., and Worthley, S. (2012). Appropriate indications for computed tomography coronary angiography. *Med J Aust* 196, 246–249. https://www.mja.com.au/journal/2012/196/4/appropriate-indications-computed-tomography-coronary-angiography

17. Answer B

Dabigatran is 80% renally cleared (Hankey and Eikelboom, 2011). Therefore, care must be taken when used in patients with impaired renal function. Reduced kidney function in an elderly patient with diabetes is the most likely explanation for the bleeding complication in the patient described. In addition, bleeding rates with dabigatran increase with advanced age. The combination of aspirin and dabigatran is associated with higher bleeding rates.

At present there are no available laboratory tests that have been validated for monitoring of dabigatran. The thrombin clotting time can be used to inform if dabigatran activity is present, but it does not reveal the extent of anti-coagulation. Unlike warfarin, one of the major drawbacks of dabigatran is the lack of an effective antidote for use in the event of a severe bleeding event.

Dabigatran is given as the prodrug dabigatran etexilate, and this prodrug is a substrate for efflux by the p-glycoprotein transporter. Inhibitors of p-glycoprotein, such as ketoconazole (most azoles), protease inhibitors, macrolides, calcineurin inhibitors, amiodarone and verapamil, can increase dabigatran plasma concentrations by decreasing the efflux of the drug into the gastrointestinal lumen. Strong inducers of p-glycoprotein, such as rifampicin, carbamazepine and phenytoin, can reduce plasma concentrations and co-administration should be avoided. No significant interaction was seen with digoxin, also a p-glycoprotein substrate.

Hankey, G.J. and Eikelboom, J.W. (2011). Dabigatran etexilate: a new oral thrombin inhibitor. *Circulation* 123, 1436–1450. http://circ.ahajournals.org/content/123/13/1436.long

18. Answer E

The ECGs show:

    A. Bifascicular block

    B. First-degree heart block

    C. Left bundle branch block

    D. Mobitz type I (Wenkebach) heart block

    E. Mobitz type II 2:1 heart block

Temporary transvenous pacing is necessary for patients with severe and symptomatic bradyarrhythmias, but should also be considered for those at high risk of developing complete heart block as a consequence of acute myocardial infarction (AMI). High (second or third)-degree AV block is associated with an increase in mortality in patients with an inferior or anterior AMI (Vardas et al., 2007).

Following an AMI, temporary transvenous pacing should be considered if there is:

- Complete (third-degree) heart block
- New or age-indeterminate bifascicular block (RBBB with LAFB or LPFB or LBBB) with PR prolongation
- Symptomatic bradycardia of any aetiology if hypotension is present and the bradyarrhythmia is not responsive to atropine
- Mobitz type II second-degree AV block
- Bradycardia-induced tachyarrhythmias.

Despite reperfusion treatment, the incidence of intraventricular conduction disturbances post acute myocardial infarction (AMI) has not changed, whereas the incidence of AV block post AMI has decreased but still remains high. AV block occurs in almost 7% of cases of AMI.

Vardas, P.E., Auricchio, A., Blanc, J.J., et al. (2007). Guidelines for cardiac pacing and cardiac resynchronization therapy: The Task Force for Cardiac Pacing and Cardiac Resynchronization Therapy of the European Society of Cardiology. Developed in collaboration with the European Heart Rhythm Association. *Eur Heart J* 28, 2256–2295.
http://eurheartj.oxfordjournals.org/content/28/18/2256.long

19. Answer D

Eisenmenger syndrome is pulmonary hypertension due to a left-to-right shunt caused by congenital heart defects such as a ventricular septal defect or a patent ductus arteriosus. Whilst rare in pregnancy (estimated incidence: 1.1 per 100 000 pregnancies), it has been associated with a high maternal mortality, estimated to be between 30% and 56% (Regitz-Zagrosek et al., 2011). Risk for fetal death and premature delivery is also very high. Maternal death occurs in the last trimester of pregnancy and in the first months after delivery because of pulmonary hypertensive crises, pulmonary thrombosis or refractory right heart failure. This occurs even in patients with little or no disability before or during pregnancy. Guidelines from the European Society of Cardiology (ESC) and the American College of Cardiology/American Heart Association (ACC/AHA) strongly discourage pregnancy and suggest consideration of termination should a pregnancy occur.

The importance of early counselling about pregnancy risks and contraception is strongly emphasised. For those who choose to continue pregnancy, obstetric care should be undertaken at a specialist centre, with access to intensive care. Even after successful delivery, maternal risk continues beyond the time of birth; therefore, close monitoring must be maintained in the postpartum period.

Regitz-Zagrosek, V., Blomstrom Lundqvist, C., Borghi, C., et al. (2011). ESC Guidelines on the management of cardiovascular diseases during pregnancy: the Task Force on the Management of Cardiovascular Diseases during Pregnancy of the European Society of Cardiology (ESC). *Eur Heart J* 32: 3147–3197.
http://eurheartj.oxfordjournals.org/content/32/24/3147.full

20. Answer E

While it has been recognised for many decades that some patients with hypertrophic cardiomyopathy die suddenly from ventricular arrhythmia, data from contemporary studies suggest that the overall risk is relatively small, with annual sudden cardiac death (SCD) rates of 1% or less in most series. The challenge for clinicians is to identify the small cohort of patients who are at risk in order to target potentially life-saving therapy with implantable cardioverter defibrillators (ICDs).

Predicting the risk of sudden cardiac death in a patient with hypertrophic cardiomyopathy is notoriously difficult, but a left ventricular wall thickness of greater than 3 cm is associated with a significantly increased risk (Christiaans et al., 2010). One study put the 20-year risk of sudden cardiac death at almost 40% for this population, even in the absence of symptoms such as angina or syncope. The use of the six major risk factors (previous cardiac arrest or sustained ventricular tachycardia, non-sustained ventricular tachycardia, extreme left ventricular hypertrophy, unexplained syncope, abnormal blood pressure response to exercise, and family history of sudden death) in risk stratification for SCD is recommended by international guidelines.

Christiaans, I., van Engelen, K., van Langen, I.M., et al. (2010). Risk stratification for sudden cardiac death in hypertrophic cardiomyopathy: systematic review of clinical risk markers. *Europace* 12, 313–321.
http://europace.oxfordjournals.org/content/12/3/313.long

21. Answer A

Staphylococcus aureus is the commonest cause of prosthetic valve endocarditis, followed by coagulase-negative staphylococcus (Wang et al., 2007). Prosthetic valve endocarditis accounts for a significant (20%) and increasing proportion of infective endocarditis cases; this is likely to increase in future years with increasing longevity and prosthetic valve insertion. The causative organisms vary with time since implantation. The most frequently encountered pathogens within 2 months of implantation are *S. aureus* (36%) and coagulase-negative staphylococci (17%); next in frequency are culture-negative (17%) and fungal infections (9%). After 2 months the pathogens involved are coagulase-negative staphylococci and *S. aureus* (18–20% each); next in frequency are no organism identified, enterococci and viridans streptococci (10–13% each).

The majority of infections occur in the first year after valve implantation, there is a strong association with in-hospital care and intravascular devices, and mortality exceeds 20%. Unfavourable features predicting mortality are older age, *S. aureus* infection and complications, including heart failure, stroke, intracardiac abscess and persistent bacteraemia.

Wang, A., Athan, E., Pappas, P.A., et al. (2007). Contemporary clinical profile and outcome of prosthetic valve endocarditis. *JAMA* 297, 1354–1361.
http://jama.jamanetwork.com/article.aspx?articleid=206241

22. Answer A

The electrocardiography showing torsades de pointes combined with the family history suggests that the patient has congenital long-QT syndrome (LQT) and the mainstay of therapy for this condition is beta-blockade (Roden, 2008).

A leading cause of sudden death in otherwise healthy young persons, LQT is characterised by abnormal QT-interval prolongation. The two common hereditary variants are Jervell and Lange–Nielsen syndrome and Romano–Ward syndrome, with the former being associated with sensorineural deafness. Based on genetic studies, there are three forms: LQT1 and LQT2 (due to mutations in potassium channels), and LQT3 (due to a sodium channel mutation), with LQT1 being the commonest. Syncope in patients with both the hereditary and acquired forms of LQT is generally attributed to a form of polymorphic ventricular tachycardia called torsades de pointes, which is characterised by twisting of the QRS complex around the isoelectric baseline.

An abnormal ECG obtained while the patient is at rest is the key to diagnosis and a detailed family history should be obtained. All persons with QT-interval prolongation should be screened for acquired causes such as hypocalcaemia, hypokalemia, hypomagnesaemia, hypothyroidism and the use of drugs that can prolong the QT interval; these drugs include anti-arrhythmic agents such as sotalol, quinidine and dofetilide, and non-cardiovascular drugs such as haloperidol, methadone, erythromycin, terfenadine and clarithromycin.

Treatment of LQT in those who have had a syncopal episode begins with a beta-blocker. If the patient has (1) syncope despite full-dose beta-blockade, (2) a successfully resuscitated cardiac arrest, or (3) a contraindication to beta-blockade and high risk of arrhythmia, a cardioverter–defibrillator should be implanted.

Roden, D.M. (2008). Clinical practice. Long-QT syndrome. *N Engl J Med* 358, 169–176.
http://www.ncbi.nlm.nih.gov/pubmed/18184962

23. Answer A

The indication for PBMV is progressive exertional dyspnoea (New York Heart Association functional class II, III or IV), associated with documented evidence of moderate or severe mitral stenosis (MS) (mitral orifice area <1.5 cm) (Nobuyoshi et al., 2009). There should be no or only mild associated mitral regurgitation. Asymptomatic patients usually do not need intervention, unless there is a history of thromboembolism, paroxysmal AF or significant pulmonary hypertension (pulmonary artery systolic pressure >50 mmHg). Patients with pliable, mobile, relatively thin valves, with no or minimal calcification, and without significant thickening and fusion of the subvalvular apparatus, are the best candidates. These comprise the majority of symptomatic younger patients. However, experienced operators can obtain acceptable results in older patients with less favourable anatomy.

Patients with pure or dominant MS requiring intervention should be referred for PBMV to a high volume centre with documented low complication rates, regardless of the anatomy of their mitral valve. Early referral is recommended for younger patients, as they have the most favourable valve morphology and the best long-term results.

A large left atrial thrombus is a contraindication to PBMV. However, it can often be performed safely in the presence of a small, stable thrombus in the left atrial appendage. PBMV is well suited to managing MS in pregnancy, where the risk of surgery and associated fetal loss is high.

Nobuyoshi, M., Arita, T., Shirai, S., et al. (2009). Percutaneous balloon mitral valvuloplasty: a review. *Circulation* 119, e211–219.
http://circ.ahajournals.org/content/119/8/e211.long

24. Answer C

Peri-infarction pericarditis usually occurs 1–2 days after an acute myocardial infarction (AMI). The presence of a pericardial friction rub is diagnostic. The incidence of peri-infarction pericarditis has decreased since the widespread use of reperfusion therapy. Peri-infarction pericarditis is associated with larger infarct size, more frequent anterior location of AMI, and lower ejection fraction. The ECG changes seen in other forms of pericarditis are usually overshadowed by the changes due to myocardial infarction.

Peri-infarction pericarditis is usually transient, unlike other viral or idiopathic pericarditis. Treatment with non-steroidal anti-inflammatory drugs is generally avoided because of the associated risks. The use of corticosteroids after AMI has been associated in some, but not all, studies with a greater incidence of ventricular aneurysm formation. Aspirin and anti-coagulation therapy is part of the standard management of AMI. There is great concern that these therapies may promote the development of haemorrhagic pericarditis. However, such concern has not been confirmed and the risk-to-benefit ratio favours the continuation of aspirin and anti-coagulation.

Post-myocardial infarction syndrome, which is also called Dressler syndrome, usually develops weeks to months after AMI. It usually presents with fever, pleuritic chest pain, and pericardial rub. Its pathogenesis involves myocardial injury that releases cardiac antigens and stimulates antibody formation. The immune complexes that are generated then deposit onto the pericardium and lead to an inflammatory response.

25. Answer C

The patient has a supraventricular tachycardia (Link, 2012). Vagal manoeuvres, including a Valsalva manoeuvre, carotid sinus massage, bearing down, and immersion of the face in ice water, can increase vagal tone and block the atrioventricular node and can be attempted. If these manoeuvres are unsuccessful, adenosine should be administered. Adenosine is a very short-acting endogenous nucleotide that blocks atrioventricular nodal conduction and terminates nearly all atrioventricular nodal re-entrant tachycardias and atrioventricular reciprocating tachycardias, as well the majority of atrial tachycardias. Since this drug can also excite atrial and ventricular tissue, rarely causing atrial fibrillation, transient heart block and non-sustained ventricular tachycardia, it should be administered with ECG monitoring and a defibrillator to hand. Adenosine should not be used in patients with asthma. Side effects include chest tightness, flushing and a sense of dread.

Although intravenous verapamil and diltiazem, which also block the atrioventricular node, can be of therapeutic use in narrow-complex tachycardias, they may cause hypotension and are longer lasting and thus are not a first choice in the emergency setting, particularly when blood pressure is already reduced. Electrical DC cardioversion is reserved for patients who are unstable or who do not respond to adenosine or other measures. Although the blood pressure of the patient is 98/68 mmHg, he is alert and has no signs of shock, so his condition is not considered unstable.

Link, M.S. (2012). Evaluation and initial treatment of supraventricular tachycardia. *N Engl J Med* 367, 1438–1448.
http://www.ncbi.nlm.nih.gov/pubmed/23050527

26. Answer D

This patient's electrocardiography, while in sinus rhythm 5 years ago, shows a classic pattern of pre-excitation – the Wolff–Parkinson–White (WPW) syndrome. He presents with symptomatic pre-excited atrial fibrillation (AF) with a rapid ventricular response, which now requires urgent treatment.

The goals of acute drug therapy for pre-excited AF are prompt control of the ventricular rate and stabilisation of the haemodynamic status. Treatment of pre-excited AF requires a parenteral drug with rapid onset of action that lengthens antegrade refractoriness and slows conduction in both the AV node/His–Purkinje system and the accessory pathway. The class IC anti-arrhythmic drugs, such as flecainide, are effective in this setting. Intravenous beta-blockers when used alone do not increase accessory pathway refractoriness. Furthermore, inhibition of AV node conduction may enhance the pre-excited ventricular rate response by decreasing the degree of concealed retrograde conduction into the accessory pathway. Intravenous digoxin is contraindicated because blockade of AV nodal conduction can lead to an unpredictable effect on accessory pathway refractoriness. Verapamil is the most dangerous AV nodal blocker to administer during pre-excited AF. Intravenous verapamil lengthens AV node refractoriness, decreases concealed conduction into the accessory pathway and has no direct effect on the accessory pathway. Myocardial contractility and systemic vascular resistance are also reduced; these effects may cause a reflex increase in already elevated sympathetic tone that further shortens accessory pathway refractoriness. Intravenous adenosine is also contraindicated because it causes an effect similar to verapamil and can precipitate ventricular fibrillation. Although not approved for acute therapy of AF, intravenous amiodarone may be effective for reverted AF in WPW or may slow the ventricular rate because of its effect on accessory pathway refractoriness and conduction (Fuster et al., 2006).

Fuster, V., Ryden, L.E., Cannom, D.S., et al. (2006). ACC/AHA/ESC 2006 guidelines for the management of patients with atrial fibrillation. *J Am Coll Cardiol* 48, 854–906.
http://www.sciencedirect.com/science/article/pii/S073510970601816X

27. Answer D

Streptococcus bovis, a non-enterococcal group D streptococcus, is a bacterium that is found among the normal flora of the human gastrointestinal tract in 5–16% of adults. In addition, *S. bovis* is commonly detected as a contaminant in packaged meat. If *S. bovis* enters the bloodstream, it can cause bacteraemia and endocarditis; approximately 12% of infective endocarditis is caused by *S. bovis*. Endocarditis caused by *S. bovis* is more common in men and in the elderly. In two studies, patients with endocarditis caused by *S. bovis* type I, recently reclassified as *Streptococcus gallolyticus*, had an increased risk of prevalent colorectal neoplasia. Nearly all patients with *S. bovis* endocarditis are older than 50 years, and there is an association with malignancy of the gastrointestinal tract. Many debate the temporality of this association. One view is that ulcerating colorectal carcinomas allow increased growth of *S. bovis*, invasion of the bloodstream and establishment of infection. Others argue that *S. bovis* is a direct cause of colon carcinogenesis. This patient's clinical picture is suggestive of endocarditis. He also has microcytic anaemia and weight loss that may be related to colorectal cancer.

Burnett-Hartman, A.N., Newcomb, P.A., and Potter, J.D. (2008). Infectious agents and colorectal cancer: A review of *Helicobacter pylori*, *Streptococcus bovis*, JC virus, and human papillomavirus. *Cancer Epidemiol Biomarkers Prev* 17, 2970–2979.
http://cebp.aacrjournals.org/content/17/11/2970.long

28. Answer E

Most patients with heart failure have a low or normal cardiac output. High-output heart failure is characterised by an elevated resting cardiac index beyond the normal range of 2.5–4.0 L/min/m^2. Chronic volume overload and chronic activation of the sympathetic nervous and renin–angiotensin–aldosterone systems gradually cause ventricular enlargement, remodelling and heart failure.

Cardiac amyloidosis is usually dominated by right heart failure and is a cause of low-output heart failure. Hyperthyroidism can cause sympatho-adrenal activation and create a hyperdynamic circulatory state.

There are multiple arteriovenous fistulas in the bony lesions in patients with Paget disease. Extensive Paget disease (>20% of the skeleton) can cause an increase in cardiac output and lead to high-output heart failure.

In dialysis patients with an arteriovenous fistula, blood from a high-pressure artery is shunted to a low-pressure vein, which decreases systemic vascular resistance. A compensatory increase in the heart rate and stroke volume ensues.

In patients with severe cirrhosis, the increased cardiac output is due to splanchnic vasodilation and the development of intrahepatic or mesenteric arteriovenous shunts.

Other causes of high-output heart failure include:
- Severe anaemia
- Vitamin B$_1$ or thiamine deficiency (beriberi heart disease)
- Psoriasis
- Severe septicaemia

- Congenital fistulas
- Acromegaly
- Pregnancy
- Polycythemia vera.

High-output states can cause or contribute to heart failure, especially in patients with underlying cardiovascular disease. The treating clinician should consider the possibility of high-output cardiac failure in patients with physical signs that suggest an increase in cardiac output, such as warm extremities, wide pulse pressure and systolic flow murmur.

Mehta, P.A. and Dubrey, S.W. (2009). High output heart failure. *QJM* 102, 235–241.
http://qjmed.oxfordjournals.org/content/102/4/235.long

29. Answer B
The following features identify high-risk patients with infective endocarditis:
- Heart failure
- Stroke, abnormal mental status
- Recurrent embolic events
- Septic shock
- Fever persisting >7–10 days
- Large or enlarging vegetation
- Perivalvular extension of infection (abscess, pseudoaneurysm, fistula)
- New heart block
- Severe left-sided regurgitation, severe prosthetic dysfunction
- Signs of increased left-cavities' filling pressure, pulmonary hypertension
- Pathogens other than viridans streptococci, especially *Staphylococcus aureus*, fungi and Gram-negative bacilli
- Acute renal failure.

Thuny, F., Grisoli, D., Collart, F., Habib, G., and Raoult, D. (2012). Management of infective endocarditis: challenges and perspectives. *Lancet* 379, 965–975.
http://www.ncbi.nlm.nih.gov/pubmed/22317840

30. Answer C
Cholesterol embolisation syndrome refers to embolisation of the contents of an atherosclerotic plaque (primarily cholesterol crystals) from a proximal large-calibre artery to distal small-to-medium arteries, causing end-organ damage by mechanical plugging and an inflammatory response. Cholesterol embolisation syndrome is generally characterised by a multitude of small emboli (showers of microemboli) occurring over time. This is in contrast to arterio-arterial thromboembolism, which is usually characterised by an abrupt release of one or a few large emboli, leading to severe ischaemia of target organs.

Cholesterol embolisation syndrome has a variety of clinical presentations. Cholesterol emboli originating in the descending thoracic and abdominal aorta may lead to renal failure, bowel ischaemia and emboli to the skeletal muscles and skin. Dermatological manifestations (most commonly livedo reticularis and blue toe syndrome) are usually confined to the lower extremities

Cholesterol crystals trigger an inflammatory response after they lodge in the small arteries of the target organ. Constitutional signs and symptoms, such as fever, weight loss, anorexia, fatigue and myalgias, are frequent manifestations of the inflammatory response. Laboratory tests may also show an abnormality in inflammatory markers such as a rise in leucocyte count, erythrocyte sedimentation rate and C-reactive protein, or a decrease in serum complement levels (hypocomplementaemia). The patient may also develop anaemia or thrombocytopenia.

Hypereosinophilia has been reported in up to 80% of the patients with cholesterol embolisation syndrome. The duration and magnitude of hypereosinophilia in cholesterol embolisation syndrome are variable. Hypereosinophilia often occurs only during the first few days, and the proportion of eosinophils may vary from 6% to 18% of the total leucocyte count. The exact mechanism of hypereosinophilia in cholesterol embolisation syndrome is not known; it is believed that cholesterol embolisation syndrome is a form of cytokine-mediated eosinophilic disorder. One of the cytokines may be interleukin 5 derived from vascular endothelium. It is important to emphasise that hypereosinophilia is not pathognomonic for cholesterol embolisation syndrome because it may occur in a variety of other disorders, such as systemic vasculitides, acute interstitial nephritis and radiographic contrast-induced renal injury. Because none of the aforementioned clinical or laboratory findings is specific for cholesterol embolisation syndrome, a high degree of clinical suspicion is required in establishing the diagnosis, particularly if the patient has recently undergone a vascular procedure such as cardiac catheterisation.

Kronzon, I. and Saric, M. (2010). Cholesterol embolization syndrome. *Circulation* 122, 631–641.
http://circ.ahajournals.org/content/122/6/631.long

31. Answer E
This patient has ongoing ventricular fibrillation despite defibrillation. The next line of therapy is amiodarone. According to the 2010 American Heart Association (AHA) Guidelines and the Australian Resuscitation Council Guidelines (www.resus.org.au), intravenous anti-arrhythmic therapy should be considered in cases that remain in ventricular fibrillation (VF) or ventricular tachycardia (VT) despite defibrillation or recur promptly after successful defibrillation. Anti-arrhythmic drugs that may be used include amiodarone, lidocaine and magnesium sulphate, with amiodarone being the preferred agent. In the ALIVE trial of 347 patients with out-of-hospital sudden cardiac arrest and persistent or recurrent VF despite three defibrillation shocks and intravenous epinephrine (adrenaline),

survival to hospital admission was significantly higher in the amiodarone group compared to the lignocaine group (23% versus 12%) (Dorian et al., 2002). Magnesium sulphate is indicated *only* in the treatment of VF or pulseless VT arrest due to the drug-induced prolonged QT interval associated with torsades de pointes.

Although the 2010 AHA guidelines concluded that a single dose of vasopressin may be administered in place of the first or second dose of epinephrine (adrenaline) in the treatment of VF or pulseless VT arrest, clear evidence that this is a superior approach is lacking.

Dorian, P., Cass, D., Schwartz, B., Cooper, R., Gelaznikas, R., and Barr, A. (2002). Amiodarone as compared with lidocaine for shock-resistant ventricular fibrillation. *N Engl J Med* 346, 884–890.
http://www.ncbi.nlm.nih.gov/pubmed/11907287

32. Answer D

Uncontrolled heart failure is the most important risk factor for cardiac death or complications. A history of functional limitation appears to be the most helpful of all the historical points in this assessment. Patients who can perform activities that require four metabolic equivalents (METs) have a good chance of survival for most surgical procedures; such patients require no further testing. One MET represents metabolic demand at rest, climbing two flights of stairs demands four METs and strenuous sports such as swimming needs more than 10 METs. The use of echocardiography as a predictive tool is controversial. Although many experts advocate echocardiography as a good tool for assessing heart failure control, the procedure may provide little prognostic information beyond that available from a careful history and physical examination. The most important preoperative use of echocardiography is in the differentiation of systolic dysfunction from diastolic dysfunction in patients with new-onset heart failure. The distinction is important, because data clearly show that systolic dysfunction, in a patient with substantial clinical manifestations (i.e. overt congestive failure), adds significantly to the risk of surgery. On the other hand, there are no data showing that echocardiographic evidence of systolic dysfunction in a patient without symptoms or signs of heart failure have any prognostic implications. There are also no good data indicating that diastolic dysfunction increases risk significantly. The preoperative evaluation of the patient with established or probable coronary artery disease (CAD) is of great importance. Recent myocardial infarction is second only to decompensated heart failure as a risk factor for perioperative complications. Decisions regarding the evaluation of chest pain in patients without a history of CAD can be difficult under any circumstance.

The American College of Physicians clinical guidelines on the perioperative assessment and management of risk from CAD state that most patients who do not have an independent clinical need for coronary revascularisation can proceed to surgery without further cardiac investigation. In other words, if there is no prior reason to perform coronary artery bypass surgery, further cardiac investigation usually does not need to be carried out for the anticipated surgery, unless there is some other overriding consideration.

Cardiac complications after non-cardiac surgery depend not only on specific risk factors but also on the type of surgery and the circumstances under which it takes place. The high-risk group consists of major vascular interventions. Abdominal surgery, head and neck surgery, urological surgery and major orthopaedic surgery, such as hip and spine surgery, belong in an intermediate-risk group.

 Fleisher L.A., Beckman J.A., Brown K.A., et al (2007). ACC/AHA 2007 Guidelines on Perioperative Cardiovascular Evaluation and Care for Noncardiac Surgery: A Report of the American College of Cardiology/American Heart Association Task Force on Practice Guidelines (Writing Committee to Revise the 2002 Guidelines on Perioperative Cardiovascular Evaluation for Noncardiac Surgery). *Circulation* 116, e418–e500.
http://circ.ahajournals.org/content/116/17/e418.full

33. Answer B
Transplant coronary artery disease (TCAD) remains the most significant cause of morbidity and mortality after orthotopic heart transplantation (OHT) (Zimmer and Lee, 2010). Transplant coronary artery disease is largely an immunological phenomenon, driven by an inflammatory milieu consisting of multiple cell types that contribute to fibromuscular and smooth muscle cell proliferation with subsequent coronary obstruction. Multiple clinical factors contribute to the development of TCAD.

The gold standard for diagnosing and monitoring TCAD is coronary angiography. Although angiography is particularly useful for discerning focal lesions, which are commonly seen in native coronary artery disease, TCAD often presents as diffuse concentric disease without discrete stenosis, making angiography a less sensitive modality for diagnosis in these cases.

Clinical history is generally unreliable in the diagnosis of TCAD, because of the denervation of the allograft, although paediatric patients have indicated that symptoms such as abdominal, chest and/or arm pain are strongly associated with the presence of TCAD.

Intravascular ultrasound (IVUS) can evaluate all layers of the vessel wall as well as the lumen, and an intimal thickness of greater than 0.5 mm in a single transplant coronary artery. IVUS can subsequently confer prognostic information for cardiovascular complications associated with TCAD, as evidenced by findings that severe and rapid increases in intimal thickness, particularly an increase of 0.5 mm or greater within the first year after OHT, are strongly correlated with the future development of angiographic disease up to 5 years after OHT and are also associated with increased mortality, myocardial infarction and the need for repeat revascularisation. Limitations of IVUS include higher cost compared with angiography, lack of general expertise in its use, requirement for concurrent invasive angiography, decreased ability to examine secondary and tertiary vessels because of the larger size of the catheter, and higher risk of complications compared with routine angiography.

Myocardial contrast echocardiography can adequately detect the presence of TCAD but is unable to identify the extent of disease compared with angiography.

Current treatments for TCAD include pharmacotherapy, percutaneous coronary intervention and repeat transplantation; other novel therapies are emerging. Although percutaneous coronary intervention has generally demonstrated high procedural success rates, it has been plagued by a high incidence of in-stent restenosis. Drug-eluting stents reduce in-stent restenosis compared with bare metal stents. Repeat transplantation is the only definitive treatment.

Zimmer, R.J. and Lee, M.S. (2010).Transplant coronary artery disease. *JACC Cardiovasc Interv* 3, 367–377.
http://www.sciencedirect.com/science/article/pii/S193687981000169X

34. Answer A

In this scenario, the dyspnoea and peripheral oedema can be caused by any form of cardiomyopathy. The rise in jugular venous pressure (JVP) with inspiration suggests either constrictive or restrictive cardiomyopathy. Echocardiography showing no pericardial effusion and stiffness suggests restrictive rather than constrictive cardiomyopathy. The transmitral Doppler on the echocardiography may show an increased E:A ratio (E: early diastolic filling; A: atrial filling), decreased E-deceleration time (90 ms) and decreased isovolumetric relaxation time (40 ms), which may suggest a restrictive picture.

Restrictive cardiomyopathy is characterised by increased stiffness of the ventricles leading to compromised diastolic filling with preserved systolic function (Mogensen et al., 2009). These changes may develop in association with inflammatory, infiltrative or storage disease. Infiltrative pathology includes sarcoidosis, amyloidosis, post-irradiation therapy, myeloma, lymphoma or connective tissue disease. Inflammatory disease can be endomyocardial fibrosis or Löffler cardiomyopathy, while storage diseases include haemochromatosis, glycogen storage disease and Fabry disease.

Differentiation of restrictive cardiomyopathy from constrictive pericarditis is important because patients with the latter condition may recover completely following surgical removal of the fibrotic pericardium. However, the distinction between the two may be difficult.

Mogensen, J., Arbustini, E. (2009). Restrictive cardiomyopathy. *Curr Opin Cardiol* 24, 214–220.
http://qrs.ly/m52zfpa

35. Answer A

Patients with fulminant myocarditis typically present in acute heart failure up to 2 weeks after a viral prodrome. Many symptomatic cases of myocarditis present with a syndrome of dilated cardiomyopathy and heart failure (Gupta et al., 2008).

Chest pain may be seen if there is concomitant pericarditis. Myocarditis may present with arrhythmias leading to palpitations and hypotension. Troponins are raised in up to one-third of cases and ECG may show changes of myocardial ischaemia, arrhythmias or conduction disturbances.

In the developed world, myocarditis is most commonly associated with viral infections with Coxsackie being the commonest pathogen. Other causes include bacteria, protozoa, spirochaetes, rickettsia, cardiotoxic agents (anthracyclines, cyclophosphamide, cocaine and alcohol), hypersensitivity reactions (penicillins, cephalosporins, sulphonamides, diuretics, lithium, clozapine and methyldopa) and systemic disorders (sarcoidosis, inflammatory bowel disease, celiac disease, Wegener's disease and Kawasaki disease).

Acute myocarditis should always be suspected when a young patient with no significant medical history presents with a new onset cardiac abnormality such as heart failure, myocardial infarction, arrhythmias or conduction defects.

Gupta, S., Markham, D.W., Drazner, M.H., and Mammen, P.P. (2008). Fulminant myocarditis. *Nat Rev Cardiovasc Med* 5, 693–706.
http://www.nature.com/nrcardio/journal/v5/n11/full/ncpcardio1331.html

36. Answer E

Weight reduction can achieve important reductions in blood pressure in patients with hypertension and, if combined with a DASH diet, can achieve impressive average reductions in blood pressure, equal or exceeding that seen with single anti-hypertensive agents. The effect of adding weight loss to the DASH diet was evaluated in the Exercise and Nutrition Interventions for Cardiovascular Health (ENCORE) study. Participants were randomised to a control diet, to the DASH diet alone or to a reduced-calorie modification of the DASH diet. At 4 months, blood pressure was reduced by 3.4/3.8 mmHg in the control group, by 11.2/7.5 mmHg in the group given the DASH diet alone and 16.1/9.9 mmHg with the DASH diet plus weight management.

The most carefully studied and established healthy dietary patterns are the DASH diet and variations of the Mediterranean diet. In the original DASH trial, adults whose systolic blood pressure was less than 160 mmHg and whose diastolic blood pressure was 80–95 mmHg, 133 of whom had hypertension, were randomised to a control diet typical of the average US diet, a diet rich in fruits and vegetables, or a combination diet rich in fruits, vegetables and low-fat dairy products and relatively low in saturated and total fat. In hypertensive adults, the diet rich in fruits and vegetables reduced systolic and diastolic blood pressure by 7.2 and 2.8 mmHg more, respectively, than the control diet and the combination diet resulted in even greater reductions (11.4 and 5.5 mmHg). In a subsequent trial, the effect of sodium intake was studied in the context of the DASH diet. Patients were randomised to either the DASH 'combination' diet or a control diet. Participants were then given a diet with high, intermediate and low levels of sodium (3.5, 2.3 and 1.2 g/day, respectively). Reducing sodium intake resulted in a significant incremental reduction in systolic and diastolic blood pressure in both groups. The DASH diet is characterised by a relatively high potassium content (Sacks and Campos, 2010).

Sacks, F.M. and Campos, H. (2010). Dietary therapy in hypertension. *N Engl J Med* 362, 2102–2112.
http://www.ncbi.nlm.nih.gov/pubmed/20519681

37. Answer B

This patient has had an asymptomatic heart murmur for a long time, and he now presents with clinical features consistent with infectious endocarditis. Ventricular septal defects (VSDs) are among the most common congenital cardiac disorders seen at birth, but are less frequently seen as an isolated lesion in adulthood. This is because most VSDs in infants either are large and lead to heart failure, necessitating early surgical closure, or are small and close spontaneously. With the exception of patients who contract infective endocarditis or those with Eisenmenger syndrome, adults with VSD are asymptomatic. The classic physical finding of a VSD is a harsh, pan-systolic murmur heard best at the left lower sternal border and usually accompanied by a palpable thrill. Aortic regurgitation may be present if the VSD undermines the valvular annulus.

With a large defect, there is electrocardiographic evidence of left atrial and ventricular enlargement. If pulmonary hypertension occurs, the QRS axis shifts to the right and right atrial and ventricular enlargement is noted. Echocardiography is the procedure of choice for determining the location, size and haemodynamic significance of a VSD. The physiological consequences of a VSD are determined by the size of the defect.

Eisenmenger syndrome is a serious complication of long-standing left-to-right cardiac shunts in which severe, irreversible pulmonary hypertension develops. The presence of cyanosis is characteristic; symptoms such as dyspnoea and chest discomfort can be seen.

Patients with large VSD defects who survive to adulthood usually have left ventricular failure or pulmonary hypertension with associated right ventricular failure. Surgical closure of the defect is recommended if the magnitude of pulmonary vascular obstructive disease is not prohibitive (i.e. the ratio of pulmonary-to-systemic vascular resistance is <0.7).

38. Answer A

Atrial septal defects (ASDs) occur in three main locations: the region of the fossa ovalis (termed ostium secundum ASDs; 75% of ASDs); the inferior portion of the atrial septum near the tricuspid valve annulus (ostium primum ASDs; 15%); and the superior portion of the atrial septum (sinus venosus ASDs; 10%). The last two are considered to be part of the spectrum of AVSDs. Ostium secundum defects are associated with mitral valve prolapse, ostium primum defects with mitral regurgitation and sinus venosus defects with partial anomalous drainage of the pulmonary veins.

Most patients with ostium secundum ASDs with small defects are asymptomatic through young adulthood. As the patient reaches middle age, compliance of the left ventricle may decrease, increasing the magnitude of left-to-right shunting. A symptomatic patient with an ASD typically reports fatigue or dyspnoea on exertion. Alternatively, patients may present with complications such as supraventricular arrhythmias, right heart failure, paradoxical embolism or recurrent pulmonary infections.

The hallmark of the physical examination in ASD is the wide and fixed splitting of the second heart sound because phasic changes in systemic venous return to the right atrium during respiration are accompanied by reciprocal changes in the volume of shunted blood from the left atrium to the right atrium, thereby minimising the respiratory changes in right and left ventricular stroke volumes that are normally responsible for physiological splitting. A systolic murmur (from increased pulmonary flow) is common. On electrocardiography, the QRS axis is usually normal in patients with ostium secundum ASD but may have right axis deviation and incomplete right bundle branch block. The chest X-ray reveals an enlarged right atrium, right ventricle and main pulmonary artery. The diagnosis is confirmed by echocardiography. An ASD with a ratio of pulmonary-to-systemic flow of 1.5 or more should be closed surgically to prevent right ventricular dysfunction. Surgical closure is not recommended for patients with irreversible pulmonary vascular disease and pulmonary hypertension. Prophylaxis against infective endocarditis is not recommended for patients with ASD, repaired or unrepaired, unless there is a concomitant valvular abnormality such as mitral valve prolapse.

39. Answer H

In this patient, the findings on physical examination are consistent with coarctation of the aorta. Coarctation is an important cause of secondary hypertension. Although lower-extremity claudication may occur, patients are commonly asymptomatic. Coarctation may occur in conjunction with gonadal dysgenesis, bicuspid aortic valve, ventricular septal defect, patent ductus arteriosus, mitral stenosis or regurgitation or aneurysm of the circle of Willis.

The main feature on physical examination is the differences in pulses and blood pressures above the coarctation as compared to below the coarctation. In coarctation of the aorta, the femoral pulse will occur later than the radial pulse and it is often lower in amplitude. Because of variations in anatomy, blood pressure should be evaluated in both arms and in either leg when evaluating for coarctation of the aorta. When the coarctation is distal to the origin of the left subclavian artery, both arms will be in the high-pressure zone and both legs in the low-pressure zone. However, some coarctations are proximal to the left subclavian. Thus, the left arm and both legs will be in the low-pressure zone, and the diagnosis may be missed if only the left arm is used for measuring blood pressure. In addition to differential blood pressures, physical examination may also reveal a murmur across the coarctation that can be best heard in the left infrascapular area.

ECG usually shows left ventricular hypertrophy. Dilatation of the aorta proximal and distal to the coarctation site may lead to a so-called '3 sign' on chest X-ray. Rib notching is often present; this term refers to apparent effacement or so-called scalloping of the lower edges of ribs because of large, high-flow intercostal collateral vessels that develop as a compensatory mechanism to bypass the narrowing at the coarctation site. Computed tomography or magnetic resonance imaging provides precise anatomical information regarding the location and length of the coarctation.

Complications of aortic coarctation include left ventricular failure, aortic dissection, premature coronary artery disease, infective endocarditis and haemorrhagic stroke from rupture of intracerebral aneurysm. Surgical repair should be considered for patients with a transcoarctation pressure gradient of greater than 30 mmHg. Survival after repair is influenced by the age of patient at the time of surgery.

40. Answer F
This patient presents with a systolic murmur that increases on inspiration. This makes it likely that the aetiology is right sided. Given the location, pulmonary stenosis is more likely than tricuspid regurgitation. These murmurs vary with respiration because filling of the right heart is significantly affected by inspiration (as blood is returning from outside the chest and is therefore influenced by the negative thoracic pressure). In patients with moderate-to-severe pulmonary stenosis, a right ventricular impulse is palpable at the left sternal border and a thrill may also be present at the second left intercostal space.

Obstruction of right ventricular outflow is valvular in 90% of patients and the remainder is either supravalvular or subvalvular. Severe pulmonary stenosis is characterised by a valve area of less than $5 \, cm^2/m^2$ of body surface area, a transvalvular gradient of greater than 80 mmHg or a right ventricular systolic pressure of greater than 100 mmHg. With moderate-to-severe pulmonary stenosis, the electrocardiogram shows right axis deviation and right ventricular hypertrophy. When the stenosis is severe, dyspnoea on exertion or fatigability may occur. Eventually right ventricular failure may develop and if the foramen ovale is patent, shunting of blood from right to left may occur, resulting in cyanosis and clubbing.

Treatment for this disorder is most commonly by percutaneous balloon valvuloplasty. Valvular replacement is required if the leaflets are dysplastic or calcified or if marked regurgitation is present.

Brickner, M.E., Hillis, L.D., and Lange, R.A. (2000). Congenital heart disease in adults. First of two parts. *N Engl J Med* 342, 256–263.
http://www.ncbi.nlm.nih.gov/pubmed/10648769

Brickner, M.E., Hillis, L.D., and Lange, R.A. (2000). Congenital heart disease in adults. Second of two parts. *N Engl J Med* 342, 334–342.
http://www.ncbi.nlm.nih.gov/pubmed/10655533

Rouine-Rapp, K., Russell, I.A., and Foster, E. (2012). Congenital heart disease in the adult. *Int Anesthesiol Clin* 50, 16–39.
http://www.ncbi.nlm.nih.gov/pubmed/22481554

 Therrien, J. and Webb, G. (2003). Clinical update on adults with congenital heart disease. *Lancet* 362, 1305–1313.
http://www.ncbi.nlm.nih.gov/pubmed/14575977

2 Respiratory and sleep medicine

Questions

BASIC SCIENCE

Answers can be found in the Respiratory and sleep medicine Answers section at the end of this chapter.

1. The majority of the carbon dioxide in blood is carried in the form of:
   A. Carbamino compounds bound to haemoglobin
   B. Bicarbonate ions
   C. Carbon monoxide
   D. Carbonic acid
   E. Dissolved in plasma

2. Which one of the following statements concerning the diaphragm is correct?
   A. It is innervated by the phrenic nerves that arise from nerve roots C1–3
   B. In diaphragmatic paralysis, the abdomen may be seen to move outwards on inspiration
   C. A common cause of diaphragmatic paralysis is phrenic nerve injury at cardiothoracic surgery
   D. In bilateral diaphragmatic paralysis vital capacity is unaffected
   E. Sleep-disordered breathing is rare among patients with diaphragmatic dysfunction

3. The oxygen dissociation curve is characterised by:
   A. A shift to the right by carbon monoxide
   B. A shift to the right by carbon dioxide, leading to enhanced oxygen release
   C. A shift to the left by acidosis, leading to enhanced oxygen release
   D. A shift to the left by 2, 3-bisphosphoglycerate (2, 3-BPG)
   E. The percentage saturation of haemoglobin (y axis) at various partial pressures of carbon dioxide (x axis)

4. Which one of the following acute physiological cardiovascular effects occurs in obstructive sleep apnoea?
   A. Decreased left ventricular afterload
   B. Decreased venous return to the right ventricle

Passing the FRACP Written Examination: Questions and Answers, First Edition. Jonathan Gleadle, Tuck Yong, Jordan Li, Surjit Tarafdar, and Danielle Wu.
© 2013 John Wiley & Sons, Ltd. Published 2013 by John Wiley & Sons, Ltd.

   C. Increased left ventricular preload
   D. Increased stroke volume during apnoea
   E. Increased sympathetic activity

5. The role of oxygen in cellular respiration is:
   A. The metabolism of glucose to acetyl CoA
   B. A cofactor in the citric acid cycle
   C. The terminal electron acceptor in the electron transport chain
   D. The production of ATP by glycolysis
   E. Conversion of pyruvate to lactate

6. Rapid eye movement (REM) behaviour sleep disorder is associated with:
   A. No therapeutic response to clonazepam
   B. Obstructive sleep apnoea
   C. Increased female incidence
   D. An epileptiform electroencephalogram (EEG) tracing
   E. An increased incidence of subsequent parkinsonism

7. Which of the following structures is devoid of cartilage?
   A. Primary bronchus
   B. Larynx
   C. Respiratory bronchiole
   D. Trachea
   E. Segmental bronchus

8. Vital capacity is the sum of:
   A. Tidal volume and expiratory reserve volume
   B. Tidal volume and inspiratory reserve volume
   C. Tidal volume, inspiratory reserve volume and expiratory reserve volume
   D. Tidal volume and residual volume
   E. Inspiratory reserve volume and expiratory reserve volume

9. Which one of the following changes in sleep pattern occurs in the elderly?
   A. Longer duration of sleep during the night
   B. Increased duration of non-rapid eye movement (REM) sleep
   C. Increased duration of slow wave sleep
   D. Increased sleep onset latency
   E. Decreased frequency of nocturnal awakenings

10. In familial pulmonary arterial hypertension, which gene is commonly mutated?
   A. Bone morphogenetic protein receptor II
   B. Endothelin receptor type A
   C. Endothelin receptor type B
   D. Matrix protein fibrillin
   E. Polycystin

11. A 40 year-old man has experienced increasing breathlessness on exertion for the last few weeks. His arterial blood gases whilst breathing room air are given below. What is the alveolar–arterial oxygen gradient?

	Value	Reference range
pH	7.47	7.35–7.45
$PaCO_2$ (mmHg)	49	35–45
PaO_2 (mmHg)	56	80–110
Bicarbonate (mmol/L)	33	22–35
Base excess	8.8	
Oxygen saturation (%)	89	>93

A. 33
B. 12
C. 56
D. 89
E. 8

12. Which one of the following is associated with narcolepsy?
A. Increased daytime sleep latency
B. Reduced levels of cerebrospinal fluid (CSF) hypocretin
C. Improvement in symptoms with clonazepam
D. Temporal lobe abnormalities
E. HLA-B29

13. A 65-year-old woman with severe kyphoscoliosis undergoes a preoperative pulmonary function test. Which one of the following components of the lung function test is likely to be maximally impacted by the above disorder?
A. Increased total lung capacity (TLC)
B. Increased functional residual capacity (FRC)
C. Increased maximal inspiratory pressure (MIP)
D. Decreased vital capacity (VC)
E. Reduced forced expiratory volume in 1 s (FEV_1)-to-forced vital capacity (FVC) ratio

14. Omalizumab is the first monoclonal antibody used in the treatment of asthma. The mechanism of action of omalizumab is best explained by:
A. Binding to immunoglobulin E (IgE) with reductions in serum IgE and reduced IgE binding to the IgE receptor on basophils and mast cells
B. Blockage of the binding of leukotrienes to type 1 cysteinyl leukotriene receptor
C. Binding to tumour necrosis factor (TNF)
D. Inhibition of IgE synthesis
E. Inhibition of degranulation of mast cells

Theme: Arterial blood gases (for Questions 15–17)

	pH (7.35–7.45)	P_aO_2 (80–110 mmHg)	P_aCO_2 (35–45 mmHg)	Bicarbonate (23–33 mmol/L)
A	7.50	55	33	25
B	7.50	100	33	25
C	7.45	100	24	18
D	7.40	100	40	25
E	7.33	61	75	38
F	7.20	54	55	16
G	7.26	128	16	7
H	7.15	96	33	11

Values provided are those measured on room air.

For each patient described below, select the most likely arterial blood gas findings.

15. A 20-year-old woman was brought in after ingesting a hundred 300 mg aspirin tablets. She is semi-conscious but responding to painful stimuli. Her blood pressure is 125/80 mmHg, pulse rate of 100 beats/min and respiratory rate of 36 breaths/min.

16. A 63-year-old man has long-term chronic obstructive pulmonary disease (reformed smoker) and is currently on domiciliary oxygen. He has previously been admitted to hospital with acute exacerbation of his respiratory symptoms and required non-invasive ventilation.

17. A 19-year-old pregnant woman with type 1 diabetes presents with a 2-day history of polyuria, dysuria and general unwellness. There is a history of poor compliance with medical therapy. On examination, she is afebrile and her blood pressure is 110/60 mmHg. Chest examination is normal. The results of investigations are given below.

	Value	Reference range
Sodium (mmol/L)	135	137–145
Potassium (mmol/L)	4.8	3.2–4.3
Chloride (mmol/L)	101	100–109
Bicarbonate (mmol/L)	10	22–32
Urea (mmol/L)	8.1	2.7–8.0
Creatinine (μmol/L)	90	50–110
Glucose (mmol/L)	24.0	3.2–5.5

Urinalysis results: +++ ketones, ++++ glucose.

CLINICAL

18. Which one of the following features excludes a diagnosis of chronic obstructive pulmonary disease (COPD)?
   A. FEV_1/FVC <0.70 post bronchodilator
   B. FEV_1/FVC >0.70 post bronchodilator
   C. Non-smoker
   D. Weight loss
   E. Improvement with pulmonary rehabilitation programmes

19. Which one of the following treatment modalities for cystic fibrosis is described correctly?
   A. Bronchodilator therapy is helpful in the majority of patients
   B. Nebulised dornase alpha can improve the viscosity of the mucus
   C. Oral azithromycin is used to eradicate *Staphylococcus aureus*
   D. Regular use of oral corticosteroids reduces the frequency of infective exacerbations
   E. A course of a single intravenous antibiotic is adequate in the treatment of a severe exacerbation

20. A 58-year-old woman develops a moderate pleural effusion following a right lower lobe pneumonia. Thoracocentesis reveals straw-coloured fluid with Gram-positive diplococci on Gram stain, pH 6.9, glucose 2.2 mmol/L and lactate dehydrogenase 1400 U/L. Which one of the following is the best next step?
   A. Continue current antibiotics for pneumonia
   B. Intravenous ceftriaxone for 5 days
   C. Tube thoracostomy to drain the effusion
   D. Administer streptokinase intrapleurally
   E. Repeat chest X-ray in 2 weeks to evaluate the size of the effusion

21. Which one of the following does not preclude an attempt at curative lobectomy for bronchogenic non-small cell lung carcinoma?
   A. Pulmonary osteoarthropathy
   B. Hoarseness of voice
   C. Superior vena cava obstruction
   D. Blood-stained pleural effusion
   E. Preoperative forced expiratory volume in 1 s (FEV_1)of 1.0 L

22. Which one of the following is correct in patients with malignant mesothelioma?
   A. A median survival from diagnosis of 30 months
   B. Positron emission tomography (PET) scanning is not helpful in diagnosis
   C. Mesothelioma does not affect the peritoneum
   D. It is associated with prior exposure to amphibole asbestos fibres
   E. Imatinib therapy significantly improves survival

23. Which one of the following findings indicates a high risk of adverse outcomes in a patient with newly diagnosed acute pulmonary embolism?
  A. Normal troponin
  B. Hypertension
  C. Normal C-reactive protein
  D. Westermark's sign on chest X-ray
  E. Right ventricular dysfunction on echocardiography

24. A 58-year-old man has worked as a miner for 20 years. He presents with a 3-month history of cough and breathlessness. Chest X-ray shows diffuse interstitial shadowing. A sputum sample is positive for acid-fast bacilli. Which one of the following dusts is most likely to have predisposed the patient to tuberculosis?
  A. Beryllium
  B. Cadmium
  C. Coal dust
  D. Copper dust
  E. Silica

25. Which one of the following antibiotics has been found to have potential immunomodulatory benefits in the treatment of non-cystic fibrosis bronchiectasis?
  A. Azithromycin
  B. Tobramycin
  C. Amoxycillin with clavulanic acid
  D. Vancomycin
  E. Metronidazole

26. Which one of the following is commonly associated with secondary pneumothorax?
  A. Bronchiectasis
  B. Cystic fibrosis
  C. Wegener granulomatosis
  D. Osteogenesis imperfecta
  E. *Pneumocystis jirovecii* pneumonia in patients with human immunodeficiency virus (HIV) infection

27. A 56-year-old woman with a history of depression and chronic back pain is admitted to an Acute Medical Unit after her daughter found her unresponsive on the floor with shallow breathing. She was well 2 h before her daughter left to go shopping. Her arterial blood gas on room air is shown below. What is the most likely explanation for her presentation?

	Value	Reference range
pH	7.23	7.35–7.45
P_aCO_2 (mmHg)	68	35–45
P_aO_2 (mmHg)	60	80–110
Bicarbonate (mmol/L)	26	22–32
Anion gap (mmol/L)	12	8–14

A. Lactic acidosis
B. Opioid overdose
C. Distal renal tubular acidosis
D. Proximal renal tubular acidosis
E. Ethylene glycol poisoning

28. A 38-year-old Aboriginal man presents with a 4-week history of low-grade fever, weight loss and cough. As the treating medical practitioner, you are considering the possibility of active pulmonary tuberculosis. Which one of the following is the most sensitive test to confirm the diagnosis?
A. Tuberculin skin test
B. Sputum smear
C. Rapid polymerase chain reaction (PCR) test
D. Sputum mycobacterial culture
E. Interferon-gamma release assay

29. A 72-year-old woman with a known history of sarcoidosis presents with hypercalcaemia (total calcium 3.10 mmol/L; reference range: 2.10–2.55 mmol/L) and renal impairment (creatinine 219 μmol/L; reference range: 50–100 μmol/L). Which one of the following best explains the mechanism of hypercalcaemia in sarcoidosis?
A. Chronic renal failure with secondary hyperparathyroidism
B. Increased formation of 1, 25-alpha hydroxy vitamin D
C. Milk alkali syndrome
D. Immobility
E. Ectopic calcitonin formation

30. A 65-year-old Caucasian man with a 60-pack year smoking history and previous asbestos exposure presents with dyspnoea. He has a past medical history of congestive cardiac failure with a recent echocardiogram showing impairment of LV function with an ejection fraction of 28%. Chest X-ray shows a large right-sided pleural effusion. A pleural tap reveals fluid with an LDH of 150 U/L (with a serum LDH of 300 U/L) and a pleural fluid protein of 12 g/L (with a concurrent serum protein of 40 g/L). These results are most consistent with which one of the following as the cause of the effusion?
A. Congestive cardiac failure
B. Mesothelioma
C. Pulmonary embolism
D. Carcinoma of the bronchus
E. Tuberculosis

31. Which one of the following has been found to reduce lung function decline and mortality rates in patients with chronic obstructive pulmonary disease (COPD)?
A. Budesonide
B. Salbutamol
C. Cessation of cigarette smoking
D. Long-term antibiotics
E. Ipratropium

32. A 25-year-old pregnant woman was found to have pulmonary embolism on investigation for dyspnoea during her third trimester (week 39). Which one of the following treatment options is the most appropriate in this setting?
   A. Warfarin
   B. Low molecular weight heparin
   C. Aspirin
   D. Intravenous unfractionated heparin
   E. Graduated compression stockings

33. A 70-year-old man presents with a history of progressive dyspnoea for the past several years. He has chronic obstructive pulmonary disease (COPD) resulting from a 45-pack year smoking history but quit about 4 years before his current presentation. He is currently on combination budesonide 160 μg and formoterol 4.5 μg per dose, two inhalations twice a day; and salbutamol 100 μg per dose, two inhalations every 4–6 h as required. The results of his investigations are shown below. Which one of the following treatments is the most likely to improve his long-term survival?

	Value	Reference range
Arterial blood gas on air at rest:		
pH	7.40	7.35–7.45
P_aCO_2 (mmHg)	40	35–45
P_aO_2 (mmHg)	53	80–110
Spirometry:		
FEV$_1$/FVC (%)	43	
FEV$_1$ (% of predicted value)	30	

   A. Pulmonary rehabilitation
   B. Ambulatory oxygen therapy for 18 h/day
   C. Lung volume reduction surgery
   D. Lung transplantation
   E. Theophylline sustained-release 200 mg once a day

34. Which one of the following is a major risk factor for chronic allograft dysfunction due to bronchiolitis obliterans after lung transplantation?
   A. Silent aspiration
   B. Acute cellular rejection
   C. Use of azithromycin
   D. Cyclosporine
   E. Nissen fundoplication

35. A 55-year-old woman has had six admissions in the past 12 months for infective exacerbations of her bronchiectasis. A trial of long-term oral macrolides is being considered. Prior to commencing the macrolide, which one of the following investigations must be undertaken?
   A. Sputum specimen to exclude non-tuberculous mycobacterial infection
   B. Chest X-ray to exclude a pleural effusion

    C. High-resolution computed tomography of the chest to evaluate the extent of disease

    D. Spirometry to assess the forced expiratory volume in 1 s (FEV_1)

    E. Transthoracic echocardiography to estimate pulmonary arterial pressure

Theme: Chronic infiltrative lung disease (for Questions 36–39)

    A. Bronchiolitis obliterans organising pneumonia (BOOP)

    B. Desquamative interstitial pneumonitis (DIP)

    C. Idiopathic pulmonary fibrosis (IPF)

    D. Acute interstitial fibrosis (Hamman–Rich syndrome)

    E. Allergic bronchopulmonary aspergillosis

    F. Alveolar proteinosis

    G. Löffler syndrome

    H. Lymphangioleiomyomatosis

For each of the following scenarios, select the most likely diagnosis.

36. A 43-year-old woman who has had asthma for 15 years presents with progressive dyspnoea, chills and productive cough. Physical examination reveals a thin woman in moderate respiratory distress. She is afebrile but has mild tachypnoea and tachycardia. Lung examination reveals moderate air movement, diffuse wheezes and egophony in the left upper lung zone without change in tactile fremitus. The chest X-ray is shown below. Which of the following diagnoses best explains the constellation of clinical findings and radiological changes?

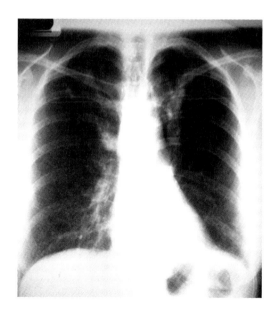

37. A 64-year-old Caucasian man presents with a 1-year history of worsening dyspnoea on exertion and mild non-productive cough. He reports previous asbestos exposure when he was working in a shipyard. The patient has never smoked. He has been treated with several inhaled beta-agonists, without any improvement. The physical examination is significant for dry inspiratory crackles and clubbing of his digits. A chest X-ray shows a diffuse infiltrative process, without lymphadenopathy or effusions. The patient undergoes an open lung biopsy, which shows minimal inflammatory round cell infiltrate, widening of alveolar septa and fibrosis with fibroblastic foci. What is the most likely diagnosis for this patient?

38. A 34-year-old man presents with a cough of abrupt onset, fever and chest pain. He has no significant medical history. He is admitted to the intensive care unit, where his respiratory distress worsens to the point that he requires intubation. The patient's chest radiograph shows diffuse, patchy ground-glass opacities and intralobular septal thickening. Bronchoscopy with bronchoalveolar lavage (BAL) show copious amounts of grossly turbid exudates in the airways with material that tests positive with periodic acid–Schiff (PAS) reagent on pathological examination. What is the most likely diagnosis for this patient?

39. A 32-year-old woman presents with dyspnoea, non-productive cough and a previous history of left-sided spontaneous pneumothorax. Bronchoscopic biopsy revealed proliferation of atypical pulmonary interstitial smooth muscle cells. What is the diagnosis for this patient?

Answers

BASIC SCIENCE

1. Answer B

The majority of the carbon dioxide in blood is carried as bicarbonate ions. The solubility of carbon dioxide in blood is about 20 times greater than that of oxygen. It diffuses into the red blood cell and is rapidly hydrated to carbonic acid (H_2CO_3) by intracellular carbonic anhydrase. The carbonic acid then dissociates into the hydrogen ion and bicarbonate that enters the plasma.

Some of the carbon dioxide in the red blood cell reacts with haemoglobin to form carbamino compounds. This binding stabilises the deoxy form of haemoglobin, leading to a decrease in its affinity for oxygen and a shift of the oxygen dissociation curve to the right.

Seventy to 80% of carbon dioxide in the blood is carried as bicarbonate ion, while 5–10% is carried as carbamino compounds bound to haemoglobin. Another 5–10% of the carbon dioxide circulates dissolved in the plasma.

2. Answer C

The diaphragm is innervated by the phrenic nerves that arise from the nerve roots at C3–C5. Normal diaphragmatic contraction leads to an outward motion of the abdomen, but in diaphragmatic paralysis there is a paradoxical inward motion of the abdomen during inspiration (abdominal paradox). The accessory inspiratory muscles contract, lifting the rib cage and lowering the intrathoracic pressure and causing the flaccid diaphragm to move in a cephalad direction and the anterior abdominal wall to move inward. Damage to the phrenic nerve may occur in up to 2% of patients undergoing cardiothoracic surgery and is one of the commonest causes of diaphragmatic paralysis (McCool and Tzelepis, 2012).

Diaphragmatic dysfunction is an underdiagnosed cause of breathlessness and should be considered in the differential diagnosis of unexplained dyspnoea. In bilateral diaphragmatic paralysis, there is usually moderate-to-severe restriction in total lung capacity. In both unilateral and bilateral diaphragmatic paralysis, the restrictive dysfunction becomes more severe when the patient is lying down. A decrease in vital capacity of 30–50% when the patient is supine supports the diagnosis of bilateral diaphragmatic paralysis.

Sleep-disordered breathing is common among patients with diaphragmatic dysfunction, since reduced activity of accessory inspiratory muscles during rapid eye movement (REM) sleep can lead to hypoventilation. Non-invasive positive-pressure ventilation can improve symptoms.

McCool, F.D. and Tzelepis, G.E. (2012). Dysfunction of the diaphragm. *N Engl J Med* 366, 932–942.
http://www.ncbi.nlm.nih.gov/pubmed/22397655

3. Answer B
Carbon dioxide, acidosis and 2, 3-bisphosphoglycerate(2, 3-BPG) decrease the oxygen affinity of haemoglobin, which manifests as the oxygen dissociation curve shifting to the right.

Haemoglobin consists of four globin chains, each of which is linked to a haem molecule. Haem is a complex of protoporphyrin IX and the ferrous iron which binds oxygen. While binding of the first oxygen molecule to the first haem is difficult, subsequent binding to the remaining haems in the haemoglobin becomes progressively easier. The net effect is that the affinity of haemoglobin for the fourth oxygen to be bound is approximately 300 times greater than its affinity for the first oxygen to be bound. This positive cooperative binding leads to the sigmoidal shape of the oxygen-binding curve of haemoglobin.

The oxygen dissociation curve is a graph that shows the percentage saturation of haemoglobin (y axis) at various partial pressures of oxygen (x axis). In the lungs with higher partial pressures of oxygen, haemoglobin binds to oxygen to form oxyhaemoglobin. As the red blood cells travel to tissues with reduced oxygen tension, oxyhaemoglobin releases oxygen to form deoxyhaemoglobin.

Carbon dioxide and acidosis stabilise the deoxyhaemoglobin form preferentially and consequently haemoglobin releases its oxygen, a desired effect in the peripheral tissues. This effect is known as the Bohr effect.

2, 3-BPG, which is an intermediate in the glycolytic pathway, also stabilises the deoxyhaemoglobin form and thus shifts the oxygen dissociation curve to the right. The concentration of 2, 3-BPG is raised in the red blood cells in response to chronic hypoxia, such as is seen in COPD or at high altitude.

The adult haemoglobin consists of two α- and two β-globin chains. 2, 3-BPG binds to a pocket in the centre of the deoxyhaemoglobin tetramer, formed by the two β-chains.

Carbon monoxide (CO) binds to haemoglobin with an avidity that is 220 times greater than oxygen. Binding of CO to one or more of the four binding sites of haem causes the remaining haem sites to bind oxygen with increased affinity. This leads to oxygen being effectively trapped within the haemoglobin and hence the oxygen dissociation curve shifts to the left.

4. Answer E
A variety of adverse physiological effects occur as a result of the repetitive obstructive apnoea and hypopnoeas that characterise obstructive sleep apnoea (OSA) (Hamilton et al., 2004).

The following acute physiological effects on the cardiovascular system can be observed in OSA:

1. Exaggerated negative intrathoracic pressure with airway obstruction results in:
- Initial inhibition, then progressive increase in sympathetic outflow
- Increased venous return to the right ventricle
- Decreased left ventricular preload
- Increased left ventricular afterload

- Decreased stroke volume during apnoea
- Increased stroke volume with relief of obstruction.
2. Hypoxia resulting in:
   - Either vagal (without airflow) or sympathetic stimulation (with airflow)
   - Ischaemia that leads to reperfusion injury of endothelial cells.
3. Arousal from sleep resulting in increased sympathetic activity.
4. Variations in blood pressure:
   - During apnoea, blood pressure decreases with varying effect on heart rate
   - Following apnoea, blood pressure and heart rate increase significantly.

The following chronic physiological effects of OSA are also observed:
- Increase in 24-h sympathetic nervous system activity
- Decrease in heart rate variability
- Endothelial damage and dysfunction
- Platelet activation and increase in blood coagulability
- Insulin resistance.

Treatment of OSA with continuous positive airway pressure (CPAP) has been shown to improve hypertension and left ventricular ejection fraction in those with congestive cardiac failure.

Hamilton, G.S., Solin, P., and Naughton, M.T. (2004). Obstructive sleep apnoea and cardiovascular disease. *Intern Med J 34*, 420–426.
http://www.sleepgroup.com.au/wp-content/uploads/2012/03/OSA-CVS-disease.pdf

5. Answer C

Cellular respiration is the set of metabolic reactions that take place in the cells of organisms to convert biochemical energy from nutrients to adenosine triphosphate (ATP). Oxygen is the terminal electron acceptor in the electron transport chain, which enables the oxidation of reducing equivalents such as NADH, establishing a proton gradient (chemiosmotic potential) which leads to the mitochondrial generation of ATP.

6. Answer E

Rapid eye movement (REM) sleep behaviour disorder (RBD) is a parasomnia in which vivid, often frightening, dreams are associated with simple or complex motor behaviour during REM sleep. Patients appear to 'act out' their dreams, often with a fighting or chasing theme at their centre. Sleep study features of RBD include increased electromyographic tone and dream enactment behaviour during REM sleep. There is a marked male predominance; it may be an early feature of neurodegenerative diseases such as Parkinson disease, Lewy body dementia and multisystem atrophy. There is often a good response to clonazepam treatment (Boeve, 2010).

Boeve, B.F. (2010). REM sleep behavior disorder: Updated review of the core features, the REM sleep behavior disorder-neurodegenerative disease association, evolving concepts, controversies, and future directions. *Ann N Y Acad Sci 1184*, 15–54.
http://www.ncbi.nlm.nih.gov/pmc/articles/PMC2902006/

7. Answer C
Respiratory bronchioles are the terminal division of the bronchi and are devoid of cartilage.

The trachea, which is about 10-12 cm in length and is situated slightly to the right of the midline, divides at the carina (junction at the level of manubrium sternum and second right costal cartilage) into the right and left main bronchi. The right main bronchus, which is the straighter of the two divides into the upper lobe bronchus and intermediate lobe bronchus and then further subdivides into the middle and lower lobe bronchi. The left main bronchus divides into the upper and lower lobe bronchi only. The lobar bronchi divide into tertiary bronchi, also known as segmental bronchi, each of which supplies a bronchopulmonary segment. Bronchopulmonary segments are separated from each other by connective tissue septum. There are ten segments on the right lung and eight on the left. The segmental bronchi divide into many primary bronchioles, which further divide into terminal bronchioles, each of which then gives rise to several respiratory bronchioles, which drain into and form multiple alveoli.

There are about 25 divisions between the trachea and the alveoli. The first seven divisions have cartilage and smooth muscles in their walls, while the remaining divisions lack cartilage and have a muscular layer that becomes progressively thinner.

8. Answer C
Vital capacity is the largest volume of air that can be expired after a maximal inspiratory effort. The amount of air that moves into the lungs with each inspiration (or moves out with each expiration) is the tidal volume (TV). The air inspired with a maximal inspiratory effort in excess of the tidal volume is the inspiratory reserve volume (IRV). The air expelled by an active expiratory effort after passive expiration is the expiratory reserve volume (ERV). The air left in the lungs after a maximal expiratory effort is the residual volume (RV). Total lung capacity is the sum of vital capacity and residual volume. Vital capacity is the sum of TV, IRV and ERV.

9. Answer D
Elderly persons tend to achieve less total night time sleep compared with younger people. They experience more night time arousals and awakenings. Increased daytime sleepiness may be the effect of such a pattern. Overall, the sleep–wake cycle in the elderly may be fragmented, with interrupted night-time sleep and daytime wakefulness interrupted by naps. The deepest stages of non-REM sleep are frequently reduced or non-existent in elderly persons; however, REM sleep tends to be preserved. Although a mild deterioration in sleep quality may be normal in the ageing process, an elderly patient's complaint of significantly disrupted night-time sleep or impaired daytime functioning because of excessive sleepiness must be evaluated.

Another common age-associated sleep change relates to the circadian rhythm of the typical sleep period. Although exceptions exist, elderly persons tend to go to sleep earlier in the evening and to awaken earlier in the morning. Early-morning awakening is a common complaint in the elderly. Slow-wave sleep (SWS), often referred to as deep sleep, consists of stage 3 and 4 of non-REM sleep, and is shorter in older adults than in children and young adults. The elderly may not go into SWS at all during many nights of sleep.

Non-drug therapies are first line for treating primary insomnia in the elderly. Melatonin prolonged-release tablets have been approved for short-term treatment (up to 3 weeks) of primary insomnia characterised by poor quality of sleep in people aged 55 years or older. (These drugs are currently not listed on the Australian Pharmaceutical Benefit Scheme).

10. Answer A

Mutations in two receptors of the transforming growth factor-beta family [bone morphogenetic protein receptor type-2 (BMPR2) and activin-like kinase type-1 (ALK1)] have been shown to be present in the majority of cases of inherited (familial) pulmonary arterial hypertension (PAH) (Machado et al., 2009). Exonic mutations in BMPR2 are found in about 50% of patients with familial PAH, and ALK1 mutations are found in a minority of patients with hereditary haemorrhagic telangiectasia and co-existent PAH. Because familial PAH is highly linked to chromosome 2q33, it is likely that the remaining 50% of family cases without exonic mutations have either intronic BMPR2 abnormalities or alterations in the promoter or regulatory genes. Also, about 10% of patients with 'sporadic' idiopathic PAH have identifiable BMPR2 mutations. Mutations in BMPR2 confer a 15–20% chance of developing PAH in a carrier's lifetime. Thus, there must be genetic or epigenetic or gene–environmental interactions that either enhance or prevent the development of the vascular disease in persons carrying a mutation.

Mutations in the FBN1 gene, which encodes the matrix protein fibrillin-1, are the predominant cause of classic Marfan syndrome. Polycystin genes are mutated in autosomal-dominant polycystic kidney disease.

Machado, R.D., Eickelberg, O., Elliott, C.G., et al. (2009). Genetics and genomics of pulmonary arterial hypertension. *J Am Coll Cardiol* 54, S32–42.
http://www.ncbi.nlm.nih.gov/pubmed/19555857

11. Answer A

The alveolar-to-arterial (A–a) oxygen gradient is the difference between the concentration (or partial pressure) of the oxygen in the alveoli, which is the alveolar oxygen tension (PAO_2), and the concentration of oxygen dissolved in the plasma (PaO_2). The A–a gradient is helpful in determining the source of hypoxaemia. The A–a oxygen gradient = $PAO_2 - PaO_2$. PaO_2 is measured by arterial blood gas measurements, while PAO_2 is calculated using the alveolar gas equation:

$$PAO_2 = (FiO_2 \times [P_{atm} - PH_2O]) - (PaCO_2/R)$$

where F_iO_2 is the fraction of inspired oxygen, P_{atm} is the atmospheric pressure (760 mmHg at sea level), PH_2O is the partial pressure of water (47 mmHg at 37°C), $PaCO_2$ is the arterial carbon dioxide tension and R is the respiratory quotient, which is approximately 0.8 at steady state, but varies according to the relative utilisation of carbohydrate, protein and fat.

On room air $F_iO_2 = 0.21$ (or 21%) and at sea level $P_{atm} = 760$ mmHg. A simplified version of the equation is:

$$A - a \text{ gradient} = [150 - 5/4(PCO_2)] - PaO_2$$

So in this example:

$$A - a \text{ gradient} = [150 - 5/4(49)] - 56 = 33 \text{ mmHg}$$

The normal A–a gradient varies with age and can be approximated by the following equation, assuming the patient is breathing room air:

$$A - a \text{ gradient} = 2.5 + 0.21 \text{ x age in years}$$

Causes of hypoxemia *with* increased A–a gradient are diffusion defect, ventilation–perfusion (V/Q) mismatch and shunting.

Causes of hypoxemia *without* increased A–a gradient are alveolar hypoventilation and low FiO_2 ($FiO_2 < 21\%$).

12. Answer B

Narcolepsy is a severe sleep disorder affecting 0·02% of adults. It is characterised by severe, irresistible daytime sleepiness and often by cataplexy (sudden loss of muscle tone following emotional or other provocation). Sleep monitoring shows rapid sleep onset (latency) and rapid onset of shortened rapid eye movement (REM) sleep. The onset of narcolepsy with cataplexy is usually during teenage and young adulthood and persists throughout life. The disease is associated with the loss of neurons in the hypothalamus that produce hypocretin, a wakefulness-associated neurotransmitter present in cerebrospinal fluid (CSF) and CSF levels are depressed in narcolepsy. The cause of neural loss may be autoimmune since most patients have the HLA DQB1*0602 allele (Dauvilliers et al., 2007).

Dauvilliers, Y., Arnulf, I., and Mignot, E. (2007). Narcolepsy with cataplexy. *Lancet* 369, 499–511.
http://www.ncbi.nlm.nih.gov/pubmed/17292770

13. Answer D

Kyphoscoliosis is associated with a restrictive pattern on pulmonary function testing (Donath and Miller, 2009). There is a decrease in vital capacity (VC) and total lung capacity (TLC) in proportion to the spinal deformity. Forced expiratory volume in the 1 s (FEV_1) and forced vital capacity (FVC) are proportionately decreased. Hence the ratio of FEV_1:FVC remains normal or is increased.

Functional residual capacity (FRC) is decreased because of reduced compliance of the chest wall. Lung compliance eventually decreases due to progressive atelectasis and air trapping. This reduced compliance increases the work of breathing. In addition, chest wall compliance decreases with age, further increasing work of breathing and risk of respiratory muscle fatigue in elderly patients. Consequently, these patients tend to breathe with lower tidal volumes and increased respiratory rate. Although this breathing pattern decreases respiratory effort, dead space fraction may be increased, and alveolar hypoventilation may ensue with resultant hypercapnia. Hypoxaemia without hypercapnia is also seen in moderate-to-severe kyphoscoliosis and ventilation–perfusion (V/Q) mismatch has been reported with severe kyphoscoliosis. Pulmonary hypertension develops in some patients as a result of persistent hypoxaemia.

Maximal inspiratory pressure (MIP) and maximal expiratory pressure (MEP) are decreased either because of muscle weakness or mechanical disadvantage from the rib cage distortion.

Donath, J. and Miller, A. (2009). Restrictive chest wall disorders. *Semin Respir Crit Care Med* 30, 275–292.
http://www.ncbi.nlm.nih.gov/pubmed/19452388

14. Answer A

Omalizumab is a humanised IgG monoclonal antibody that binds to IgE, reducing serum levels of IgE and decreases IgE binding to the high-affinity IgE receptors on mast cells and basophils (Fanta, 2009). There is also down-regulation of the IgE receptors on immune cells.

The pathogenesis of asthma involves elaboration of specific IgE molecules after allergen exposure. On re-exposure these IgE molecules bind to high-affinity IgE receptors on mast cells and basophils, leading to their degranulation with release of bronchoconstricting agents such as histamine, certain prostaglandins and leukotrienes. By preventing the binding of IgE to the receptors on mast cells and basophils, omalizumab prevents the release of these bronchoconstricting agents.

Omalizumab is indicated for the treatment of moderate and severe persistent asthma when inhaled corticosteroids, long-acting beta-agonists and leukotriene modifiers have not provided adequate control or cannot be used because of intolerable adverse effects. It is administered by subcutaneous injection and there have been occasional reports of anaphylaxis. The cysteinyl leukotriene-receptor antagonists, montelukast and zafirlukast, block the action of leukotriene C_4, D_4 and E_4 at the type 1 cysteinyl leukotriene receptor.

Fanta, C.H. (2009). Asthma. *N Engl J Med* 360, 1002–1014.
http://www.ncbi.nlm.nih.gov/pubmed/19264689

15. Answer C

With salicylate intoxication, the patient has a primary respiratory alkalosis due to salicylate-induced hyperventilation and a metabolic acidosis due to salicylate interference with intermediary metabolism, which results in the over-production of organic acids.

16. Answer E

It is likely that this patient has a chronic respiratory acidosis with low PaO_2 from decreased respiratory exchange; hence he is on domiciliary oxygen. The elevated serum bicarbonate is due to renal compensation.

17. Answer G

The diagnosis here is obvious from the history: diabetic ketoacidosis (DKA). The underlying problem seems to be poor compliance but other precipitants should be actively searched for, especially infection. There is little clinical evidence of a respiratory or skin infection. A suitable urine specimen should be sent for micro-scopy and culture.

   A pH of 7.26 is an acidaemia so a net acidosis must be present. Both the $PaCO_2$ (16 mmHg) and the bicarbonate (7.1 mmol/L) are decreased significantly. This is consistent with the presence of a metabolic acidosis. The anion gap is elevated at 25 mmol/L. The lactate level was not measured here so a contribution from lactic acidosis cannot be fully excluded.

CLINICAL

18. Answer B

A clinical diagnosis of COPD should be considered in any patient with breathlessness, chronic cough and/or sputum production, and confirmed by spirometry showing an obstructive defect with an $FEV_1:FVC$ of <0.70 post bronchodilator.

Although cigarette smoking is the leading risk factor for the development of COPD, there is substantial evidence that non-smokers develop COPD. Additional risk factors include genetic predisposition, such as alpha-1 anti-trypsin deficiency, particulate exposure, indoor pollution from heating, fires and stoves, asthma and childhood respiratory infections. Weight loss is a common feature of severe COPD and can indicate a poor prognosis. Pulmonary rehabilitation is an important part of treatment and has been shown to improve exercise capacity, perception of breathlessness and quality of life, and to reduce hospitalisation.

 Global Strategy for Diagnosis, Management, and Prevention of COPD 2013. http://www.goldcopd.org/uploads/users/files/GOLD_Report_2013.pdf

19. Answer B

The most common colonised pathogen in sputum of cystic fibrosis (CF) patients is *Pseudomonas aeruginosa*. For mild exacerbation, oral ciprofloxacin for 2 weeks and nebulised aminoglycosides, such as tobramycin, for 2–4 weeks are used. Nebulised colistin can be used as an alternative to tobramycin. If the patient's sputum does not show *P. aeruginosa* colonisation, a course of dicloxacillin or amoxicillin/clavulanic acid may be used to cover for *Staphylococcus aureus* infection. Other pathogens such as *Stenotrophomonas maltophilia* and *Haemophilus influenzae* are sometimes isolated and need targeted cover with sulfamethoxazole/trimethoprim and amoxycillin, respectively. For more severe infective exacerbations, a combination of a beta-lactam-derived antibiotic and an aminoglycoside is recommended as previous sputum sensitivities are not a useful guide to choosing therapy. A single antibiotic agent is inadequate treatment for severe exacerbations. Rotating nebulised tobramycin or colistin over some months to years is commonly used without strong evidence for the benefit of this practice (Masel, 2012). In a randomised, double-blind, placebo-controlled trial, treatment of CF patients chronically infected with *P. aeruginosa* with azithromycin for 24 weeks resulted in improved pulmonary function and nutritional status, decreased pulmonary exacerbation rate and slightly improved quality of life.

A bronchodilator is helpful in 30% of patients. Many CF patients exhibit a paradoxical response with worsening of expiratory flow rates. Therefore, patients should be objectly evaluated and periodically monitored for improvement while receiving bronchodialator. Mucolytics such as nebulised dorhase alpha are given to improve the viscosity of mucus and aids its clearance, but response is variable. Patients with abnormal lung function, such as a forced vital capacity of less than

80% of predicted, and chronic purulent sputum are most likely to benefit from this treatment. Clinical evidence is lacking to support regular use of an oral corticosteroid.

 Masel, P. (2012). Management of cystic fibrosis in adults. *Aust Prescr* 35, 118–121.
http://www.australianprescriber.com/magazine/35/4/118/21

20. Answer C

Para-pneumonic effusions occur in 20–40% of patients who are hospitalised with pneumonia (Light, 2006). The mortality rate in patients with a para-pneumonic effusion is higher than that in patients with uncomplicated pneumonia. Characteristics of patients with para-pneumonic effusion that indicate that an invasive procedure will be necessary for resolution include: the effusion occupying more than 50% of the hemithorax or one that is loculated, and features of empyema [a positive Gram stain or culture of the pleural fluid; and a purulent pleural fluid that has a pH below 7.20 or a glucose below 3.33 mmol/L, or has a lactate dehydrogenase (LDH) level of more than three times the upper normal limit for serum]. Patients with pneumonia and an effusion of more than minimal size should have a therapeutic thoracocentesis. If the fluid cannot be drained with a therapeutic thoracocentesis, a chest tube should be inserted and consideration given to the intrapleural instillation of fibrinolytics and DNAse (Rahman et al., 2011). Previously, fibrinolysis with streptokinase was not associated with clinical benefit, but more recent study using both DNAse and tissue plasminogen activator intrapleurally has been associated with improved outcomes. If the loculated effusion persists, the patient should be referred for video-assisted thoracoscopic surgery, and if the lung cannot be expanded with this procedure, a full thoracotomy with decortication should be considered.

 Light, R.W. (2006). Parapneumonic effusions and empyema. *Proc Am Thorac Soc* 3, 75–80.
http://pats.atsjournals.org/content/3/1/75.long

 Rahman, N.M., Maskell, N.A., West, A., *et al.* (2011). Intrapleural use of tissue plasminogen activator and DNase in pleural infection. *N Engl J Med* 365, 518–526.
http://www.ncbi.nlm.nih.gov/pubmed/21830966

21. Answer A

Pulmonary osteoarthropathy is a paraneoplastic manifestation that does not reflect the operability of a bronchogenic carcinoma.

When a patient develops obstruction of the superior vena cava or hoarseness of the voice, the disease has become locally advanced with invasion of adjacent structures, and this usually indicates inoperability.

Performing a lobectomy or pneumonectomy on a patient with very poor pulmonary function reserve would be risky and this may also be indicative of advanced disease. Guidelines from the American College of Chest Physicians and the British Thoracic Society suggest that patients with a preoperative FEV_1 of greater than 1.5 L are generally able to tolerate lobectomy. A blood-stained pleural effusion indicates pleural involvement and makes any attempted resection merely palliative.

The options for management of patients with poor lung function may include bronchoplastic and angioplastic sleeve resections, and sublobar resection (wedge resection or segmentectomy) is occasionally offered. With advances in stereotactic radiotherapy and with the introduction of radiofrequency ablation, patients with poor lung function can be offered a wider range of therapeutic modalities (Goldstraw et al., 2011).

Goldstraw, P., Ball, D., Jett, J.R., Le Chevalier, T., Lim, E., Nicholson, A.G., and Shepherd, F.A. (2011). Non-small-cell lung cancer. *Lancet* 378, 1727–1740. http://www.ncbi.nlm.nih.gov/pubmed/21565398

22. Answer D

There are two principal forms of asbestos: long, thin fibres known as amphiboles (blue asbestos) and feathery fibres known as chrysotile (white asbestos). Amphibole fibres are the major cause of mesothelioma but chrysotile fibres may also be oncogenic.

Peritoneal malignant mesothelioma can produce ascites, abdominal pain and occasionally bowel obstruction. In addition to the pleura and the peritoneum, mesotheliomas can rarely occur on other serosal surfaces, such as the pericardium and the tunica vaginalis. Because malignant mesothelioma develops within body cavities, patients usually have fairly extensive tumour involvement by the time they develop symptoms. Malignant mesothelioma is usually associated with prior exposure to asbestos, which may have happened decades earlier. Common initial presenting symptoms include dyspnoea due to pleural effusion and chest wall pain. As the disease progresses, patients may experience a 'cancer syndrome', such as lethargy, loss of appetite, weight loss, cachexia, fevers, night sweats, thrombocytosis, elevated erythrocyte sedimentation rate (ESR), anaemia and hypoalbuminaemia.

Poor prognostic factors for malignant mesothelioma include male sex, extensive disease, anaemia, poor functional status, high standardised uptake value ratios on positron-emission tomography (PET), increased white-cell counts, thrombocytosis, sarcomatoid histological findings, expression of cyclooxygenase-2, expression of vascular endothelial growth factor (VEGF), hypermethylation of the P16 INK4a gene, presence of Simian virus 40 and increased vascularity (Robinson and Lake, 2005).

From diagnosis, the median survival of patients with malignant mesothelioma is 12 months. Currently, there is no curative treatment for malignant mesothelioma.

In rare cases of localised tumours, surgical treatment such as extrapleural pneumonectomy can be performed in selected patients. Subcutaneous masses are almost always associated with prior medical procedures and occur along needle or intercostal tube tracks. Targeted radiotherapy to surgical sites prevents seeding of tumour, and radiotherapy can provide palliative relief of somatic chest-wall pain. Chemotherapy is not recommended as it has not shown significant improvement in survival rate or quality of life at this stage. PET can be used to distinguish benign from malignant pleural masses. It can detect extrathoracic disease, particularly lymph-node involvement, and hence has a role in staging.

Robinson, B.W. and Lake, R.A. (2005). Advances in malignant mesothelioma. *N Engl J Med* 353, 1591–1603.
http://www.ncbi.nlm.nih.gov/pubmed/16221782

23. Answer E

Patients with acute pulmonary embolism should be stratified according to the risk of an adverse outcome during hospitalisation (Agnelli and Becattini, 2010; Goldhaber and Bounameaux, 2012). Risk stratification should be done promptly because fatal pulmonary embolism generally occurs early after hospital admission. Risk stratification is based on clinical features and markers of myocardial dysfunction or injury.

Right ventricular dysfunction on echocardiography has been associated with increased mortality among patients with acute pulmonary embolism. Right ventricular hypokinesis and dilatation have been shown to be independent predictors of 30-day mortality among haemodynamically stable patients.

Shock and sustained hypotension also identify patients at high risk of an adverse outcome. The death rate is nearly 58% among haemodynamically unstable patients and about 15% among those who are haemodynamically stable.

Risk stratification of patients with acute pulmonary embolism has clinical implications. The absence of right ventricular dysfunction and a normal troponin level can identify patients who are eligible for early discharge and outpatient treatment. Haemodynamically stable patients with right ventricular dysfunction or injury should be admitted. An ongoing study is assessing the benefit of thrombolysis as compared with anti-coagulation in haemodynamically stable patients with evidence of right ventricular dysfunction and an elevated troponin level.

The Westermark sign represents a focus of oligaemia (vasoconstriction) distal to a pulmonary embolism (PE). While the chest X-ray is normal in the majority of PE cases, the Westermark sign is seen in 2% of patients. The Westermark sign, like Hampton's hump (a wedge-shaped, pleural-based consolidation associated with PE), has a low sensitivity (11%) and high specificity (92%) for the diagnosis of PE.

Agnelli, G. and Becattini, C. (2010). Acute pulmonary embolism. *N Engl J Med* 363, 266–274.
http://www.ncbi.nlm.nih.gov/pubmed/20592294

Goldhaber, S.Z. and Bournameaux, H. (2012). Pulmonary embolism and deep vein thrombosis. *Lancet* 379, 1835–1846.
http://www.ncbi.nlm.nih.gov/pubmed/22494827

24. Answer E

Occupational exposure to silica dust occurs in many industrial operations. Slate workers, stone masons and miners are exposed to silica dust. Silicosis impairs macrophage function and, in particular, predisposes to tuberculosis infection (Leung et al., 2012). In addition to silicosis, silica exposure is associated with other mycobacterial, fungal and bacterial lung infections, chronic obstructive pulmonary disease, malignant disease, including lung, gastric and oesophageal cancers, autoimmune diseases, namely scleroderma and rheumatoid arthritis, and chronic kidney disease. Tuberculosis risk increases with severity of silicosis, and in acute and accelerated silicosis. Silica exposure increases tuberculosis risk even without silicosis. Additionally, active tuberculosis at baseline predicts radiological progression of silicosis. Smoking is another aggravating factor. Major morbidities and mortalities result when these epidemics of silicosis, tuberculosis and smoking coexist.

Beryllium, which is used in the aerospace industry and in beryllium copper alloy machining, can cause granulomatous disease. Cadmium, which is used in electronics, metal plating and batteries, can cause emphysema. Coal dust causes emphysema with nodular fibrosis. Copper causes nasal ulceration and perforation of the septum.

Leung, C.C., Yu, I.T., and Chen, W. (2012). Silicosis. *Lancet* 379, 2008–2018.
http://www.ncbi.nlm.nih.gov/pubmed/22534002

25. Answer A

About one-third of patients with bronchiectasis are chronically colonised with *Pseudomonas aeruginosa*. During acute exacerbation, patients should be treated aggressively with ciprofloxacin for 14 days. In patients with resistance to ciprofloxacin, the combination of ciprofloxacin and nebulised aminoglycoside, such as tobramycin, should be considered. Recent data have found that long-term, low-dose oral azithromycin reduces the frequency of exacerbation and sputum microbiology/volume, and improves forced expiratory volume in 1 s (FEV_1). Azithromycin has an inhibitory effect on biofilm formation, production of immunostimulatory cytokines and the inflammatory response to *P. aeruginosa*. Azithromycin also improves gut motility and has been associated with reduced levels of aspiration markers (Livnat and Bentur, 2009). Prior to the institution of azithromycin therapy and every 6 months thereafter, patients should be screened for mycobacteria to avoid the emergence of macrolide-resistant non-tuberculous mycobacteria.

Management strategies for non-cystic fibrosis bronchiectasis are largely derived from cystic fibrosis, including antibiotics, anti-inflammatory, airway clearance therapies, immunisation and pulmonary rehabilitation.

Livnat, G. and Bentur, L. (2009). Non-cystic fibrosis bronchiectasis: review and recent advances. *F1000 Med Rep* 1.
http://www.ncbi.nlm.nih.gov/pmc/articles/PMC2948306

26. Answer E

Pneumothoraces are classified as either spontaneous or traumatic (Sahn and Heffner, 2000). Traumatic pneumothoraces result from direct or indirect injury to the chest and are further classified as iatrogenic or non-iatrogenic. Spontaneous pneumothoraces are further classified into primary (no obvious lung disease is identified) and secondary (as a result of a clinically apparent lung condition). Primary spontaneous pneumothorax is common in young men, aged between 10 and 30 years, who are thin and tall, and is rarely observed in persons older than 40 years old. Other risk factors for spontaneous pneumothorax include a history of smoking and a family history of spontaneous pneumothorax. Although in patients with primary spontaneous pneumothorax there is no clinically apparent pulmonary disease, subpleural bullae are found during video-assisted thoraco-scopic (VAT) surgery in 76–100% of patients and in virtually all patients during thoracotomy.

Chronic obstructive pulmonary disease (COPD) and *Pneumocystis jiroveci* pneumonia related to human immunodeficiency virus (HIV) infection are the most common conditions associated with secondary pneumothorax. The rate of spontaneous pneumothorax in patients with HIV infection is between 2% and 6%, and around 80% of these cases are associated with *Pneumocystis jiroveci* pneumonia with a high mortality rate. COPD patients with a forced expiratory volume in 1 s (FEV_1) of less than 1 L are at the highest risk of secondary pneumothorax. Early clinical suspicion and diagnosis is critical in the management of tension pneumothorax, which if untreated is associated with high mortality. Patients who present with tachycardia of more than 135 beats/min, hypotension or cyanosis should raise the suspicion of a tension pneumothorax.

Secondary spontaneous pneumothorax can be life-threatening because patients usually have limited pulmonary reserve associated with underlying primary lung disease.

Sahn, S.A. and Heffner, J.E. (2000). Spontaneous pneumothorax. *N Engl J Med* 342, 868–874.
http://www.ncbi.nlm.nih.gov/pubmed/10727592

27. Answer B

The clinical presentation is consistent with opioid overdose which suppresses the medullary respiratory centre, leading to hypoventilation and hypercapnia. Renal compensation for respiratory acidosis takes hours to start and days to complete. In this case, there is inadequate time for renal compensation to develop and for compensatory rise of plasma bicarbonate. Therefore, the arterial blood gases show an acute, uncompensated respiratory acidosis. The other potential causes lead to metabolic acidosis and would tend to promote hyperventilation rather than carbon dioxide retention. Lactic acidosis and ethylene glycol poisoning would lead to high anion gap acidosis, unlike the normal anion gap acidosis seen in this case.

28. Answer D

Tuberculosis (TB) is estimated to infect a third of the world's population, but the overall incidence of TB is low in Australia; about 1000 cases are diagnosed nationally each year and the incidence is 5–6 per 100 000 population (Horsburgh and Rubin, 2011; Johnson, 2011).

Populations at increased risk of TB include:
- Elderly patients, particularly post World War II European migrants
- Refugees from the Vietnam War
- Aboriginal Australians
- Torres Strait Island residents
- Migrants or refugees from high TB-burden countries, particularly refugees from sub-Saharan Africa and students from India, China and other Asian countries
- Healthcare workers.

This patient has symptoms to suggest active TB. Culture is the most sensitive test. Acid-fast microscopy is rapid (within 24 h) and inexpensive, but approximately 5000 bacilli/ml of sputum are required for a positive smear. Molecular assays detect DNA specific for *Mycobacterium tuberculosis* (MTB). In smear-positive samples, they are highly sensitive, but in smear-negative specimens, sensitivity drops to 50%. Recently, a new rapid polymerase chain reaction (PCR) test that is not prone to contamination has improved the sensitivity. Chest X-ray is essential for assessment of active TB.

Latent TB infection is diagnosed by detecting specific immunological responses to MTB proteins. The tuberculin skin test (TST) or Mantoux test assesses inflammation in the dermis following intradermal injection of tuberculin protein. The test needs to be read 48–72 h after administration. The diameter of induration gives a semi-quantitative assessment of the likelihood of latent TB. False positives can result from previous bacilli Calmetre-Guèrin (BCG) vaccination and exposure to environmental Mycobacterium spp. Interferon gamma release assays (IGRAs) utilise the ability of human lymphocytes to survive for a short period in a test tube. If primed by previous TB infection, lymphocytes will produce detectable amounts of gamma interferon. IGRAs are unaffected by previous BCG vaccination. A positive IGRA suggests that the patient's immune system recognises TB antigens. This may be due to either current infection or a remote past infection.

Horsburgh, C.R., Jr. and Rubin, E.J. (2011). Latent tuberculosis infection in the United States. *N Engl J Med* 364, 1441–1448.
http://www.ncbi.nlm.nih.gov/pubmed/21488766

Johnson, P.D. (2011). Extensively resistant tuberculosis in the lands Down Under. Med J Aust *194*, 565-566.
http://www.ncbi.nlm.nih.gov/pubmed/21644866

29. Answer B

In sarcoidosis, hypercalciuria and hypercalcaemia are common (Iannuzzi et al., 2007). There is enhanced 1-alpha hydroxylation of 25-hydroxy vitamin D by macrophages in granulomatous tissue (also seen in other granulomatous conditions) generating active 1, 25-hydroxy vitamin D. This promotes intestinal calcium bone absorption and increases bone resorption. Increased sunlight exposure in the summer months can provoke hypercalcaemia further. Whilst chronic renal failure can be a feature of sarcoidosis, secondary hyperparathyroidism is associated with depressed serum calcium levels. Immobility and milk alkali syndrome are important potential causes of hypercalcaemia, but are not specifically linked to sarcoidosis or calcitonin production, which tends to suppress calcium levels.

Iannuzzi, M.C., Rybicki, B.A., and Teirstein, A.S. (2007). Sarcoidosis. *N Engl J Med* 357, 2153–2165.
http://www.nejm.org/doi/full/10.1056/NEJMra071714

30. Answer A

The most widely used criteria to distinguish between a transudative and exudative fluid are the Light criteria (Light, 2011). For a fluid to be labelled an exudate, it must meet at least one of the following criteria (transudates meet none of these criteria):

- Pleural fluid/serum protein ratio more than 0.5
- Pleural fluid/serum lactate dehydrogenase (LDH) ratio more than 0.6
- Pleural fluid LDH greater than two-thirds the upper limit of normal for serum LDH.

In this case the fluid is a transudate and most likely a feature of cardiac failure. The most common causes of a transudate pleural effusion are cardiac failure and cirrhosis. Less commonly, nephrotic syndrome can lead to increased loss of albumin and resultant hypoalbuminaemia and thus reduced colloid osmotic pressure. Pulmonary embolism was once thought to give a transudative picture but has been recently shown to be exudative. Transudate is produced through pressure filtration by systemic factors that alter the pleural equilibrium (or Starling forces) without capillary injury, while exudate is 'inflammatory fluid' leaking between cells. Pleural infections and malignancy produce exudative pleural effusions.

Light, R.W. (2011). Pleural effusions. *Med Clin North Am* 95, 1055–1070.
http://www.ncbi.nlm.nih.gov/pubmed/22032427

31. Answer C
An important goal of COPD management is to reduce disease progression, prevent exacerbations and reduce the mortality rate. Cessation of cigarette smoking has been shown to reduce lung function decline and mortality. Long-term oxygen and some non-invasive ventilation might also improve survival in patients with COPD who have chronic hypercapnic respiratory failure.

In large interventional trials of lung function decline, no effect on disease progression was noted with inhaled corticosteroids when used alone compared with placebo.

32. Answer D
Pregnancy is a hypercoagulable state (Marik and Plante, 2008). The risk of venous thromboembolism (VTE) in pregnant women is four times as great as the risk in the non-pregnant population. Warfarin crosses the placenta and the use of warfarin between 6 and 9 weeks of gestation is associated with midface hypoplasia, stippled chondral calcification, scoliosis, short proximal limbs and short phalanges. Fetal intracranial haemorrhage has been reported in the second and early third trimesters. As a result, warfarin is contraindicated in pregnancy. Low molecular weight heparin could be used during pregnancy for treatment as well as prophylaxis for VTE. However, this woman is very close to the time of delivery and the timing of delivery is very unpredictable. Intravenous unfractionated heparin is the agent of choice because of its reversibility. Once the woman has gone into active labour, the heparin should be stopped and reversed with protamine if necessary to avoid excessive bleeding related to labour, induction of labour or Caesarean section. Aspirin is not an adequate treatment for confirmed VTE. Graduated compression stockings are recommended for thromboprophylaxis for all women with previous VTE antepartum and postpartum. However, compression stockings are not sufficient for treatment of confirmed pulmonary embolism.

 Marik, P.E. and Plante, L.A. (2008). Venous thromboembolic disease and pregnancy. *N Engl J Med* 359, 2025–2033.
http://www.ncbi.nlm.nih.gov/pubmed/18987370

33. Answer B
Randomised trials have found ambulatory oxygen therapy for 15–18 h/day to reduce the rate of death in patients with severe chronic obstructive pulmonary disease (COPD) and persistent hypoxaemia (Niewoehner, 2010). Indications for long-term oxygen therapy include chronic hypoxaemia with PaO_2 of 55 mmHg or less or arterial oxygen saturation of 88% or less or chronic hypoxaemia with a PaO_2 of 55–60 mmHg in the presence of right-sided heart failure or polycythaemia.

Pulmonary rehabilitation can significantly improve both functional exercise capacity (assessed by 6-min walk test) and respiratory quality of life (evaluated with the Chronic Respiratory Questionnaire), but data on its effect on mortality are lacking. Lung volume reduction surgery is not associated with overall reduction in mortality compared with the use of optimal medical therapy. Nonetheless, this type of surgery improves lung function, exercise capacity and respiratory quality of life. Lung transplantation offers the only opportunity for severely disabled patients with COPD to resume normal daily activities, but the median survival rate after lung transplantation is about 5 years, well below the median survival rate following transplantation of other solid organs. It is not known whether lung transplantation in COPD reduces mortality, as compared with optimal medical therapy.

Niewoehner, D.E. (2010). Clinical practice. Outpatient management of severe COPD. *N Engl J Med* 362, 1407–1416.
http://www.ncbi.nlm.nih.gov/pubmed/20393177

34. Answer B
In lung transplantation, chronic allograft dysfunction because of bronchiolitis obliterans syndrome (BOS) is a major impediment to long-term graft and patient survival. Bronchiolitis obliterans is a fibroproliferative process that narrows and ultimately obliterates the lumens of small airways, resulting in progressive and largely irreversible airflow obstruction. The characteristic histology is difficult to demonstrate by transbronchial biopsy, the forced expiratory volume in 1 s (FEV_1) is used as a surrogate marker and the term BOS is applied to this functionally-defined disorder. Approximately 50% of lung transplant recipients develop BOS by 5 years and 75% by 10 years.

Acute cellular rejection and lymphocytic bronchiolitis have been consistently identified as the major risk factors for BOS. Additional alloimmune, autoimmune and non-immunological factors have also been implicated. Gastro-oesophageal reflux or silent aspiration is one of the non-immunological factors that is present in some patients and may be contributory to the pathophysiology of BOS.

The natural history of BOS is highly variable; those with early or abrupt onset generally experience more rapid decline in lung function and higher mortality. Previous treatment strategies focused on augmentation of immunosuppression, but the benefits of such an approach are questionable and the risk of infection is considerable. A possible therapeutic role of macrolides to suppress airway inflammation has led to observations of improvement in FEV_1 in several retrospective studies. Aerosolised cyclosporine has also shown potential efficacy in preventing BOS. Surgical fundoplication to control gastro-oesophageal reflux has been associated with improvement in lung function in some patients with BOS. Re-transplantation remains the only definitive treatment for advanced BOS.

Kotloff, R.M. and Thabut, G. (2011). Lung transplantation. *Am J Respir Crit Care Med* 184, 159–171.
http://ajrccm.atsjournals.org/content/184/2/159.long

35. Answer A

Prolonged oral or inhaled antibiotic treatments are sometimes used to improve quality of life and to prevent exacerbations in patients with chronic suppurative lung disease (CSLD) or bronchiectasis, although the evidence is limited and the possibility of developing antibiotic resistance is of concern (Chang et al., 2010). There is increasing interest in macrolides for this purpose. However, further studies are required to establish their role in CSLD/bronchiectasis.

In addition, before using macrolides long-term, the presence of non-tuberculous mycobacteria should be excluded in adults and older children capable of providing sputum samples.

 Chang, A.B., Bell, S.C., Byrnes, C.A., et al. (2010). Chronic suppuratives lung disease and bronchiectasis in children and adults in Australia and New Zealand: A position statement from the Thoracic Society of Australia and New Zealand and the Australian Lung Foundation.
http://lungfoundation.com.au/wp-content/uploads/2012/06/bronchiectasis.pdf

 Doucet-Populaire, F., Buriankova, K., Weiser, J., and Pernodet, J.L. (2002). Natural and acquired macrolide resistance in mycobacteria. *Curr Drug Targets Infect Disord* 2, 355–370.
http://www.ncbi.nlm.nih.gov/pubmed/12570741

36. Answer E

Allergic bronchopulmonaryaspergillosis (ABPA), which is also associated with asthma, is a hypersensitivity disease that primarily affects the central airways (Agarwal, 2009). Immediate and delayed hypersensitivity to *Aspergillus fumigatus* are involved in the pathogenesis of this disorder. Onset of disease occurs most often in the fourth and fifth decades, and virtually all patients have long-standing atopic asthma. Clinically, a patient presents with chronic asthma, recurrent pulmonary infiltrates and bronchiectasis. The typical patient has a long history of intermittent wheezing, after which the illness evolves into a more chronic and more highly symptomatic disorder with fever, chills, pulmonary infiltrates and productive cough. The chest X-ray may show a segmental infiltrate or segmental atelectasis, most commonly in the upper lobes. In the patient with typical symptoms, the branching, finger-like shadows from mucoid impaction of dilated central bronchi are pathognomonic of ABPA.

The disorder needs to be detected before bronchiectasis has developed because the occurrence of bronchiectasis is associated with poorer outcomes. Because many patients with ABPA may be minimally symptomatic or asymptomatic, a high index of suspicion for ABPA should be maintained while managing any patient with bronchial asthma, whatever the severity or the level of control.

37. Answer C

This patient's history and presentation is classic for idiopathic pulmonary fibrosis (IPF) – an insidious loss of pulmonary function and the absence of signs or symptoms of a systemic process (King et al., 2011). His biopsy specimen report describes usual interstitial pneumonitis (UIP), which is characteristic of IPF. Besides a chest X-ray, high-resolution CT of the chest and pulmonary function testing are useful non-invasive ways to evaluate patients; however, an open lung biopsy is ultimately needed for diagnosis in the majority of patients. Older patients may be spared the morbidity of open lung biopsy if they have a classic presentation and features suggestive of IPF on transbronchial biopsy. Survival is usually 2–3 years after diagnosis. Although multiple medicinal therapies have been tried, none to date has improved survival in this patient population. Lung transplantation is a good option, and patients should be referred once the diffusing capacity of the lung for carbon monoxide (DLco) has dropped below 40%. Patients with desquamative interstitial pneumonia (DIP) are usually younger; biopsy in these patients reveals a homogeneous pattern of involvement and characteristic pigmented alveolar macrophages. In patients with Hamman–Rich syndrome, cough and dyspnoea rapidly progress to significant respiratory compromise. The onset of bronchiolitis obliterans organising pneumonia (BOOP) is more acute, and systemic symptoms such as fever and malaise are not uncommon; microscopic findings are distinct in BOOP.

38. Answer F
Clinical presentations of patients with pulmonary alveolar proteinosis (PAP) can vary considerably (Borie et al., 2011). The condition may progress, remain stable or resolve spontaneously. Some patients are asymptomatic; others have severe respiratory insufficiency. Most patients present with gradually progressive exertional dyspnoea and cough that is usually unproductive. Diagnosis is made with bronchoalveolar lavage (BAL), which shows grossly turbid exudates in the airways and periodic acid–Schiff (PAS)-positive material on pathological examination. Löffler syndrome is characterised by transient and migratory infiltrates on chest X-ray and a predominance of eosinophils on BAL. Diffuse alveolar haemorrhage is associated with a history of haemoptysis or is evidenced by bleeding at the time of BAL. Lymphangioleiomyomatosis affects women only.

PAP is a rare pulmonary disease characterised by alveolar accumulation of surfactant. It may result from mutations in surfactant proteins or granulocyte macrophage–colony stimulating factor (GM-CSF) receptor genes, it may be secondary to toxic inhalation or haematological disorders or it may be autoimmune, with anti-GM-CSF antibodies blocking activation of alveolar macrophages. Autoimmune alveolar proteinosis is the most frequent form of PAP, representing 90% of cases. Although not specific, high-resolution computed tomography shows a characteristic 'crazy paving' pattern. In most cases, BAL findings establish the diagnosis. Whole lung lavage is the most effective therapy, especially for autoimmune disease. Novel therapies targeting alveolar macrophages (recombinant GM-CSF therapy) or anti-GM-CSF antibodies (rituximab and plasmapheresis) are being investigated.

39. Answer H
Pulmonary lymphangioleiomyomatosis (or lymphangiomyomatosis; LAM) is an uncommon disease in women that is characterised by smooth muscle cell infiltra-

tion and cystic destruction of the lung (McCormack, 2008). LAM occurs in about 30% of women with the tuberous sclerosis complex (TSC-LAM), a genetic disorder of highly variable penetrance associated with seizures, brain tumours and cognitive impairment, and also in women who do not have TSC [i.e. sporadic LAM (S-LAM)]. Both S-LAM and TSC-LAM are associated with mutations in tuberous sclerosis genes, which regulate signalling through critical cellular pathways that control energy and nutrient resources in the cell.

Clinically, LAM is characterised by progressive dyspnoea on exertion, recurrent pneumothoraces, abdominal and thoracic lymphadenopathy, and abdominal tumours, including angiomyolipomas and lymphangiomyomas. The pulmonary manifestations of LAM usually predominate, but occasionally LAM presents exclusively in the abdomen and mimics lymphoma or ovarian cancer. LAM lesions express markers of smooth muscle and melanocytic differentiation, which are useful diagnostically. There are no proven therapies for LAM, but an improved understanding of the molecular pathogenesis of the disease has identified several promising molecular targets, such as mammalian target of rapamycin (mTOR) which can be inhibited by sirolimus.

References for Questions 36–39:

 Agarwal, R. (2009). Allergic bronchopulmonary aspergillosis. *Chest* 135, 805–826.
http://journal.publications.chestnet.org/article.aspx?articleid=1089694

 Borie, R., Danel, C., Debray, et al. (2011). Pulmonary alveolar proteinosis. *Eur Respir Rev* 20, 98–107.
http://err.ersjournals.com/content/20/120/98.long

 King, T.E., Jr., Pardo, A., and Selman, M. (2011). Idiopathic pulmonary fibrosis. *Lancet* 378, 1949–1961.
http://www.ncbi.nlm.nih.gov/pubmed/21719092

 McCormack, F.X. (2008). Lymphangioleiomyomatosis: a clinical update. *Chest* 133, 507–516.
http://journal.publications.chestnet.org/article.aspx?articleid=1085685

3 Gastroenterology

Questions

BASIC SCIENCE

Answers can be found in the Gastroenterology Answers section at the end of this chapter.

1. Which one of the following cell types has a role in determining the body iron content and distribution?
   A. Gastric parietal cells
   B. Microfold cells
   C. Goblet cells of the small intestine
   D. Reticuloendothelial macrophages
   E. Cardiac myocytes

2. The absorption of which one of the following is affected by the resection of the distal ileum?
   A. Bile salts
   B. Calcium
   C. Folate
   D. Iron
   E. Vitamin C

3. Which one of the following is true of fructose?
   A. Intake worldwide is reducing
   B. It is less prone to promote hypertension than glucose
   C. Fructose intolerance can present as a metabolic disorder in infancy
   D. It is not malabsorbed
   E. It is not as sweet tasting as glucose

4. Which one of the following is a stimulus for gastrin secretion?
   A. Calcitonin
   B. Epinephrine (adrenaline)
   C. Glucagon

Passing the FRACP Written Examination: Questions and Answers, First Edition. Jonathan Gleadle, Tuck Yong, Jordan Li, Surjit Tarafdar, and Danielle Wu.
© 2013 John Wiley & Sons, Ltd. Published 2013 by John Wiley & Sons, Ltd.

D. Somatostatin
E. Vasoactive inhibitory peptide (VIP)

5. Which one of the following hormones increases appetite?
  A. Glucagon
  B. Leptin
  C. Glucagon-like peptide 1
  D. Ghrelin
  E. Lipase

6. A 35-year-old immigrant has had a hepatitis serology test for investigation of abnormal liver function tests. He has a positive hepatitis B surface antigen (HBsAg) and has IgM antibodies to hepatitis B core (anti-HBc). What is the most likely stage of infection for this patient?
  A. Acute hepatitis B infection
  B. Chronic hepatitis B infection
  C. High levels of hepatitis B virus DNA in the blood
  D. Inactive carrier
  E. Post-vaccination changes

7. A 35-year-old woman presents with jaundice and lethargy. Her blood tests are shown below. Anti-mitochondrial antibody is positive. What is the liver biopsy likely to show?

	Value	Reference ranges
Serum bilirubin (mmol/L)	110	2–24
Alkaline phosphatase (U/L)	650	30–110
Aspartate aminotransferase (U/L)	240	<45

  A. Granulomatous changes of hepatocytes
  B. Fatty changes of the liver parenchyma
  C. Piecemeal necrosis and fibrosis around portal veins
  D. Collagen layering around bile ducts
  E. Lymphocyte infiltrates causing biliary duct destruction

8. Which one of the following best describes the faecal immunochemical test (FIT)?
  A. The antibodies in this test bind to the haem portion of human haemoglobin
  B. FIT has a higher clinical sensitivity in detecting occult blood at lower concentrations compared to the guaiac-based faecal occult blood test (gFOBT)
  C. Digested blood from the upper gastrointestinal tract is often detected by FIT

    D. Patients have to observe dietary restrictions before collecting a stool sample

    E. FIT has a higher false-positive rate than gFOBT

Theme: Pathological and clinical features of chronic liver disease (for Questions 9 and 10)

    A. Alcoholic hepatitis
    B. Autoimmune hepatitis
    C. Chronic hepatitis B
    D. Haemochromatosis
    E. Hepatocellular carcinoma
    F. Primary biliary cirrhosis
    G. Primary sclerosing cholangitis
    H. Wilson disease

For each patient with abnormal liver biochemistry and biopsy, select the most likely diagnosis.

9. A 42-year-old woman presented with fatigue, nausea, abdominal pain and arthralgia. She does not drink any alcohol. Her aspartate and alanine aminotransferase are markedly elevated, above three times the upper limit of normal. Her viral hepatitis serology is negative. Caeruloplasmin level is normal. Her liver biopsy shows dense portal and periportal predominance of plasma cell infiltrate with some lymphocytes.

10. A 35-year-old woman with a history of hypothyroidism, on adequate thyroxine replacement, presented with fatigue and pruritus. She has jaundice and enlarged liver on examination. Her alkaline phosphatase has been elevated for more than 6 months. Her liver biopsy shows portal inflammation and destruction of the intrahepatic bile ducts.

Theme: Nutritional issues after bariatric surgery
(for Questions 11 and 12)

    A. Thiamine
    B. Folic acid
    C. Vitamin A
    D. Vitamin B_{12}
    E. Vitamin C
    F. Vitamin D
    G. Vitamin E
    H. Vitamin K

Deficiency of which micronutrient is the most likely cause of the following clinical scenarios?

11. A 45-year-old man presents with confusion and nausea. He had a Roux-en-Y gastric bypass surgery 2 years prior to this presentation. He has not been adherent to nutritional recommendations after the surgery. On examination he has tachycardia and bilateral pitting oedema of his legs.

12. A 50-year-old woman presents with visual disturbance 8 years after having a Roux-en-Y gastric bypass surgery for morbid obesity. She does not have type 2 diabetes. On examination she has reduced visual acuity and bilateral conjunctival keratinisation with superficial punctuate keratopathy in the cornea.

CLINICAL

13. A 38-year-old woman has had a 10-year history of heartburn but has not received any treatment. Over the past 4 months, she has had progressive difficulty swallowing large bits of solid food. She has no difficulty with soft foods or liquids, and she has not lost weight. Which one of the following is the most likely explanation for her symptoms?
   A. Adenocarcinoma in the lower third of the oesophagus
   B. Barrett oesophagus in the distal oesophagus
   C. Stricture of the distal oesophagus
   D. Schatzki ring of the distal oesophagus
   E. Squamous carcinoma in the mid-third of the oesophagus

14. A 65-year-old woman with recently diagnosed renal cell cancer presents to hospital with abdominal pain and abdominal distension. She states that her abdomen has become more distended and painful over a 3-week period and that she was afraid to come into hospital as she thought this was further spread of the cancer. On examination she has a tender distended abdomen with moderate hepatomegaly and evidence of ascites. The hepatojugular reflux is absent. The abdominal veins are dilated in the flanks and over the back, along with pedal oedema. Which one of the following diagnoses is the most likely?
   A. Alpha-1-anti-trypsin deficiency
   B. Budd–Chiari syndrome
   C. Constrictive pericarditis
   D. Cytomegalovirus hepatitis
   E. Epstein–Barr virus infection

15. A 28-year-old woman was found to have an elevated total bilirubin level on her pre-operative blood test. She has no other significant medical history. She is only taking an oral contraceptive pill and no other over-the-counter medications. Her physical examination is unremarkable. Her hepatitis A, B and C serology are all negative. Her other investigation results are shown below. Which is the most appropriate next step in her management?

	Value	Reference ranges
Haemoglobin (g/L)	139	120–140
Serum bilirubin (mmol/L)	39	2–24
Alkaline phosphatase (U/L)	65	30–110
Aspartate aminotransferase (U/L)	34	<45

   A. Investigation for the presence and cause of haemolysis
   B. An abdominal ultrasonography before surgery
   C. Discontinuation of the oral contraceptive pill permanently
   D. Half of the recommended paracetamol dose post surgery
   E. Recommended dose of morphine peri-operatively

16. Which one of the following is a predictor of a favourable response to pegylated interferon (PEG-IFN) plus ribavirin therapy in previously untreated immunocompetent patients with chronic hepatitis C infection?
- **A.** HCV genotype 1
- **B.** High hepatitis C RNA levels
- **C.** Absence of cirrhosis
- **D.** Age over 50 years
- **E.** Normal aminotransferase levels

17. A 27–year-old woman who has not travelled abroad in the last 2 years presents with a 8-month history of abdominal discomfort and diarrhoea up to 4 times a day. There is no history of rectal bleeding or weight loss. Her full blood examination, C-reactive protein, electrolytes and coeliac serology are normal. She has tried a lactose-free diet for the last 2 months with no improvement. What is the next most appropriate step?
- **A.** Colonoscopy
- **B.** Hydrogen breath test
- **C.** Pancreatic function testing
- **D.** Trial of anti-spasmodic therapy
- **E.** Computed tomography of the abdomen and pelvis

18. A 60-year-old woman has epigastric pain for several months and is referred for endoscopy. Gastric biopsy confirms mucosa-associated lymphoid tissue (MALT) lymphoma and the presence of *Helicobacter pylori*. Further evaluation confirms only gastric involvement. What is the next most appropriate treatment?
- **A.** Amoxycillin, clarithromycin and omeprazole
- **B.** Oral cyclophosphamide
- **C.** Radiotherapy
- **D.** Rituximab therapy
- **E.** Total gastrectomy

19. A 52-year-old woman presents with an 8-month history of chronic non-bloody watery diarrhoea. Faecal leucocytes are present but stool cultures are negative. C-reactive protein is mildly elevated. Barium enema and colonoscopy were normal but biopsy reveals increased intraepithelial lymphocytes within the surface epithelium. What is the most likely diagnosis?
- **A.** Microscopic colitis
- **B.** Crohn disease
- **C.** Ulcerative colitis
- **D.** Pseudomembranous colitis
- **E.** Irritable bowel syndrome

20. A 60-year-old man presents with a 1-week history of non-specific epigastric pain. His medical history includes hypertension, gout, hypercholesterolemia and obesity with a BMI of 38 kg/m². He is currently taking ramipril 10 mg daily, allopurinol 300 mg daily and atorvastatin 40 mg daily. He does not drink any alcohol. His physical examination is normal and liver function test results are within the normal reference ranges. Liver ultrasound revealed features of hepatic steatosis. What is the next appropriate step in his management?

A. Liver biopsy
B. Commence metformin
C. Commence ursodeoxycholic acid
D. Immediate referral for bariatric surgery
E. Continue atorvastatin

21. A 73-year-old man presents with a 2-month history of regurgitating food and foul-smelling breath. He describes the regurgitated food as slightly changed but denies any blood or pain when he eats. He has not lost any weight recently. He is otherwise fit and well. Which of the following diagnoses is most likely?

A. Gastric outlet obstruction
B. Mallory–Weiss tear
C. Oesophageal carcinoma
D. Pharyngeal pouch
E. Plummer–Vinson syndrome

22. The earliest phenotypic manifestation of idiopathic hereditary haemochromatosis is:

A. Post-prandial increase in serum iron concentration
B. Elevated serum ferritin level
C. Slate-grey pigmentation of skin
D. Increased transferrin saturation
E. Jaundice

23. A 45-year-old man presents with lethargy, abdominal discomfort, jaundice and pruritus. The results of investigations are shown below. Anti-nuclear antibody and anti-mitochondrial antibody is negative. Ultrasound of the abdomen shows normal intrahepatic and extrahepatic bile ducts. The gallbladder is mildly enlarged and liver parenchyma show prominent periportal echogenicity. Which one of the following is the likely diagnosis?

	Value	Reference range
Bilirubin (μmol/L)	86	2–24
Albumin (g/L)	35	34–48
Alkaline phosphatase (U/L)	1200	30–110
Alanine aminotransferase (U/L)	150	<55

A. Autoimmune hepatitis
B. Cholangiocarcinoma
C. Chronic active viral hepatitis

D. Primary biliary cirrhosis
E. Primary sclerosing cholangitis

24. Which of the following patients with acute non-typhoid Salmonella gastro-enteritis requires antibiotic treatment?
A. Has fever for more than 48 h
B. Has diarrhoea for more than 48 h
C. Has constant abdominal pain for 24 h
D. Has sickle-cell disease
E. International travel a month prior to presentation

25. A 50-year-old man with a 7-year history of cirrhosis caused by hepatitis C and alcohol is seen regularly in the liver clinic. What is the most appropriate surveillance for hepatocellular carcinoma?
A. Aminotransferase measurements every 3 months
B. Serum alpha-fetoprotein every 6 months
C. Liver ultrasonography every 12 months
D. Serum alpha-fetoprotein and liver ultrasonography every 6–12 months
E. Computed tomography of the abdomen every 12 months

26. A 62-year-old man presented with melaena, dizziness and abdominal dis-comfort. On examination, his blood pressure was 85/40 mmHg and heart rate was 105 beats/min. After initial resuscitation and assessment, he underwent an urgent endoscopy which revealed a duodenal ulcer and a non-bleeding vessel was visible. He was treated with epinephrine (adrenaline) injection and thermal therapy. Gastric biopsy was positive for *H. pylori* infection. Which one of the following statements concerning his management is correct?
A. The risk of further bleeding is high because he did not receive pre-endoscopic pantoprazole
B. He should receive oral pantoprazole 40 mg twice a day for 3 days
C. He should have a repeat endoscopy 24 h after initial endoscopic haemo-static therapy
D. He should be fasted for 72 h after endoscopy
E. After confirmation of eradication of *H. pylori*, long-term usage of panto-prazole is not recommended

27. A 45-year-old woman has rectal bleeding during bowel movements for 10 weeks. She has intermittent diarrhoea and severe lower abdominal pains. Her appetite is poor and she has also lost 7 kg in weight. On examination she has a tender left lower abdomen and active bowel sounds. Rectal examination reveals a small streak of blood. Her investigations results are shown below. A rigid sig-moidoscopy shows inflammatory changes with multiple ulceration and numerous areas of petechial haemorrhages. Elevated sessile reddish nodules (small and multiple) appear on the flat surface. There are multiple confluent ulcers leading to denudation of the mucosa.

Which treatment should be administered?

	Value	Reference ranges
Haemoglobin (g/L)	111	135–175
White cell count (cells/L)	13.5×10^9	$4.0–11.0 \times 10^9$
Platelet count (cells/L)	600×10^9	$150–450 \times 10^9$
Urea (mmol/L)	6.0	2.7–8.0
Creatinine (μmol/L)	100	50–100
C-reactive protein (mg/L)	80	<10

A. Intravenous hydrocortisone
B. Intravenous metronidazole
C. Intravenous 5-aminosalicylate
D. Intravenous anti-TNF-α antibody infusion
E. Intravenous gamma globulin infusion

28. A 65-year-old man complains of fevers, weight loss, joint pains and diarrhoea. A jejunal biopsy reveals flattened mucosa containing periodic acid–Schiff (PAS) positive macrophages. What is the most likely diagnosis?
A. *Campylobacter jejuni* infection
B. Coeliac disease
C. Giardiasis
D. Small bowel amyloidosis
E. *Tropheryma whipplei* infection

29. Which one of the following tests provides the most useful early information about possible ascitic fluid infection in a patient with cirrhosis, abdominal pain and fever?
A. Gram stain of ascitic fluid
B. Neutrophil count of ascitic fluid
C. Albumin gradient of ascitic fluid compared to serum
D. Total protein in ascitic fluid
E. Bacterial culture of ascitic fluid

30. Which one of the following laboratory results is most likely to be observed in patient with severe small intestinal bacterial overgrowth?

	Mean corpuscular volume	Folate level	Vitamin B_{12} level
A	High	Low	Low
B	Normal	High	Normal
C	Normal	Normal	High
D	High	High	Low
E	High	Low	High

Theme: Treatment of inflammatory bowel disease
(for Questions 29–33)

    A. Azathioprine
    B. Cholestyramine
    C. Infliximab
    D. Mesalazine suppository
    E. Methotrexate
    F. Metronidazole
    G. Oral mesalazine
    H. Prednisolone

For each of the following scenarios, select the most appropriate treatment.

31. A 24-year-old woman with a 6-month history of severe diarrhoea is newly diagnosed with primary eosinophilic colitis.

32. A 52-year-old man with Crohn disease has recently been diagnosed with an enteroenteric fistula. He is already being treated with azathioprine.

33. A 38-year-old woman with ulcerative colitis presents with mild bloody diarrhoea and is found to have mild-to-moderate proctitis only on colonoscopy.

34. A 65-year-old man with a long-standing history of Crohn disease, which has been in remission for the past 10 years, presents with acute diarrhoea. Exotoxin from an anaerobic Gram-positive rod is detected in his stool specimen.

35. A 46-year-old woman with a 10-year history of Crohn disease presents with a non-healing leg wound. She has been on a course of prednisolone for a month and maintenance dose of azathioprine.

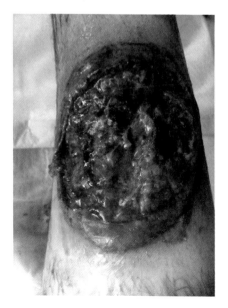

Answers

BASIC SCIENCE

1. Answer D
The four major cell types that determine the body iron content and distribution are:
- Duodenal enterocytes affecting dietary iron absorption
- Erythroid precursors affecting iron utilisation
- Reticuloendothelial macrophages affecting iron storage and recycling
- Hepatocytes affecting iron storage and endocrine regulation.

Duodenal enterocytes absorb approximately 1–2 mg of iron/day to offset losses. Absorbed iron circulates bound to transferrin and is used primarily by erythroid precursors in the synthesis of haem. Reticuloendothelial macrophages clear senescent red blood cells and release the iron from haem to export it to the circulation or store it in ferritin. Hepatocytes are another site of iron storage as ferritin and the principal site of production of the peptide hormone hepcidin. Hepcidin blocks the release of iron from enterocytes and reticuloendothelial macrophages by degrading the iron exporter ferroportin. Microfold cells are epithelial cells that overlie Peyer's patches and other large lymphatic aggregations. They are relatively flat and their surface is thrown into folds, rather than microvilli. They endocytose antigens and transport them to the underlying lymphoid cells where immune responses to foreign antigens can be initiated (Fleming and Ponka, 2012).

Fleming, R.E. and Ponka, P. (2012). Iron overload in human disease. *N Engl J Med* 366, 348–359.
http://www.ncbi.nlm.nih.gov/pubmed/22276824

2. Answer A
Bile salts aid fat absorption in the duodenum and jejunum and are reabsorbed in the distal ileum as part of enterohepatic circulation, so that usually only approximately 0.5 g/day are lost in the faeces. One of the consequences of surgical resection of the distal ileum is the reduced absorption of bile salts.

Iron, folate, vitamin C and calcium are absorbed mainly in the proximal jejunum. The only vitamin absorbed in the distal ileum is vitamin B_{12}, which also requires the presence of intrinsic factor, a glycoprotein produced by gastric parietal cells.

3. Answer C
Fructose is a simple sugar, a monosaccharide that is present primarily in added dietary sugars, honey and fruit. Fructose is absorbed by facilitated diffusion utilising the sodium-independent insulin-independent transporter (GLUT-5). Worldwide, dietary fructose intake is increasing. It is obtained primarily from added sugars, including sucrose and high fructose corn syrup, and this correlates epidemiologically with the rising prevalence of metabolic syndrome and hypertension world-

wide (Madero et al., 2011). The administration of fructose to animals and humans increases blood pressure and the development of metabolic syndrome. These changes occur independently of caloric intake because of the effect of fructose on adenosine triphosphate (ATP) depletion and uric acid generation. Fructose ingestion may also be a risk factor for kidney disease with glomerular hypertension, renal inflammation and tubulointerstitial injury seen in animals. Fructose intolerance is due to fructose-1-phosphate aldolase deficiency and can present in infancy with hypoglycaemia and vomiting. Fructose malabsorption may play a role in the symptoms of coeliac disease and, potentially, irritable bowel syndrome.

 Madero, M., Perez-Pozo, S.E., Jalal, D., Johnson, R.J., and Sanchez-Lozada, L.G. (2011). Dietary fructose and hypertension. *Curr Hypertens Rep* 13, 29–35. http://link.springer.com/article/10.1007%2Fs11906-010-0163-x

4. Answer B

Gastrin is a peptide hormone that stimulates secretion of gastric acid by the parietal cells of the stomach and aids in gastric motility. It is released by G cells in the antrum of the stomach, duodenum and pancreas. It binds to cholecystokinin B receptors to stimulate the release of histamines in enterochromaffin-like cells, and it induces the insertion of potassium–hydrogen (K^+/H^+)-ATPase pumps into the apical membrane of parietal cells, which in turn increases hydrogen ion (H^+) release.

The major stimuli for gastrin secretion are:
- L-Amino acids (i.e. phenylalanine, tryptophan, cysteine, tyrosine)
- Vagal stimulation
- Gastric distension
- Epinephrine (adrenaline)
- Calcium
- Acetylcholine.

The major inhibitors of gastrin secretion are:
- Gastric pH <2
- Somatostatin
- Calcitonin
- Gastric inhibitory polypeptide (GIP)
- Glucagon
- Vasoactive inhibitory peptide (VIP).

5. Answer D

Ghrelin functions as an appetite stimulatory hormone, chiefly by its actions on the hypothalamic appetite centre (Dong and Brubaker, 2012).

Leptin and ghrelin are two hormones that are now recognised to have a major influence on energy balance. Ghrelin attenuates leptin-induced reduction in food intake and body weight by modulating the expression of various hypothalamic peptides.

The secretion of ghrelin by the stomach depends largely on the nutritional state. Ghrelin levels show preprandial increases and postprandial decreases. Ghrelin stimulates the activity of neurones expressing appetite stimulating neuropeptide Y (NPY), agouti-related peptide (AgRP) and orexin, while it has an inhibitory effect on pro-opiomelanocortin (POMC) neurones, which produce the appetite suppressant peptide α-melanocyte stimulating hormone (α-MSH). These actions are the opposite of leptin.

It has been demonstrated that circulating ghrelin levels increase when obese humans lose weight, and because obese mice show an increase in sensitivity to ghrelin upon weight loss, inhibition of ghrelin prevents weight regain after weight loss. There is considerable interest in the potential of the ghrelin system as a therapeutic target for obesity treatment.

Glucagon increases glucose production by stimulating both glycogenolysis and gluconeogenesis.

Glucagon-like peptide-1 (GLP-1) causes glucose-dependent secretion of insulin, slows gastric emptying, suppresses inappropriately elevated levels of glucagon and leads to weight loss.

Dong, C. X. and Brubaker, P. L. (2012). Ghrelin, the proglucagon-derived peptides and peptide YY in nutrient homeostasis. *Nat Rev Gastroenterol Hepatol* 9, 705–715.
http://www.nature.com/nrgastro/journal/v9/n12/full/nrgastro.2012.185.html

6. Answer A

Test	Result	Typical interpretation
HBsAg	Negative	Susceptible (needs vaccination)
Anti-HBc	Negative	
Anti-HBs	Negative	
HBsAg	Negative	Resolved HBV infection
Anti-HBc	Positive	
Anti-HBs	Positive	
HBsAg	Negative	Vaccinated
Anti-HBc	Negative	
Anti-HBs	Positive	
HBsAg	Positive	Active HBV infection (*usually* chronic)
Anti-HBc*	Positive	*If IgM anti-HBc is present, this may represent acute HBV
Anti-HBs	Negative	infection
HBsAg	Negative	Various possibilities, including:
Anti-HBc	Positive	• Distant resolved infection (*most common*)
Anti-HBs	Negative	• Recovering from acute infection
		• False positive
		• 'Occult' HBV (*determined by positive HBV DNA viral load*)

A positive anti-HBc (IgM) and HBsAg suggest acute infection. When the infection resolves, HBsAg becomes negative and anti-HBc (IgG) positive. In patients who have been vaccinated, HBsAg is negative and anti-HBs is positive (Dienstag, 2008; Liaw and Chu, 2009) (see table above).

Viral proteins of clinical importance include the envelope protein, hepatitis B surface antigen (HBsAg); a structural nucleocapsid core protein, hepatitis B core antigen (HBcAg); soluble nucleocapsid protein; and hepatitis Be antigen (HBeAg). Hepatitis B virus (HBV) relies on a retroviral replication strategy (reverse transcription from RNA to DNA), and eradication of HBV infection is rendered difficult because stable, long-enduring, covalently closed circular DNA (ccDNA) becomes established in hepatocyte nuclei and HBV DNA becomes integrated into the host genome.

Dienstag, J.L. (2008). Hepatitis B virus infection. *N Engl J Med* 359, 1486–1500.
http://www.ncbi.nlm.nih.gov/pubmed/18832247

Liaw, Y.F. and Chu, C.M. (2009). Hepatitis B virus infection. *Lancet* 373, 582–592.
http://www.ncbi.nlm.nih.gov/pubmed/19217993

7. Answer E

This patient is likely to have primary biliary cirrhosis. Inflammatory changes with biliary destruction are suggestive of primary biliary cirrhosis. Granulomatous changes would suggest sarcoidosis or Wegener granulomatosis. Piecemeal necrosis and fibrosis suggest chronic hepatitis.

Primary biliary cirrhosis is now diagnosed earlier in its clinical course than it was in the past; 50–60% of patients are asymptomatic at diagnosis. Fatigue and pruritus are the most common presenting symptoms, occurring in about 21% and 19% of patients, respectively. Overt symptoms develop within 2–4 years in the majority of asymptomatic patients, although one-third of patients may remain symptom-free for many years (Kaplan and Gershwin, 2005).

Primary biliary cirrhosis is divided into four histological stages. However, the liver is not affected uniformly, and a single biopsy may demonstrate the presence of all four stages at the same time. Stage 1 is defined by the localisation of inflammation to the portal triads. In stage 2, the number of normal bile ducts is reduced, and inflammation extends beyond the portal triads into the surrounding parenchyma. In stage 3, fibrous septa link adjacent portal triads. Stage 4 represents end-stage liver disease, characterised by frank cirrhosis with regenerative nodules.

Kaplan, M.M. and Gershwin, M.E. (2005). Primary biliary cirrhosis. *N Engl J Med* 353, 1261–1273.
http://www.ncbi.nlm.nih.gov/pubmed/16177252

8. Answer B

The faecal immunochemical test (FIT) uses antibodies that bind the globin portion of haemoglobin with high specificity. This means that patients do not have to observe drug or dietary restrictions before collecting a stool sample. Patient adherence is likely to be higher with FIT. Digested blood from the upper gastrointestinal tract is not usually detected by FIT, making the test highly specific for occult lower GI bleeding.

In comparison to the guaiac-based faecal occult blood test (gFOBT), studies have shown that FIT detects lower concentrations of occult blood with higher clinical sensitivity and specificity (Young, 2011). The major advantage of FIT is the decreased number of false-positive results. However, FIT is more costly than gFOBT, but this can be offset by the fewer colonoscopies required.

Young, G.P. (2009). Population-based screening for colorectal cancer: Australian research and implementation. *J Gastroenterol Hepatol* 24 Suppl 3, S33–42.
http://onlinelibrary.wiley.com/doi/10.1111/j.1440-1746.2009.06069.x/pdf

9. Answer B

Autoimmune hepatitis (AIH) is an inflammatory liver disease that mainly affects females. It is characterised histologically by interface hepatitis, biochemically by increased aspartate and alanine aminotransferase levels, and serologically by the presence of autoantibodies and increased levels of immunoglobulin G (Mieli-Vergani and Vergani, 2011). Interface hepatitis is typical of, though not exclusive to, AIH. It is characterised by necroinflammatory change, sometimes referred to as 'lymphocytic' piecemeal necrosis. It initially destroys the limiting plate of liver cells (i.e. is periportal). In the untreated patient, there is continuous erosion of the hepatic parenchyma. The necroinflammatory changes are followed by fibrosis. Interface hepatitis may not involve all portal areas equally in a given case and can affect a segment or the entire perimeter of a portal area. It can continue unabated in the cirrhotic liver, complicating chronic hepatitis and, thus, contributing to the activity of the cirrhotic process. A predominance of plasma cells in portal areas and in foci and zones of necrosis is characteristic of chronic AIH and is most helpful for distinguishing it from chronic hepatitis C, in which the predominant cell is the lymphocyte. However, their presence in low numbers does not exclude the diagnosis of AIH. An abundance of plasma cells can also be found in chronic hepatitis B and some cases of drug-induced chronic hepatitis.

When AIH presents acutely and during episodes of relapse, a common histological picture is pan-lobular hepatitis with bridging necrosis and, if the disease takes a fulminant course, massive necrosis and multilobular collapse.

Mieli-Vergani, G. and Vergani, D. (2011). Autoimmune hepatitis. *Nat Rev Gastroenterol Hepatol* 8, 320–329.
http://www.ncbi.nlm.nih.gov/pubmed/21537351

10. Answer F

Histopathologically, primary biliary cirrhosis (PBC) is characterised by portal inflammation and immune-mediated destruction of the intrahepatic bile ducts (Kaplan and Gershwin, 2005). These changes occur at different rates and with varying degrees of severity in different patients. The loss of bile ducts leads to decreased bile secretion and the retention of toxic substances within the liver, resulting in further hepatic damage, fibrosis, cirrhosis and, eventually, liver failure.

PBC is a slowly progressive autoimmune disease of the liver that primarily affects women. Its peak incidence occurs in the fifth decade of life, and it is uncommon in persons under 25 years of age. Other common findings in PBC include hyperlipidaemia, hypothyroidism, osteopenia and coexisting autoimmune diseases, including Sjögren syndrome and scleroderma. PBC is characterised serologically by the presence of anti-mitochondrial antibodies, which are present in 90–95% of patients and are often detectable years before clinical signs appear.

Kaplan, M.M. and Gershwin, M.E. (2005). Primary biliary cirrhosis. *N Engl J Med* 353, 1261–1273.
http://www.ncbi.nlm.nih.gov/pubmed/16177252

11. Answer A

Bariatric surgery remains an important treatment option for patients with a body mass index (BMI) of $40 \, kg/m^2$ or greater (or those with a BMI of $\geq 35 \, kg/m^2$ and co-morbidities) in whom lifestyle intervention and pharmacotherapy result in inadequate weight loss. The type of surgery that is chosen is a major determinant of the risk of future nutritional deficiencies (Bal et al., 2012). Unfortunately, surgical options that are more effective for inducing weight loss are more likely to lead to nutritional deficiencies. After bariatric surgery, protein is the major macronutrient associated with malnutrition. The guidelines of The Endocrine Society suggest that bariatric patients should ingest 60–120 g of protein/day.

Thiamine, or vitamin B_1, is a coenzyme for the essential enzymes transketolase, pyruvate dehydrogenase and pyruvate carboxylase in the early stages of the tricarboxylic acid cycle and in the pentose phosphate pathway. Thiamine deficiency after Roux-en-Y gastric bypass surgery (RYGB) is quite common. Manifestations of thiamine deficiency include:

- Neuropsychiatric: aggression, hallucinations, confusion, ataxia, nystagmus, paralysis of the motor nerves of the eye
- Neurological or 'dry' beriberi: convulsions, numbness, muscle weakness and/or pain in the lower and upper extremities, brisk tendon reflexes
- High-output cardiac or 'wet' beriberi: tachycardia or bradycardia, lactic acidosis, dyspnoea, leg oedema, right ventricular dilatation
- Gastrointestinal: slow gastric emptying, nausea, vomiting, jejunal dilatation or megacolon, constipation.

Oral thiamine (100 mg twice daily) is a standard therapy for thiamine deficiency. The presence of small intestinal bacterial overgrowth should be considered if a patient has refractory thiamine deficiency. Patients presenting with symptoms of Wernicke encephalopathy or acute psychosis – the neuropsychiatric types of beriberi – should be considered medical emergencies; they require hospitalisation with supportive care and they should receive a minimum of 300 mg of thiamine daily, given intramuscularly or intravenously for at least 3–5 days; intravenous infusions are given over 3–4 h to reduce the risk of an anaphylactic reaction. Within several days after initiation of parenteral thiamine administration, patients should report symptomatic improvement. Patients with Wernicke disease can also present with acute bilateral blindness. For the treatment of this serious disorder, intravenous thiamine can result in symptom resolution.

12. Answer C
After bariatric surgery, vitamin A, including β-carotenes, carotenoids and retinols, deficiency has been identified in patients with a short common channel [biliopancreatic diversion, duodenal switch or extended Roux-en-Y gastric bypass (RYGB)]. Given that fat and fat-soluble vitamin absorption require micelle formation with bile acids, potential origins of vitamin A deficiency include a relative deficiency of bile acids in the bypassed duodenojejunal segment, as well as deconjugation of bile acids by upper gut bacterial overgrowth.

Vitamin A deficiency can result in decreased vision, poor night vision (nyctalopia), xerosis, corneal ulceration and keratomalacia, retinopathy, itching (pruritus) and dry hair. Initial treatment of mild vitamin A deficiency is oral vitamin A supplementation (10 000 IU daily). For severe cases with visual impairment, parenteral vitamin A replacement may be required.

 Bal, B.S., Finelli, F.C., Shope, T.R., and Koch, T.R. (2012). Nutritional deficiencies after bariatric surgery. *Nat Rev Endocrinol* 8, 544–556.
http://www.ncbi.nlm.nih.gov/pubmed/22525731

CLINICAL

13. Answer C

This patient has classic symptoms of mechanical dysphagia, as she has difficulty with larger boluses of solid food but not softer foods or liquids. Mechanical dysphagia may follow many years of reflux and is often indicative of a peptic stricture that has developed as a result of fibrosis after a long period of chronic inflammation due to gastro-oesophageal reflux disease (GORD) (Kahrilas, 2008). These benign strictures can usually be dilated endoscopically. An intensive regimen of proton-pump inhibitors should then be instituted to reduce the frequency of recurrence.

Although chronic acid reflux can predispose for Barrett oesophagus and then subsequently adenocarcinoma, Barrett oesophagus is a mucosal change that causes luminal narrowing only. Furthermore, adenocarcinoma is very unusual in a patient this young.

Schatzki ring is unlikely, since it typically produces episodic mechanical dysphagia rather than the progressive mechanical dysphagia described in this question. Squamous carcinoma in the mid-third of the oesophagus can produce mechanical dysphagia. However, this patient is far younger than the usual patient with squamous carcinoma, and she has no risk factors, such as smoking, drinking, or upper oesophageal web (Plummer–Vinson syndrome).

Kahrilas, P.J. (2008). Gastroesophageal reflux disease. *N Engl J Med 359*, 1700–1707.
http://www.ncbi.nlm.nih.gov/pmc/articles/PMC3058591/

14. Answer B

Budd–Chiari syndrome is characterised by hepatic venous outflow obstruction at the level of the hepatic venules, the large hepatic veins, the inferior vena cava or the right atrium (Menon et al., 2004). Approximately one-third of cases have no identifiable cause; however, associations between hypercoagulable states have been well described in the literature. The oral contraceptive pill, polycythaemia rubra vera as well as haematological and intra-abdominal malignancy may all predispose to this catastrophic syndrome. Renal cell carcinoma can cause Budd–Chiari syndrome by direct tumoural invasion.

Diagnosis is usually by venous phase CT scan, which delineates the filling defect in the hepatic vein and even inferior vena cava. Ultrasound of the liver may be a useful non-invasive investigation to demonstrate retrograde flow in the portal system due to outflow obstruction and hence strengthen the diagnosis. Medical management of Budd–Chiari syndrome consists of controlling further development of ascites, using anti-coagulant therapy to prevent further extension of venous thrombosis and treating detectable underlying causes.

Viral hepatitis may present similarly, but usually with jaundice and right upper quadrant pain with or without a palpable liver. Gross ascites and signs of portal hypertension do not usually manifest without chronic liver disease and this goes against an acute infectious cause. Epstein–Barr virus infection can cause hepatomegaly and may occur post infectious mononucleosis but, as with viral hepatitis, does not usually cause a picture of chronic liver disease. The absence of hepatojugular reflux with the application of abdominal pressure also rules out a cardiac cause of ascites. α1-Anti-trypsin deficiency affects both lungs and liver, causing emphysema and chronic liver disease. α1-Anti-trypsin is a protease involved in downregulating inflammatory cascades and plays an especially important role in the protection of alveoli from protease damage in the lungs. It is associated with chronic liver disease and hepatocellular carcinoma in adults in approximately a quarter of all α1-anti-trypsin deficient patients.

Menon, K.V., Shah, V., and Kamath, P.S. (2004). The Budd-Chiari syndrome. *N Engl J Med* 350, 578–585.
http://www.ncbi.nlm.nih.gov/pubmed/14762185

15. Answer E

This patient has an incidental finding of hyperbilirubinaemia and she is otherwise asymptomatic. She does not have anaemia and her liver function is normal. This is consistent with Gilbert syndrome (Hirschfield and Alexander, 2006).

Gilbert syndrome, a mild form of unconjugated hyperbilirubinaemia, is a relatively common and often accidental finding in healthy individuals and patients with unrelated diseases (affects 3–10% of the general population). The clinical importance of this frequently encountered entity is unclear. Gilbert syndrome is caused by impaired bilirubin conjugation in the liver. It was also noted that, although overt haemolysis is not a typical feature of Gilbert syndrome, the lifespan of erythrocytes is shorter than normal in about 50% of affected individuals. This may suggest that a certain degree of a mild, compensated haemolytic state may be present and can further increase the bilirubin load.

Gilbert syndrome is usually a benign and clinically inconsequential entity that requires neither treatment nor long-term medical attention. Its clinical importance lies in the fact that the mild hyperbilirubinaemia may be mistaken for a sign of occult, chronic or progressive liver disease.

Since the UDP-GT (uridine diphosphate glucuronyl transferase) system plays an important role in the elimination not only of endogenous metabolites but also of xenobiotics, such as drugs that undergo glucuronidation, their metabolism could be impaired in patients with genetic hyperbilirubinaemia. Many drugs are direct substrates of the various isoforms of UDP-GT: paracetamol (UGT1A6, UGT1A9), morphine, oxazepam, temazepam, (UGT2B7) and amitryptiline (UGT1A4). Since Gilbert syndrome occurs quite frequently among the general population, it would seem conceivable that drugs that undergo glucuronidation will display a different pharmacokinetic profile in affected individuals and these patients may be at a potentially higher risk for certain drug toxicities. However, there is no clear indication that therapeutic doses of paracetamol are associated with an increased risk for hepatic or systemic toxicity in subjects with Gilbert syndrome.

Hirschfield, G.M. and Alexander, G.J. (2006). Gilbert's syndrome: an overview for clinical biochemists. *Ann Clin Biochem* 43, 340–343.
http://www.ncbi.nlm.nih.gov/pubmed/17022875

16. Answer C

Treatments of patients with chronic hepatitis C infection usually include combination pegylated interferon (PEG-IFN) alpha by subcutaneous injection once a week and oral ribavirin daily (Rosen, 2011). However, an increasing number of anti-viral agents are emerging, including the protease inhibitors, telaprevir and boceprevir, asunaprevir and the NS5A replication complex inhibitor daclatasvir. Randomised controlled trials (RCTs) have shown that combination PEG-IFN alpha and ribavirin therapy can achieve a sustained virological response (SVR) in 54–56% of patients: 42–52% of patients with genotype 1 and 76–84% of those with genotypes 2 and 3. Predictors of response to therapy in these large RCTs are summarised below:

- Non-genotype 1
- Low HCV RNA levels
- Absence of cirrhosis/bridging fibrosis
- Duration of therapy (for genotype 1)
- Age 40 years or younger
- Adherence
- Absence of steatosis on liver biopsy.

Rosen, H.R. (2011). Chronic hepatitis C infection. *N Engl J Med* 364, 2429–2438.
http://www.ncbi.nlm.nih.gov/pubmed/21696309

17. Answer D

This clinical picture is consistent with a diagnosis of irritable bowel syndrome (IBS) and low doses of anti-diarrhoeals, anti-spasmodics or peppermint oil may provide helpful relief (Ford and Talley, 2012). IBS is characterised by chronically recurring abdominal pain or discomfort and altered bowel habits. The female-to-male ratio is 2:1 and symptoms develop in approximately 10% of adult patients after bacterial or viral enteric infections; risk factors for the development of post-infectious IBS include female sex, a longer duration of gastroenteritis and the presence of psychosocial factors (including a major life stress at the time of infection).

IBS can generally be diagnosed without additional testing beyond a careful history taking, general physical examination and routine laboratory studies (not including colonoscopy) in patients who have typical symptoms and who do not have warning signs such as rectal bleeding, anaemia, weight loss, fever, family history of colon cancer, onset of the first symptom after 50 years of age and a major change in symptoms.

On the basis of bowel habits and stool characteristics, patients can be sub-classified as having diarrhoea-predominant IBS, constipation-predominant IBS or mixed bowel habits. Symptomatic treatment with osmotic laxatives or fibre is often useful in the treatment of constipation, while low doses of anti-diarrhoeals seem effective in uncontrollable diarrhoea. Patients should be encouraged to exercise regularly and, although data on the efficacy of tricyclic anti-depressants in patients with IBS are inconsistent, they are often used by physicians in low doses.

Ford, A.C. and Talley, N.J. (2012). Irritable bowel syndrome. *BMJ* 345, e5836.
http://www.bmj.com/content/345/bmj.e5836?view=long&pmid=22951548

18. Answer A

Mucosal-associated lymphoid tissue (MALT) lymphoma represents about 7% of all non-Hodgkin lymphomas and can arise at any extranodal site; however, at least one-third of MALT lymphomas present as a primary gastric lymphoma (Zucca and Dreyling, 2010). Most cases of MALT lymphoma affecting the stomach are associated with *Helicobacter pylori* infection. The most common presenting symptoms of gastric MALT lymphoma are non-specific upper gastrointestinal complaints that often lead to an endoscopy, usually revealing non-specific gastritis or peptic ulcer with mass lesions being unusual. Diagnosis is based on the histopathological evaluation of the gastric biopsies. The presence of active *H. pylori* infection must be determined by histochemistry or urea breath test. Eradication of *H. pylori* with antibiotics should be employed as the sole initial treatment of localised (i.e. confined to the stomach) *H. pylori*-positive gastric MALT lymphoma. Any of the highly effective anti-helicobacter antibiotic regimens proposed can be used. In case of unsuccessful *H. pylori* eradication, a second-line therapy should be attempted with alternative triple- or quadruple-therapy regimens of proton-pump inhibitor plus antibiotics. *H. pylori* eradication can induce lymphoma regression and long-term clinical disease control in most patients. The length of time necessary to obtain a remission can span from a few months to more than 12 months. Patients with systemic disease should be considered for systemic chemotherapy and/or immunotherapy with anti-CD-20 monoclonal antibodies (rituximab).

Zucca, E. and Dreyling, M. (2010). Gastric marginal zone lymphoma of MALT type: ESMO Clinical Practice Guidelines for diagnosis, treatment and follow-up. *Ann Oncol* 21 Suppl 5, v175–176.
http://annonc.oxfordjournals.org/content/21/suppl_5/v175.long

19. Answer A

Microscopic colitis (MC) is a clinical syndrome characterised by chronic watery diarrhoea, grossly normal appearing colonic mucosa and abnormal histological features (Chetty and Govender, 2012). Two entities have been described – collagenous colitis (CC) and lymphocytic colitis (LC). However, it is unclear if these two entities are clinically distinct or represent the spectrum of one disease.

MC involves the colon discontinuously and the patchy involvement necessitates a minimum of four biopsy samples. One of the features of LC is an increase in intraepithelial lymphocytes within the surface epithelium. The essential distinction between LC and CC is the presence of collagen deposition immediately beneath the basement membrane in CC.

Patients with MC can initially be treated with dietary changes by avoiding caffeine, alcohol and dairy products, and they should stop medications associated with this condition (e.g. aspirin, lansoprazole, ranitidine, NSAIDs, acarbose and sertraline). Some do well on anti-diarrhoeals or cholestyramine alone. Budesonide has been shown to be effective in treating lymphocytic colitis. Bismuth and sulphasalazine have also been shown to be effective. Some patients may respond to methotrexate or azathioprine.

Chetty, R. and Govender, D. (2012). Lymphocytic and collagenous colitis: an overview of so-called microscopic colitis. *Nat Rev Gastroenterol Hepatol* 9, 209–218.
http://www.ncbi.nlm.nih.gov/pubmed/22349169

20. Answer E

In the absence of alcohol intake and other known causes of liver disease, the hepatic steatosis is most likely related to non-alcoholic fatty liver disease (NAFLD) in the setting of obesity (Chalasani et al., 2012). This patient has no liver-related symptoms or signs and has normal liver biochemistries. Therefore, a liver biopsy is not recommended. If a biopsy is performed, it usually shows the presence of hepatic steatosis with no evidence of fibrosis or hepatocellular injury in the form of ballooning of the hepatocytes.

The risk of progression to cirrhosis and liver failure is minimal. On the other hand, in non-alcoholic steatohepatitis (NASH), there is hepatic steatosis and inflammation with hepatocyte injury (ballooning) with or without fibrosis. This can progress to cirrhosis, liver failure and, rarely, hepatocellular carcinoma.

Weight loss generally reduces hepatic steatosis, achieved either by hypocaloric diet alone or in conjunction with increased physical activity. Loss of at least 3–5% of body weight appears necessary to improve steatosis, but a greater weight loss (up to 10%) may be needed to improve necro-inflammation. Metformin has no significant effect on liver histology and is not recommended as a specific treatment for NAFLD or NASH. Ursodeoxycolic acid is not recommended for the treatment of NAFLD. Bariatric surgery is an option in eligible obese individuals with NAFLD but this is not the first-line treatment. Given the lack of evidence to show that patients with NAFLD and NASH are at increased risk for serious drug-induced liver injury from statins, statins can be used to treat dyslipidaemia in patients with NAFLD and NASH.

Chalasani, N., Younossi, Z., Lavine, J.E., et al. (2012). The diagnosis and management of non-alcoholic fatty liver disease: practice guideline by the American Gastroenterological Association, American Association for the Study of Liver Diseases, and American College of Gastroenterology. *Gastroenterology* 142, 1592–1609.
http://www.ncbi.nlm.nih.gov/pubmed/22656328

21. Answer D

Pharyngeal pouches occur more commonly in men than in women and in the elderly. The features described above are classically associated with the presence of a pharyngeal pouch. It typically causes halitosis and regurgitation of saliva and food particles consumed several days earlier. It is also associated with chronic cough and aspiration. The aetiology remains unknown but theories centre upon a structural or physiological abnormality between the inferior pharyngeal muscle complex posteriorly, known as Killian's dehiscence. Diagnosis is easily established on barium studies where the pouch is clearly delineated. When a pharyngeal pouch fills with food, it may produce dysphagia by compressing the oesophagus. Treatment is surgical via an endoscopic or external cervical approach and should include a cricopharyngeal myotomy. Unfortunately, pharyngeal pouch surgery has long been associated with significant morbidity, partly due to the surgery itself and also to the fact that the majority of patients are elderly and often have general medical problems. External approaches are associated with higher complication rates than endoscopic procedures. Recently, treatment by endoscopic stapling diverticulotomy has become increasingly popular as it has distinct advantages. The small risk of developing carcinoma within a pouch that is not excised remains a contentious issue and is an argument for long-term follow-up or treatment of the condition by external excision, particularly in younger patients.

Plummer–Vinson syndrome describes iron-deficiency anaemia and dysphagia caused by the formation of a keratinised web. Features associated with iron deficiency such as koilonychias (spoon-shaped nails) and atrophic glossitis may be rarely seen. The post-cricoid web is a direct but very rare consequence of severe iron-deficiency anaemia. Gastric outlet obstruction can cause bloating and regurgitation of newly ingested food. Mallory–Weiss tear often follows a large meal and binge drinking, leading to a small linear tear in the oesophageal mucosa. Oesophageal carcinoma presents with progressive dysphagia for solids and then liquids, often with florid constitutional symptoms and signs of cancer.

22. Answer D

The majority of cases of haemochromatosis are due to mutations in the HFE gene. Increased transferrin saturation is the earliest phenotypic manifestation of haemochromatosis because most C282Y homozygotes with iron overload have high transferrin saturation (>45% in women and >50% for men) (Adams and Barton, 2007). However, there is biological variability in transferrin saturation within individuals both with and without haemochromatosis, which leads to occasional missed diagnoses and some false-positive results. High transferrin saturation suggests a diagnosis of HFE-related haemochromatosis, but normal transferrin saturation does not exclude iron overload, especially if due to genetic causes other than mutations in the HFE gene.

Magnetic resonance imaging can be useful in the diagnosis of moderate-to-severe non-HFE iron overload. In HFE-associated haemochromatosis, liver biopsy is used more for prognostication. The progression of hepatic fibrosis can be asymptomatic until substantial liver damage has taken place. The prevalence of cirrhosis increases with increasing serum ferritin and the prognosis of haemochromatosis can be estimated from the serum ferritin concentration at diagnosis.

Adams, P.C. and Barton, J.C. (2007). Haemochromatosis. *Lancet* 370, 1855–1860.
http://www.ncbi.nlm.nih.gov/pubmed/18061062

23. Answer E

Primary sclerosing cholangitis (PSC) represents a chronic cholestatic liver disease with fibro-obliterative sclerosis of intra- and/or extra-hepatic bile ducts, eventually leading to biliary cirrhosis (Saich and Chapman, 2008). The cause of PSC is unknown, and even though it is thought that the disease may have an autoimmune origin, PSC often responds unfavourably to immunosuppressive therapy.

PSC is usually seen in males and the mean age of diagnosis is in the fifth decade of life. It is typically associated with ulcerative colitis. At presentation, approximately 15–55% of PSC patients are asymptomatic. Patients are at increased risk for developing symptoms over time. Fatigue, pruritus, jaundice or abdominal discomfort develop in 60% of cases. Symptoms such as pruritus and right upper abdominal pain are the most common intermittent symptoms, occurring with considerable individual variation and resolving spontaneously. Perinuclear anti-neutrophil cytoplasmic antibody (pANCA) is present in approximately 80% of patients, but is lacking in diagnostic specificity. The best investigation to confirm the diagnosis is endoscopic cholangiography (ERCP), which will reveal multiple strictures in the biliary system.

Saich, R. and Chapman, R. (2008). Primary sclerosing cholangitis, autoimmune hepatitis and overlap syndromes in inflammatory bowel disease. *World J Gastroenterol* 14, 331–337.
http://www.wjgnet.com/1007-9327/full/v14/i3/331.htm

24. Answer D

Acute non-typhoid salmonella gastroenteritis is usually self-limiting and resolves within 5–7 days. Consideration should be given to fluid and electrolyte replacement. Symptoms may include fever, abdominal pain and diarrhoea occurring 12–72 h after infection. A Cochrane Database Systematic Review showed that antibiotic therapy only increases the carrier rate and adverse effects (Sirinavin and Garner, 2000). Antibiotics are only indicated for those at risk of increased morbidity:

- Infants up to 2 months of age
- Elderly persons
- Immunocompromised persons
- Persons with sickle-cell disease
- Persons with prosthetic grafts or valves
- Persons with extra-intestinal findings or evidence of septicaemia.

Sirinavin, S. and Garner, P. (2000). Antibiotics for treating salmonella gut infections. *Cochrane Database Syst Rev*, CD001167.
http://www.ncbi.nlm.nih.gov/pubmed/10796610

25. Answer D

The estimated risk of hepatocellular carcinoma (HCC) is 15–20 times higher among persons infected with hepatitis C virus (HCV) compared to those who are not infected, with most of the excess risk limited to those with advanced hepatic fibrosis or cirrhosis (El-Serag, 2011). Prolonged, heavy use of alcohol is a well-established risk factor for HCC, both independently (with the risk increased by a factor of 1.5–2.0) and in combination with HCV infection and, to a lesser extent, with hepatitis B virus (HBV) infection.

Liver ultrasonography combined with measurement of serum alpha-fetoprotein levels every 6–12 months is recommended for HCC surveillance in patients with cirrhosis or advanced hepatic fibrosis, irrespective of the cause. HCC is rare in HCV-infected patients with mild or no hepatic fibrosis, and so surveillance is not recommended for this group. With a cut-off of 20 ng/mL, serum levels of alpha-fetoprotein have low sensitivity (25–65%) for the detection of HCC and are therefore considered inadequate as the sole means of surveillance. Ultrasonography has a sensitivity of approximately 65% and a specificity of greater than 90% for early detection. Computed tomography (CT) and magnetic resonance imaging (MRI) are not generally recommended for HCC surveillance (as distinct from diagnosis and staging); their sensitivity, specificity and positive and negative predictive values for this purpose are unknown, and their use is associated with high cost as well as possible harm (e.g. radiation, allergic reaction to contrast medium, contrast-induced nephropathy and nephrogenic systemic fibrosis from the use of gadolinium with MRI in patients with renal insufficiency).

El-Serag, H.B. (2011). Hepatocellular carcinoma. *N Engl J Med* 365, 1118–1127.
http://www.ncbi.nlm.nih.gov/pubmed/21992124

26. Answer E

Haemodynamic status should be assessed immediately upon presentation of overt upper gastrointestinal bleeding (UGIB) and resuscitative measures begun (Laine and Jensen, 2012). Pre-endoscopic intravenous proton-pump inhibitors (PPIs) (e.g. pantoprazole 80-mg bolus followed by 8 mg/h infusion) may decrease the proportion of patients who have higher risk stigmata of haemorrhage at endoscopy and who receive endoscopic therapy. However, PPIs do not definitely improve clinical outcomes, such as further bleeding, surgery or death. Patients with UGIB should generally undergo endoscopy within 24 h of admission, following resuscitative efforts to correct shock.

Stigmata of recent haemorrhage should be recorded as they predict risk of further bleeding and guide management decisions. The stigmata, in descending risk of further bleeding, are active spurting, a non-bleeding visible vessel, active oozing, adherent clot, flat pigmented spot and clean base. Endoscopic therapy should be undertaken in patients with active spurting or oozing bleeding or a non-bleeding visible vessel. Thermal therapy with bipolar electrocoagulation or heater probe and injection of sclerosant (e.g. absolute alcohol) are recommended because they decrease further bleeding, need for surgery and mortality. Epinephrine (adrenaline) therapy should not be used alone.

After successful endoscopic haemostasis, intravenous PPI therapy with pantoprazole 80-mg bolus followed by 8 mg/h continuous infusion for 72 h should be given to patients who have an ulcer with active bleeding, a non-bleeding visible vessel or an adherent clot. Routine second-look endoscopy, in which repeat endoscopy is performed 24 h after initial endoscopic haemostatic therapy, is not recommended. Repeat endoscopy should only be performed in patients with clinical evidence of recurrent bleeding and haemostatic therapy should be applied in those with higher-risk stigmata of haemorrhage.

Patients with high-risk stigmata (active bleeding, visible vessels and clots) should generally be hospitalised for 3 days, assuming no re-bleeding and no other reason for hospitalisation. They may be fed clear liquids soon after endoscopy. Patients with *Helicobacter pylori*-associated bleeding ulcers should receive *H. pylori* therapy. After documentation of eradication, maintenance PPI therapy is not needed unless the patient also requires non-steroidal anti-inflammatory drugs (NSAIDs) or anti-thrombotics.

Laine, L. and Jensen, D.M. (2012). Management of patients with ulcer bleeding. *Am J Gastroenterol* 107, 345–360; quiz 361.
http://www.ncbi.nlm.nih.gov/pubmed/22310222

27. Answer A
The features are consistent with severe ulcerative colitis (UC) (Danese and Fiocchi, 2011). Intravenous steroids should be used in severe cases of UC. If episodes of UC are mild, then 5-aminosalicylates such as sulfasalazine can be used. Anti-tumour necrosis factor-alpha (anti-TNFα) antibody is used for severe Crohn disease. Sulphasalazine and 5-aminosalicylates (mesalazine, olsalazine and balsalazide), given orally, rectally (by means of suppository or enema), or both, represent first-line treatment for mild UC, with an expected remission rate of about 50%. Mild-to-moderate proctitis can be treated with mesalazine suppositories (1 g/day) or enemas (2–4 g/day); clinical remission occurs in most patients

within 2 weeks, with repeated treatments as needed. If this fails, 5-aminosalicylate enemas (2–4 g/day) or glucocorticoid enemas (hydrocortisone at a dose of 100 mg/day, or new preparations such as budesonide or beclomethasone) are a next step. Patients who do not have a response to rectally administered agents may be given oral glucocorticoids (up to 40 mg of prednisone or its equivalent).

After remission has been achieved, the goal is to maintain the patient free of symptoms, which can be accomplished with various medications, with the exception of glucocorticoids, which have no role in maintenance therapy, given the marked side effects associated with long-term use. Both oral and rectal 5-aminosalicylate have greater efficacy than placebo for maintenance of remission in patients with distal disease.

Danese, S. and Fiocchi, C. (2011). Ulcerative colitis. *N Engl J Med* 365, 1713–1725.
http://www.ncbi.nlm.nih.gov/pubmed/22047562

28. Answer E

Periodic acid-Schiff (PAS)-stained macrophages on jejunal biopsy indicate a diagnosis of Whipple disease (Fenollar et al., 2007). Whipple disease, caused by *Tropheryma whipplei* is characterised by two stages – a prodromal stage and a much later steady-state stage. The prodromal stage is marked by protean symptoms, along with chronic non-specific findings, mainly arthralgia and arthritis. The steady-state stage is typified by weight loss, diarrhoea, or both, and occasionally there are other manifestations, since many organs can be involved.

The most common gastrointestinal symptom of classic Whipple disease is weight loss, often associated with diarrhoea. Occult bleeding from the intestinal mucosa is observed in 20–30% of patients. Abdominal pain may be present. Hepatosplenomegaly and occasionally hepatitis may occur. Joint involvement has been reported in 65–90% of patients with classic Whipple disease.

The classic tool for diagnosing Whipple disease is PAS staining of small bowel biopsy specimens, which on light microscopy show magenta-stained inclusions within macrophages of the lamina propria. Polymerase chain reaction (PCR) is another method used to detect *T. whipplei* in samples from a variety of tissue types and body fluids. Different antibiotic regimens have been trialled, including 2 weeks of intravenous (IV) ceftriaxone followed by 1–2 years of trimethoprim–sulphamethoxazole (bactrim).

Fenollar, F., Puechal, X., and Raoult, D. (2007). Whipple's disease. *N Engl J Med* 356, 55–66.
http://www.ncbi.nlm.nih.gov/pubmed/17202456

29. Answer B

Ascitic fluid infection can be spontaneous or secondary to an intra-abdominal infection (Wiest et al., 2012). The survival rate of patients who develop spontaneous bacterial peritonitis (SBP) depends in part on early diagnosis and treatment, and hence the decision to start empirical antibiotics should be made as soon as possible.

The ascitic fluid neutrophil count is highly sensitive in detecting bacterial infection of peritoneal fluid and the result is rapidly available. An absolute neutrophil count of 250 cells/mL or greater requires empirical antibiotic therapy. Gram stain is positive in only 5–10% of patients with SBP. An elevated white blood cell count with a predominance of lymphocytes strongly suggests peritoneal carcinomatosis or tuberculous peritonitis. The serum–ascites albumin gradient is more useful than the total protein concentration of ascitic fluid in the classification of ascites according to portal pressure. However, it does not clarify if the ascitic fluid is infected.

Wiest, R., Krag, A., and Gerbes, A. (2012). Spontaneous bacterial peritonitis: recent guidelines and beyond. *Gut* 61, 297–310.
http://www.ncbi.nlm.nih.gov/pubmed/22147550

30. Answer D
Small intestinal bacterial overgrowth is defined as the presence of greater than 10^5 CFU/mL of bacteria in the proximal small bowel or greater than 10^3 CFU/mL of isolates routinely found in colonic flora (Bures et al., 2010). Conditions that causes reduced gastric acid, structural abnormalities (e.g. small bowel diverticula) and dysmotility syndromes are associated with small intestinal bacterial overgrowth. Clinical manifestations may vary but can include diarrhoea, anorexia, nausea, weight loss and anaemia. Malabsorption can result in hypocalcaemia, night blindness due to vitamin A deficiency, vitamin K deficiency and osteomalacia. Vitamin B_{12} deficiency is common with severe overgrowth. Anaemia may be megaloblastic and macrocytic as a result of vitamin B_{12} deficiency. Luminal bacteria tend to consume cobalamin but produce folate, resulting in low vitamin B_{12} and high folate levels.

Bures, J., Cyrany, J., Kohoutova, D., et al. (2010). Small intestinal bacterial overgrowth syndrome. *World J Gastroenterol* 16, 2978–2990.
http://www.wjgnet.com/1007-9327/full/v16/i24/2978.htm

31. Answer H
Eosinophilic colitis is a rare form of primary eosinophilic gastrointestinal disease with a bimodal peak of prevalence in neonates and young adults (Nielsen et al., 2008). Typical symptoms are diarrhoea, abdominal distension, peri-umbilical pain, anorexia, vomiting and weight loss. There are no pathognomonic symptoms or markers to aid diagnosis of eosinophilic colitis and blood eosinophil counts in particular are normal in most patients. Nevertheless, the presence of eosinophils in stool samples is suggestive of eosinophilic colitis. Eosinophilic colitis has a broad differential diagnosis because colon tissue eosinophilia often occurs in parasitic

infection, drug-induced allergic reactions, inflammatory bowel disease and various connective tissue disorders, which require thorough searching for secondary causes that may be specifically treated with antibiotics or dietary and drug elimination.

No specific treatment for primary eosinophilic colitis exists. As eosinophilic colitis typically involves the entire colon, a systemic approach to treatment is required, and empirically oral glucocorticoids can be efficacious. In severe refractory cases intravenous administration of glucocorticoids and/or another immunosuppressant, such as azathioprine, may be used.

Nielsen, O.H., Vainer, B., and Rask-Madsen, J. (2008).Non-IBD and non-infectious colitis. *Nat Clin Pract Gastroenterol Hepatol* 5, 28–39.
http://www.ncbi.nlm.nih.gov/pubmed/18174905

32. Answer C

Several types of fistulas are seen in Crohn's disease:

- Perianal fistulas: Fistulas start in the rectum and open to the skin around the anus. Small fistulas may drain pus and wound exudate. Larger fistulas may drain stool.
- Enteroenteric fistulas: Fistulas start in one area of the intestine and connect to a nearby loop of bowel. Large fistulas can cause problems with malabsorption by bypassing large lengths of intestine.
- Enterocutaneous fistulas: Fistulas start in the intestine and burrow up to the skin, draining stool if the connection is large enough for stool to pass through.
- Peristomal fistulas: Fistulas form at the folded intestine that creates the stoma and erupt next to the stoma. Peristomal fistulas can make it very difficult to wear an ostomy appliance.
- Enterovaginal fistulas: Fistulas start in the intestine or rectum and connect to the vagina. Stool may drain from the vagina. Alternately, small fistulas may cause foul-smelling vaginal discharge.
- Enterovesical fistulas: Fistulas start in the intestine or rectum and connect to the bladder. Recurrent bladder infections in men and women may result.
- Perineal fistulas: Perineal fistulas refer to a connection between the intestine or rectum and the perineum. The perineum is the area between the anus and the scrotum in men, and between the anus and vagina in women.

Management of fistulising Crohn's disease requires careful assessment of the fistula location, extent and potential complications (i.e. penetration of adjacent organs or abscesses) (Baumgart and Sandborn, 2012; Talley et al., 2011). If internal fistulas and complicated perianal fistulas are suspected, imaging, magnetic resonance imaging (MRI) or ultrasound can help to guide therapy. Whereas uncomplicated perianal fistulae can be managed with seton placement, abscesses and other complications require surgical intervention in addition to medical therapy, usually a combination of anti-tumour necrosis factor (TNF), such as infliximab, with antibiotics and thiopurines.

Baumgart, D.C. and Sandborn, W.J. (2012). Crohn's disease. *Lancet* 380, 1590–1605.
http://www.ncbi.nlm.nih.gov/pubmed/22914295

Talley, N.J., Abreu, M.T., Achkar, J.P., et al. (2011). An evidence-based systematic review on medical therapies for inflammatory bowel disease. *Am J Gastroenterol* 106 Suppl 1, S2–25; quiz S26.
http://www.ncbi.nlm.nih.gov/pubmed/21472012

33. Answer D

Mesalazine is the first-line treatment for mild-to-moderately active ulcerative colitis. Oral mesalazine is available in different formulations with different release characteristics, all of which have similar effectiveness. Mild-to-moderate proctitis is best treated with 1 g/day of topical mesalazine (suppositories), which is more effective than either topical steroids or oral mesalazine. Mildly-to-moderately active proctosigmoiditis can be treated with topical or oral mesalazine, whereas extensive colitis should always receive oral mesalazine. Combined treatment (oral and topical) leads to higher remission rates than does either treatment alone.

34. Answer F

Metronidazole remains the first-line agent for treatment of mild *Clostridium difficile* infection because of its lower cost and concerns about the proliferation of vancomycin-resistant nosocomial bacteria (Kelly and LaMont, 2008).

Markers of severe *C. difficile* infection include pseudomembranous colitis, a marked peripheral leucocytosis, acute renal failure and hypotension. Based on recent trials, vancomycin has been recommended as the first-line agent in patients with severe infection because of the faster symptom resolution and a significantly lower risk of treatment failure. Despite its proven superiority, oral vancomycin may not be suitable for some patients with severe or fulminant infection because of coexisting ileus or toxic megacolon. Intravenous metronidazole is used in this situation and should, if possible, be supplemented with vancomycin administered through a nasogastric tube or by enema. Patients with severe or refractory disease should be evaluated early by a gastrointestinal surgeon, since timely subtotal colectomy can be lifesaving.

Kelly, C.P. and LaMont, J.T. (2008). Clostridium difficile-more difficult than ever. *N Engl J Med* 359, 1932–1940.
http://www.ncbi.nlm.nih.gov/pubmed/18971494

35. Answer C

Crohn's disease is often complicated by extra-intestinal manifestations, such as inflammations of skin (erythema nodosum, pyoderma gangrenosum), eyes (uveitis), or joints (arthropathy, enthesiopathy). Cutaneous manifestations, such as erythema nodosum and pyodermagangrenosum, are classically associated with inflammatory bowel disease (IBD), occurring in 3–20% and 0.5–20% of patients, respectively. In many cases, pyodermagangrenosum refractory to standard medications (oral, intravenous and intralesional corticosteroids, azathioprine, 6-mercaptopurine, antibiotics, cyclosporine and mycophenolate) has been successfully treated with anti-TNFα agents. In one small multicentre, randomised, placebo-controlled trial, a response was observed in 46% of patients receiving infliximab compared with 6% of those receiving placebo ($P = 0.0025$). Maintenance therapy with infliximab may be helpful in resolving extra-intestinal manifestations of Crohn's disease, particularly arthritis and arthralgia (Cottone and Criscuoli, 2011). A large, prospective, open-label trial demonstrated improvement of peripheral arthritis in patients with IBD who had previously been refractory to corticosteroids, 6-mercaptopurine, azathioprine or methotrexate. Ocular manifestations developed in 2–6% of patients with IBD, with the most common being episcleritis and uveitis. Many case reports and pilot studies have demonstrated that infliximab can suppress uveitis and scleritis associated with various autoimmune disorders, including IBD.

Infections, specifically tuberculosis, need to be ruled out before infliximab is administered.

Cottone, M. and Criscuoli, V. (2011). Infliximab to treat Crohn's disease: an update. *Clin Exp Gastroenterol* 4, 227–238.
http://www.ncbi.nlm.nih.gov/pmc/articles/PMC3190291/

4 Nephrology

Questions

BASIC SCIENCE

Answers can be found in the Nephrology Answers section at the end of this chapter.

1. Nephrotic syndrome is associated with:
  - **A.** Elevated serum albumin concentration
  - **B.** Reduced low-density lipoprotein cholesterol level
  - **C.** Normal glomerular filtration barrier
  - **D.** Decreased hepatic synthesis of coagulation factors
  - **E.** Increased susceptibility to infection, particularly to Gram-positive bacteria

2. Glomerular diseases include a wide range of immune and non-immune insults that may target and injure the podocyte. Which of these is true?
  - **A.** The degree of podocytopenia predicts the progression of diabetic kidney disease
  - **B.** Podocyte proliferation is a feature of minimal change disease
  - **C.** Foot process effacement is seen in membranous nephropathy
  - **D.** Expression of slit diaphragm proteins are not altered in nephrotic disorders
  - **E.** Podocytes do not undergo programmed cell death

3. About 30–40% of adult patients with idiopathic membranous nephropathy develop progressive disease. Which one of the following is a risk factor for progression?
  - **A.** Normal kidney function at presentation
  - **B.** Normal blood pressure
  - **C.** Age younger than 50 years
  - **D.** Kidney biopsy showing glomerulosclerosis and tubulointerstitial fibrosis
  - **E.** Female sex

Passing the FRACP Written Examination: Questions and Answers, First Edition. Jonathan Gleadle, Tuck Yong, Jordan Li, Surjit Tarafdar, and Danielle Wu.
© 2013 John Wiley & Sons, Ltd. Published 2013 by John Wiley & Sons, Ltd.

4. Which one of the following pathophysiological processes is observed in vascular calcification in chronic kidney disease?

    A. Vascular smooth muscle cell apoptosis driven by hypophosphataemia

    B. Osteochondrogenic metaplasia driven by hypophosphataemia

    C. Elevated klotho expression

    D. Impaired soft-tissue calcification defences

    E. Elevation in serum fetuin levels

Theme: Renal physiology and pathophysiology

(for Questions 5–9)

    A. Proximal renal tubule

    B. Thin descending limb of Henle's loop

    C. Thin ascending limb of Henle's loop

    D. Thick ascending limb of Henle's loop

    E. Distal convoluted tubule

    F. Cortical collecting duct

    G. Medullary collecting duct

    H. Papillary duct

Select the most appropriate part of the renal tubule involved in the physiological or pathophysiological processes described below.

5. Aldosterone stimulates which part of the renal tubule to reabsorb sodium?

6. Atrial natriuretic peptide (ANP) affects which part of the renal tubule to inhibit sodium reabsorption?

7. Which part of the tubule is the site for excretion of trimethoprim?

8. Dapagliflozin exerts its effect on which part of the renal tubule?

9. Where is phosphate mainly reabsorbed after being filtered by the glomerulus?

CLINICAL

10. A 60-year-old man with end-stage diabetic nephropathy received his first kidney transplant 6 months ago. Post transplantation, he had one episode of severe vascular rejection, which was treated with a course of anti-thymoglobulin (ATG). His graft function has been stabilised with serum creatinine of 190 μmol/L (50–120 μmol/L) while he is taking tacrolimus, mycophenolate and prednisolone. However, his renal function has progressively worsened in the past 2 weeks. His blood and urine BK virus polymerase chain reaction (PCR) levels are very high. His preliminary kidney biopsy result reveals significant tubulitis, interstitial lymphocyte infiltration and intranuclear inclusion bodies were present. Which one of the following is NOT a treatment option?
  A. Intravenous cidofovir to eradicate the BK virus
  B. Intravenous methylprednisolone
  C. Oral ciprofloxacin
  D. Switch mycophenolate to leflunomide
  E. Reduce tacrolimus and mycophenolate doses

11. A 72-year-old man presents with severe abdominal pain in the past 6 h. The past medical history is significant for congestive heart failure, hypertension, type 2 diabetes on insulin, stage 4 chronic kidney disease with baseline serum creatinine of 180 μmol/L (50–120 μmol/L). His medications include insulin, perindopril, atenolol, pravastatin and aspirin. He has been seen by the surgical registrar who suspects the patient is suffering from ischaemic bowel and requires urgent abdominal computed tomography (CT) with intravenous contrast. The radiology registrar is concerned about the patient's renal failure and consults you about the prevention of contrast-induced nephropathy. Which one of the following recommendation would you make?
  A. Give intravenous normal saline hydration first and delay the CT for 12 h
  B. Give oral N-acetylcystine (NAC) 600 mg twice daily for 2 days because of concern regarding the ischaemic heart disease
  C. Start intravenous normal saline hydration, proceed to CT with contrast, then start haemodialysis after the CT
  D. Stop perindopril, give intravenous normal saline hydration and use furosemide to force diuresis
  E. Give intravenous sodium bicarbonate 1 h before giving contrast and 3 h after the CT

12. A 62-year-man has had stage 4 chronic kidney disease (CKD) due to diabetic nephropathy. He is found to have anaemia secondary to CKD. His erythropoietin dose was recently reduced because his haemoglobin level was 140 g/L. However, he complains that his golf performance has deteriorated at the current dose of erythropoietin and haemoglobin level of 110 g/L. He would like to increase the erythropoietin dose and keep the haemoglobin level at 140 g/L. Which one of the

following associations has been observed with a haemoglobin target above 130 g/L?
   A. Increased risk of stroke
   B. Reduced risk of stroke
   C. Increased rate of deterioration of renal failure
   D. Improved blood pressure control
   E. Decrease in frequency of headache

13. A 56-year-old man with advanced chronic kidney disease presents with proximal muscle weakness. The serum potassium level is 6.8 mmol/L. Which one of the following treatments would lower his serum potassium most quickly?
   A. 10 mL of 10% calcium gluconate intravenously
   B. 100 mL of 8.4% sodium bicarbonate intravenously
   C. 50 mL of 50% glucose and 10 units of short-acting insulin subcutaneously
   D. 30 g of resonium orally
   E. 30 g of resonium per rectum

14. A 74-year-old man is being managed at the haematology clinic for suspected myeloma. Over the past few weeks he has had increasing shortness of breath, with increased lethargy, decreased exercise tolerance and increasing lower limb oedema.

On examination he looks pale, his blood pressure is 98/68 mmHg and his pulse rate is 89 beats/min. His heart sounds are normal, but there are bilateral crackles on auscultation of the chest and he has pitting lower limb oedema. The results of laboratory investigations are given below. The 24-h urine protein is 9 g/day. Which one of the following is the most likely cause of his underlying proteinuria?

	Value	Reference range
Haemoglobin (g/L)	102	135–180
White cell count (cells/L)	8.7×10^9	$4–10 \times 10^9$
Platelet count (cells/L)	185×10^9	$150–400 \times 10^9$
Sodium (mmol/L)	140	134–143
Potassium (mmol/L)	4.3	3.5–5.0
Creatinine (µmol/L)	135	60–120
Albumin (g/L)	15	35–45

   A. AA amyloidosis
   B. AL amyloidosis
   C. BPP (β protein precursor) amyloidosis
   D. Cystatin C amyloidosis
   E. Mesangiocapillary glomerulonephritis

15. In developed countries, which one of the following bone disorders is most frequent in patients receiving maintenance haemodialysis?
   A. Osteitis fibrosa cystica
   B. Adynamic bone disease
   C. Osteomalacia
   D. Dialysis-related amyloidosis
   E. Aluminium bone disease

16. A 28-year-old woman presents with nausea and vomiting and is found to have a platelet count of 60×10^9 cells/L ($150–450 \times 10^9$ cells/L), haemoglobin of 87 g/L (115–165 g/L) and creatinine of 285 μmol/L (60–100 μmol/L). Which one of the following is consistent with a diagnosis of atypical haemolytic uraemia syndrome?
   A. Markedly suppressed ADAMTS13 activity in blood
   B. Stool culture positive for Shiga toxin-producing *Escherichia coli* (STEC)
   C. A mutation in the gene encoding factor H
   D. A mutation in the gene encoding ADAMTS13
   E. A normal haptoglobin level

17. Which one of the following is NOT a risk factor for contrast-induced acute kidney injury?
   A. Congestive heart failure
   B. Metformin
   C. Multiple myeloma
   D. Non-steroidal anti-inflammatory drugs
   E. Sepsis

18. Which one of the following anti-hypertensive medications should NOT be used in patients with pre-eclampsia?
   A. Nifedipine
   B. Methyldopa
   C. Irbesartan
   D. Labetalol
   E. Hydralazine

19. A 26-year-old woman received a living donor kidney transplant from her aunt 2 years prior to her current presentation. Her post-transplantation course was complicated by one episode of cellular rejection. Her graft function is stable with serum creatinine 92 μmol/L. She is taking tacrolimus 2 mg twice daily, mycophenolate 500 mg twice daily and prednisolone 5 mg daily. She is not taking other medications. Her BP is 110/60 mmHg. Her spot urine protein-to-creatinine ratio is 0.1. She is very keen to start a family and plan for pregnancy. What would you do with her immunosuppression?
   A. Change tacrolimus to cyclosporine
   B. Change mycophenolate to sirolimus

C. Change mycophenolate to azathioprine
D. Stop prednisolone
E. Continue the current immunosuppression drugs

20. A 54-year-old man on regular haemodialysis presents with lower back pain and fever. You request a magnetic resonance imaging (MRI) study of the spine, but request that gadolinium not be used during the test because of concern about:
A. Contrast-induced nephropathy
B. Nephrogenic systemic fibrosis
C. High incidence of allergy reaction to gadolinium among patients on haemodialysis
D. Heavy metal toxicity
E. Systemic sclerosis

21. What is the most important risk factor for the development of post-transplant lymphoproliferative disorder (PTLD) in solid organ transplantation?
A. Kidney transplantation as opposed to other solid organ transplants
B. Epstein–Barr virus status mismatch between recipient and donor
C. Use of the monoclonal anti-CD52 antibody, alemtuzumab
D. Use of sirolimus
E. Previous infection with cytomegalovirus (CMV)

22. A 56-year-old man is admitted to the intensive care unit because of severe sepsis due to ascending cholangitis. This is complicated by acute kidney injury. Which one of the following is an indication for commencement of renal replacement therapy?
A. Oliguria, urine 0.3 mL/kg/h
B. Urea of 19 mmol/L
C. Pericardial rub
D. Serum creatinine of 400 μmol/L
E. Urinary sodium of <20 mmol/L

23. A 48-year-old man presents with severe right-sided loin pain radiating to the scrotum. A computed tomography scan demonstrates a 4-mm distal ureteric calculus. Which one of the following treatments has been shown to increase the chances of stone passage?
A. Frusemide
B. Tamsulosin
C. Atenolol
D. Intravenous saline
E. Thiazide diuretics

24. A 48-year-old man with IgA nephropathy received his first renal transplant 3 years ago. His post-transplant course was complicated by an episode of acute

cellular rejection that was successfully treated with three doses of methylprednisolone. His current graft function is reflected by a serum creatinine of 145 μmol/L (70–120 μmol/L). His medications include tacrolimus, mycophenolate and prednisolone. He presented with a 3-week history of epigastric pain. Endoscopy revealed a gastric lesion and the histology confirmed Epstein–Barr virus associated post-transplantation lymphoproliferative disorder. The computed tomography scans of his head, chest and abdomen revealed no other lesion. Which is the best initial treatment for this patient?
- **A.** Immunosuppression should be withdrawn
- **B.** Immunosuppression should be reduced
- **C.** Immunosuppression should be maintained at its current levels and rituximab should be started
- **D.** Immunosuppression should be reduced and valganciclovir started
- **E.** Immunosuppression should be reduced and gastrectomy should be performed

25. Which one of the following treatment modalities achieves the best long-term survival outcome in patients with hepatorenal syndrome?
- **A.** Terlipressin
- **B.** Norepinephrine (noradrenaline)
- **C.** Continuous renal replacement therapy
- **D.** Liver transplantation
- **E.** Transjugular intrahepatic portosystemic shunts

26. A 38-year-old woman presented with bilateral red eyes, which was diagnosed as anterior uveitis. This was treated with topical steroids and improved. One month later, she represented with acute deterioration of her renal function (creatinine 250 μmol/L, reference range: 60–100 μmol/L). Moderate proteinuria (1.5 g/24 h) and urine eosinophilia were detected. There are no significant dysmorphic red blood cells or casts in the urinary sediment. Renal ultrasound showed both kidneys were normal in size and appearance. She had a percutaneous renal biopsy. What is the biopsy likely to show?
- **A.** Membranous nephropathy
- **B.** Minimal change disease
- **C.** Tubulointerstitial nephritis
- **D.** Focal and segmental glomerulosclerosis
- **E.** IgA nephropathy

Theme: Glomerulonephritis (for Questions 27–31)
- **A.** Alport disease
- **B.** Goodpasture disease
- **C.** Idiopathic membranous nephropathy (MN)
- **D.** Immunoglobulin A nephropathy
- **E.** Membranoproliferative glomerulonephritis (MPGN)

    F. Minimal change disease (MCD)
    G. Primary focal segmental glomerulosclerosis (FSGS)
    H. Rapidly progressive glomerulonephritis
For each of the following scenarios, select the most likely type of glomerulone-phritis that is involved.

27. Which glomerulonephritis is most likely to rapidly recur in a renal allograft?

28. When a patient presents with nephrotic syndrome, which type of causative glomerulonephritis is associated with the greatest risk of a venous thrombotic event?

29. Which glomerulonephritis is associated with selective cyclo-oxygenase 2 (COX-2) inhibitor use?

30. In which glomerulonephritis are anti-phospholipase A2 receptor (anti-PLA2R) antibodies commonly detected?

31. A 45-year-old man presents with microscopic haematuria and proteinuria for investigation. His serum creatinine is $196\,\mu$mol/L. His histopathology (H&E, immun-ofluorescence and electron microscopy) is shown below. What is the most likely diagnosis?

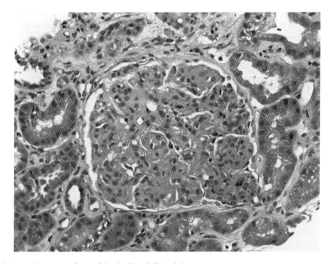

Renal biopsy: Haematoxylin and Eosin (Hand E) staining

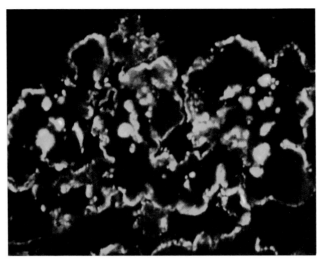

Renal biopsy: immunofluorescence with anti-IgG

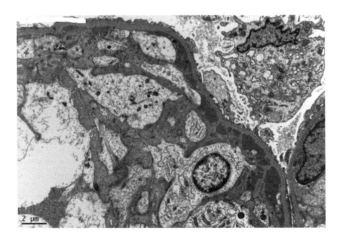

Renal biopsy: electron microscopy

Answers

BASIC SCIENCE

1. Answer E

Nephrotic syndrome is associated with hypoalbuminaemia and peripheral oedema. Hepatic cholesterol and lipoprotein synthesis are increased in nephrotic syndrome, hence an elevated total and low-density lipoprotein cholesterol level is seen. Glomerular filtration barrier is disrupted, leading to proteinuria. Nephrotic syndrome is associated with hypercoagulability from increased hepatic synthesis of coagulation factors (e.g. fibrinogen) and loss of regulatory factors (anti-thrombin III, protein C and protein S) in urine. Renal vein thrombosis complicates all forms of nephrotic syndrome, especially membranous nephropathy. Nephrotic syndrome is associated with increased susceptibility to infection, particularly to Gram-positive bacteria, especially *Streptococcus pneumoniae*. This might be caused by urinary loss of IgG and complement, and impaired cellular immunity.

2. Answer A

Clinical studies have suggested that the degree of podocytopenia predicts the progression of diabetic kidney disease (Jefferson et al., 2011). Podocyte proliferation is a feature of collapsing glomerulopathy. Foot process effacement is seen in minimal change disease. Podocytes may respond to immune complex-mediated injury by producing inflammatory mediators and oxidative injury is a prominent feature in membranous nephropathy. Expression of slit diaphragm proteins are altered in nephrotic disorders, leading to loss of slit diaphragm integrity and protein permeability. Podocytes can undergo programmed cell death or apoptosis. When podocytes are lost by detachment or apoptosis and are not replaced by adjacent viable podocytes, this leads to podocytopenia and ultimately to a leaky glomerular filtration barrier.

Jefferson, J.A., Nelson, P.J., Najafian, B., and Shankland, S.J. (2011). Podocyte disorders: Core Curriculum 2011. *Am J Kidney Dis* 58, 666–677.
http://www.ncbi.nlm.nih.gov/pmc/articles/PMC3183322/

3. Answer D

Prognostic risk factors for progression of idiopathic membranous nephropathy include:
- Greater degree and duration of proteinuria
- Impaired kidney function at presentation
- Hypertension
- Male sex and age more than 50 years
- Non-Asian race

- Biopsy features of glomerulosclerosis, stage III/IV disease, tubulointerstitial fibrosis.

A high proportion of patients with idiopathic MN have circulating antibodies to the M-type phospholipase A2 receptor (PLA2R), a transmembrane protein located on podocytes (Beck and Salant, 2010).

Beck, L.H., Jr. and Salant, D.J. (2010). Membranous nephropathy: recent travels and new roads ahead. *Kidney Int* 77, 765–770.
http://www.ncbi.nlm.nih.gov/pubmed/20182413

4. Answer D

There are five types of arterial calcification:
- Calcific aortic valve disease
- Atherosclerotic intimal calcification
- Arterial medial calcification
- Vascular calcification of chronic kidney disease (CKD; also known as CKD-mineral bone disease)
- Calcific uraemic arteriopathy (CUA; also known as calciphylaxis).

Vascular calcification in CKD involves major disturbance of the calcium phosphate homeostasis and reductions in serum fetuin and pyrophosphate levels. In terms of pathobiology, vascular smooth muscle cell (VSMC) apoptosis and osteochondrogenic metaplasia is driven by hyperphosphataemia, worsened by iatrogenic hypoparathyroidism and low-turnover bone disease. Whilst antecedent diabetes mellitus, hypertension, dyslipidaemia and the metabolic syndrome continue to contribute to arteriosclerosis, hyperphosphataemia, reduced klotho expression and impaired soft-tissue calcification defences are key pathophysiological components of this condition.

Klotho is a putative ageing suppressor gene encoding a single-pass transmembrane co-receptor that makes the fibroblast growth factor (FGF) receptor specific for FGF-23 (Thompson and Towler, 2012). Klotho is expressed in kidney distal convoluted tubules and parathyroid cells, mediating the role of FGF-23 in bone–kidney–parathyroid control of phosphate and calcium. Klotho$^{-/-}$ mice display premature ageing and chronic kidney disease-associated mineral and bone disorder (CKD-MBD)-like phenotypes mediated by hyperphosphataemia and remediated by phosphate-lowering interventions (diets low in phosphate or vitamin D; knockouts of 1α-hydroxylase, vitamin D receptor or NaPi-cotransporter). CKD can be seen as a state of hyperphosphataemia-induced accelerated ageing associated with klotho deficiency. Humans with CKD experience decreased klotho expression as early as stage 1 CKD; klotho continues to decline as CKD progresses, causing FGF-23 resistance and provoking large FGF-23 and parathyroid hormone increases, and hypovitaminosis.

Vascular calcium phosphate deposition elicits an inflammatory response which has a downstream effect of vascular mineralisation. Therefore, patients with CKD face the 'perfect storm' of vascular calcification.

Thompson, B. and Towler, D.A. (2012). Arterial calcification and bone physiology: role of the bone-vascular axis. *Nat Rev Endocrinol* 8, 529–543.
http://www.ncbi.nlm.nih.gov/pubmed/22473330

5. Answer F

In a healthy person, the proximal tubule reabsorbs 65% of the filtered sodium. The thin and thick ascending limbs of Henle's loop together reabsorb 25%, and the distal convoluted tubule and collecting duct system together reabsorb 10%. Therefore, the final urine contains less than 1% of the total filtered sodium. The reabsorption of sodium is mainly an active, transcellular process. Aldosterone mainly stimulates sodium reabsorption by the cortical collecting duct, specifically by the principal cells, the same cells acted on by anti-diuretic hormone (ADH).

6. Answer G

Many of the cells in the cardiac atria secrete a peptide hormone called atrial natriuretic peptide (ANP). ANP acts directly on the inner medullary collecting ducts to inhibit sodium reabsorption. The major stimulus for increased secretion of ANP is distension of the atria, which occurs during plasma volume expansion.

7. Answer A

Active tubular secretion in the proximal tubule is important in the elimination of many drugs, including trimethoprim. This energy-dependent process may be blocked by metabolic inhibitors. When drug concentration is high, secretory transport can reach an upper limit (transport maximum); each substance has a characteristic transport maximum. Creatinine is secreted actively by the proximal tubule and trimethoprim can inhibit this process, leading to an elevation in serum creatinine, especially in individuals with a low glomerular filtration rate.

8. Answer A

The kidneys play a major role in the regulation of glucose in humans, reabsorbing 99% of the plasma glucose that filters through the renal glomeruli tubules. The glucose transporter, SGLT2, which is found primarily in the S1 segment of the proximal renal tubule, is essential for this process, accounting for 90% of the glucose reabsorption in the kidney (Bakris et al., 2009). Evidence suggests that selective inhibition of SGLT2 induces glycosuria in a dose-dependent manner and may have beneficial effects on glucose regulation in individuals with type 2 diabetes. Preclinical data with SGLT2 inhibitors, such as dapagliflozin and sergliflozin, show that these compounds are highly selective inhibitors for SGLT2, have beneficial effects on the glucose utilisation rate and reduce hyperglycaemia, while having no hypoglycaemic adverse effects. Clinical research remains to be carried out on the long-term effects of glycosuria and other potential effects of this class of drug.

Bakris, G.L., Fonseca, V.A., Sharma, K., and Wright, E.M. (2009). Renal sodium–glucose transport: role in diabetes mellitus and potential clinical implications. *Kidney Int 75*, 1272–1277.
http://www.ncbi.nlm.nih.gov/pubmed/19357717

9. Answer A

Phosphate is one of the most abundant anions in mammals and is crucial for bone mineralisation and cellular activity (Prie and Friedlander, 2010). The kidney plays a central role in phosphate homeostasis by adjusting urinary excretion according to intake, thus maintaining the serum concentration within a narrow range. Most phosphate (85% of total body stores) resides in bones, where it associates with calcium. Phosphate in serum and extracellular fluids accounts for 1% of total body stores.

Reabsorption of phosphate filtered by the glomerulus occurs almost exclusively in the renal proximal tubule and is an active, hormonally-regulated process. The amount reabsorbed is a key determinant of the plasma phosphate concentration. When the serum phosphate concentration increases (either from high phosphate intake or reduced glomerular filtration rate), the amount reabsorbed decreases because of an increase in fibroblast growth factor 23 (FGF-23) and parathyroid hormone (PTH). FGF-23 is a hormone produced mainly by bone and connective tissue that inhibits reabsorption of phosphate by the kidney. PTH also decreases renal phosphate reabsorption.

Prie, D. and Friedlander, G. (2010). Genetic disorders of renal phosphate transport. *N Engl J Med* 362, 2399–2409.
http://www.ncbi.nlm.nih.gov/pubmed/20573928

CLINICAL

10. Answer B

The cause of rapid deterioration of graft function in this case is BK nephropathy (BKN). BK nephropathy is an important cause of premature graft failure. The risk factors associated with BKN include:

- Aggressive immunosuppressive treatment during the acute rejection, especially the usage of monoclonal antibodies such as anti-thymocyte globulin (ATG)
- Older recipient age
- Female donor
- HLA DR mismatching.

The management of BKN is challenging because no one therapeutic strategy is consistently effective. The reduction of overall immunosuppression is the cornerstone of treatment in BKN.

Cidofovir can competitively inhibit viral DNA synthesis. Cidofovir has been reported in small case series to have some benefit on BKN, but its usage has been associated with substantial nephrotoxicity.

Leflunomide is a pyrimidine synthesis inhibitor used in the treatment of rheumatoid arthritis. It is known to have both immunosuppressive and anti-viral properties. Single-centre reports of successful use of leflunomide for BKN have been published. There are no randomised, controlled trial data.

Ciprofloxacin has been used in the treatment of BKN. Quinolones may have anti-BK virus properties by inhibiting DNA topoisomerase activity and SV40 large T-antigen helicase. An observational study reported that use of a fluoroquinolone was associated with the prevention of BK viraemia after renal transplant.

Wiseman, A. (2009). Polyomavirus nephropathy: A current perspective and clinical considerations. *Am J Kidney Dis* 54, 131–142.
http://www.ncbi.nlm.nih.gov/pubmed/19394729

11. Answer E

Contrast-induced acute kidney injury (AKI) is an important complication in the use of iodinated contrast media, which is the third most common cause of hospital-acquired AKI. This patient has multiple risk factors for AKI after iodinated contrast, including chronic kidney disease, diabetes and congestive heart failure (McCullough, 2008).

Hydration with normal saline has a well-established role in the prevention of contrast-induced AKI. It is usually given 12 h before and 12 h after the procedure. However, there is an urgent need for a CT scan in this case.

Alkalinisation may protect against free radical injury, which is one of the pathological processes in contrast-induced AKI. Studies that have examined outcomes with isotonic sodium bicarbonate versus isotonic sodium chloride have noted either equivalent or better outcomes with sodium bicarbonate. Sodium bicarbonate requires pre-treatment only 1 h before contrast injection, which is more suitable for urgent CT scan.

Contrast medium is removed by haemodialysis, but there is no clinical evidence that post-exposure haemodialysis reduces the risk of AKI, even when carried out within 1 h or simultaneously with contrast administration.

Oral or intravenous N-acetylcysteine (NAC) has not been consistently demonstrated to be effective in the prevention of contrast-induced AKI, although it is safe and inexpensive.

There is no role for forced diuresis, mannitol or renal vasodilators in the prevention of contrast-induced AKI.

 McCullough, P.A. (2008). Contrast-induced acute kidney injury. *J Am Coll Cardiol* 51, 1419–1428.
http://content.onlinejacc.org/article.aspx?articleid=1138824

12. Answer A

The suggestion to set the upper haemoglobin (Hb) target to values of less than 115 g/L in adult chronic kidney disease (CKD) patients treated with an erythropoiesis-stimulating agent (ESA), and the strong recommendation not to aim for Hb increases to concentrations of greater than 130 g/L, is based on the interpretation of the combined results of recent major randomised control trials (RCTs) that there may be more harm than benefit at higher Hb concentrations, including increased risks for stroke, headache, hypertension, venous thromboembolism and vascular access thrombosis (in haemodialysis patients) (Drueke and Parfrey, 2012).

An increase of Hb above 115 g/L towards 130 g/L may be justified in individual patients with a high bleeding tendency, since this can result in lower transfusion needs. Obviously, increasing Hb above 115 g/L up to 130 g/L has to be weighed against the probability of increased harm. This perspective needs to be clearly explained to each patient who wishes to examine the possible benefits of more 'physiological' target correction.

 Drueke, T.B. and Parfrey, P.S. (2012). Summary of the KDIGO guideline on anemia and comment: reading between the (guide)line(s). *Kidney Int* 82, 952–960.
http://www.ncbi.nlm.nih.gov/pubmed/22854645

13. Answer C

Calcium gluconate is used in the treatment of hyperkalaemia because its electrophysiological effect prevents cardiac arrest. It works extremely fast but does not lower the serum potassium concentration.

Sodium bicarbonate is beneficial because it favours uptake of potassium by the cells. It is more effective when patients have severe metabolic acidosis. However, studies of sodium bicarbonate in patients with end-stage kidney disease have shown that potassium falls minimally within the first 2 h.

Insulin is effective in lowering the serum potassium concentration within minutes. Insulin acts on Na^+– K^+-ATPase to promote cellular uptake of potassium, an effect that is independent of glucose. Glucose is given concurrently with insulin to avoid hypoglycaemia.

Evans, K., Reddan, D., Szezech, L., et al. (2004). Nondialytic management of hyperkalaemia and pulmonary oedema among end-stage renal disease: An evaluation of the evidence. *Semin Dial* 17, 22–29.
http://www.ncbi.nlm.nih.gov/pubmed/14717808

14. Answer B

AL amyloidosis is associated with deposition of immunoglobulin light chains and is caused by multiple myeloma. This patient has a mixed picture of heart failure and proteinuria, which is probably caused by both cardiac and renal amyloid deposition. Given his degree of hypoalbuminaemia, light chains would probably be easily detectable in the urine. AL amyloidosis can be mimicked by hereditary causes of amyloidosis with mutations in genes encoding fibrinogen A and transthyretin.

AA amyloidosis occurs in conjunction with systemic inflammatory conditions, cystatin C amyloidosis in conjunction with Icelandic hereditary cerebral haemorrhage and amyloidosis, and β protein precursor (BPP) amyloidosis with Alzheimer disease and Down syndrome. Treatment in this case is driven by chemotherapy for the underlying myeloma.

15. Answer B

Adynamic bone disease among haemodialysis patients has become increasingly frequent in developed countries because of suppression of parathyroid hormone with calcium and potent vitamin D analogues. The degree to which it increases morbidity and mortality is unknown. Concerns in this condition relate to the inability of bone to contribute to mineral homeostasis in the absence of kidney function and the resultant risk of fractures. Dialysis-related amyloidosis (DRA) is a disorder caused by deposition of beta-2 microglobulin as amyloid deposits. The clearance of beta-2 microglobulin is diminished with decreasing renal function. DRA is relatively common in patients, especially older adults, who have been on haemodialysis for more than 5 years. Newer haemodialysis membranes, as well as peritoneal dialysis, can facilitate a greater clearance of beta-2 microglobulin, but are insufficient to keep blood levels normal. Renal transplantation can ameliorate the condition.

Carpal tunnel syndrome and shoulder pain are the most common presentations of DRA. The bone lesions are typically cystic and seen at the end of long bones. The cystic lesions contain amyloid, enlarge with time and may lead to pathological fractures of carpal bones, the femur and humeral heads, fingers, acetabulum and distal radius.

16. Answer C

Atypical haemolytic uraemic syndrome (HUS) is characterised by thrombotic microangiopathy with a fall in platelet count, haemolytic anaemia and renal impairment (Noris and Remuzzi, 2009). It is associated with deficiencies of proteins involved in complement control, including complement factor H, factor I, thrombomodulin and membrane cofactor protein. Haemolysis may manifest as anaemia, red cell fragments (schistocytes), elevated lactate dehydrogenase (LDH) and low or unde-tectable haptoglobin. Typical HUS is associated with Shiga toxin-producing *E. coli* (STEC) infection. Atypical HUS is not associated with a precipitating STEC infection (although diarrhoea can occur in some patients).

Renal failure is a common complication, but it is important to recognise that other organs may be involved, e.g. cardiomyopathy and neurological symptoms. Plasmapheresis may be utilised in treatment and there is an emerging role for the anti-C5a antibody, eculizumab.

Thrombocytopenic purpura is a related disorder with low platelets and micro-angiopathy, a tendency for a greater incidence of neurological involvement and fever, and association with deficiencies of the ADAMTS13 protease, which cleaves von Willebrand factor multimers.

Noris, M. and Remuzzi, G. (2009). Atypical hemolytic-uremic syndrome. *N Engl J Med* 361, 1676–1687.
http://www.ncbi.nlm.nih.gov/pubmed/19846853

17. Answer B

Contrast-induced acute kidney injury (AKI) is the third most common cause of hospital-acquired AKI (Mehran and Nikolsky, 2006). The incidence is low (0.6–2.3%) in the general population, but in the high-risk group the incidence may be up to 20%.

Identification of patients at high risk for the development of contrast-induced AKI is of major importance. Non-modifiable risk factors are:

- Old age
- Chronic kidney disease
- Diabetes mellitus
- Congestive heart failure
- Cardiogenic shock
- Renal transplant
- Multiple myeloma.
  Modifiable risk factors are:
- Hypotension
- Anaemia
- Dehydration
- Low serum albumin
- Angiotensin converting enzyme (ACE) inhibitors/angiotensin receptor blockers
- Diuretics
- Non-steroidal anti-inflammatory drugs
- Nephrotoxic antibiotics
- Volume of contrast agent.

Metformin is not a nephrotoxic medication; therefore, it is not a risk factor for developing contrast-induced AKI. The rationale for stopping metformin before and after contrast exposure is that the worsening of renal function may increase the blood concentration of metformin, which can rarely lead to lactic acidosis.

Mehran, R. and Nikolsky, E. (2006). Contrast-induced nephropathy: definition, epidemiology, and patients at risk. *Kidney Int* Suppl, S11–15.
http://www.ncbi.nlm.nih.gov/pubmed/16612394

18. Answer C

Hypertension affects 10–22% of pregnancies. It has been classified into four categories: chronic hypertension, gestational hypertension, pre-eclampsia/eclampsia and pre-eclampsia on chronic hypertension. Pre-eclampsia is a multisystem disorder that occurs in the second half of pregnancy and affects 5% of pregnancies. It remains the leading cause of maternal and perinatal mortality and morbidity worldwide. Impaired placental implantation, hypoxia, endothelial dysfunction and systemic inflammation are thought to have a role in the pathogenesis of pre-eclampsia.

Delivery is the only definitive management of pre-eclampsia. Blood pressure control is the essential part of the multidisciplinary treatment approach. The anti-hypertensive drugs that can be safely used are (Lowe et al., 2009):
- Labetalol (beta-blocker)
- Nifedipine (calcium channel blocker)
- Methyldopa (centrally acting)
- Hydralazine (vasodilator)

The anti-hypertensive drugs that should be avoided in pregnancy are (Lowe et al., 2009):
- All angiotensin converting enzyme (ACE) inhibitors: teratogenic in the first trimester, fetal renal dysfunction, oligohydramnios in the second and third trimesters
- All angiotensin receptor blockers: teratogenic in first trimester, fetal renal dysfunction, oligohydramnios in the second and third trimesters
- All diuretics: fetal electrolyte disturbances, reduction in maternal blood volume.

The treatment goal is usually BP less than 140/90 mmHg. Severe hypertension may require parenteral anti-hypertensive drugs, such as intravenous hydralazine.

Lowe, S.A., Brown, M.A., Dekker, G.A., et al. (2009). Guidelines for the management of hypertensive disorders of pregnancy 2008. *Aust N Z J Obstet Gynaecol* 49, 242–246.
http://www.ncbi.nlm.nih.gov/pubmed/19566552

19. Answer C

All immunosuppressants used in preventing kidney rejection have the potential to cause problems and are rated as category C or D drugs in pregnancy (see Prescribing Medicines in Pregnancy database. www.tga.gov.au/hp/medicines-pregnancy.htm).

Tacrolimus crosses the placenta and neonatal renal dysfunction has been reported. Cyclosporine has not been reported to be a teratogen but may promote pregnancy-induced hypertension and cholestasis. There is no evidence to support changing from tacrolimus to cyclosporine before pregnancy.

Structural defects have not been reported with exposure to sirolimus during pregnancy, but it has been associated with embryotoxicity and fetotoxicity in animal studies. Currently, there is no recommendation to switch mycophenolate to sirolimus before pregnancy. Mycophenolate is listed as a category D drug. It increases first-trimester pregnancy loss and congenital malformation, including cleft lip and palate, and anomalies in distal limbs and heart, and should be discontinued.

Although azathioprine was found to be teratogenic in animal studies, many pregnancies have been successfully completed in women who continue taking azathioprine.

It is suggested that the safest immunosuppression for a woman who wishes to become pregnant is the combination of calcineurin inhibitor, azathioprine and prednisolone (Maynard and Thadhani, 2009).

Maynard, S.E. and Thadhani, R. (2009). Pregnancy and the kidney. *J Am Soc Nephrol* 20, 14–22.
http://jasn.asnjournals.org/content/20/1/14.full

20. Answer B

Nephrogenic systemic fibrosis (NSF) is seen only in patients with kidney failure and is characterised by symmetrical skin involvement with extensive waxy thickening and hardening of the extremities and torso (Kribben et al., 2009). Although originally named nephrogenic fibrosing dermopathy because of the characteristic skin lesions, it was soon realised that some patients had fibrosis of deeper structures, including the lung, heart, fascia and muscles. Histologically it is characterised by marked expansion and fibrosis of the dermis with CD34-positive fibrocytes.

This condition is associated with exposure to gadolinium, which is a hyperosmolar contrast agent used primarily during magnetic resonance imaging (MRI) or angiography (MRA) studies. Free gadolinium is highly toxic and insoluble in water and so it has to be chelated for human administration. These gadolinium chelates are excreted almost exclusively by the kidneys. Gadolinium should be avoided in patients with a glomerular filtration rate (GFR) of less than 30 mL/min.

The latent period between gadolinium exposure and disease onset is usually 1–4 weeks. Skin changes and joint contractures can occur. Since the recognition of the dangers of gadolinium in patients with impaired renal function, the incidence of NSF has dramatically declined.

In patients with significant renal impairment (GFR <30 mL/min) in whom the use of gadolinium is imperative, such as liver transplant work-up, haemodialysis after the exposure should be considered. Gadolinium chelates have a molecular weight of 500–1000 kDa and are removed by haemodialysis. A single conventional haemodialysis will remove 75% of a dose. A second treatment will remove 93% of a dose. Minimum adequate doses of gadolinium should be used.

Kribben, A., Witzke, O., Hillen, U., Barkhausen, J., Daul, A.E., and Erbel, R. (2009). Nephrogenic systemic fibrosis: pathogenesis, diagnosis, and therapy. *J Am Coll Cardiol* 53, 1621–1628.
http://www.ncbi.nlm.nih.gov/pubmed/19406336

21. Answer B

The incidence of post-transplant lymphoproliferative disorder (PTLD) according to type of transplanted organ has been reported as follows: haematopoietic stem cell (0.5–1%), kidney (1%), pancreas (2.1%), heart (2.3%), lung (2.5%), liver (4.3%), heart–lung (10–20%) and bowel (10–20%).

PTLD is an uncommon but severe complication of solid organ transplant with an overall incidence of about 2%. In about 85–90% of cases, PTLD is Epstein–Barr (EBV) related. The most important risk factor is an EBV status mismatch, e.g. recipient seronegative/donor seropositive at the moment of transplant, leading to a 10–75 times greater incidence of PTLD compared to matched recipients. This at least partially explains the higher incidence of PTLD in childhood (Dierickx et al., 2011).

Dierickx, D., Tousseyn, T., De Wolf-Peeters, C., Pirenne, J., and Verhoef, G. (2011). Management of posttransplant lymphoproliferative disorders following solid organ transplant: an update. *Leuk Lymphoma* 52, 950–961.
http://informahealthcare.com/doi/abs/10.3109/10428194.2011.557453

22. Answer C

Oliguria alone or serum creatinine alone is not an indication for renal replacement therapy (RRT) in acute kidney injury. The indications for RRT are the life-threatening complications of renal failure, which include severe refractory hyperkalaemia, resistant fluid overload (e.g. unresponsive to intravenous diuretics) or pulmonary oedema, and severe metabolic acidosis. Pericarditis due to uraemia is also an absolute indication for urgent dialysis, as is uraemic encephalopathy. If a patient is oliguric, consider the following first:

• Exclude obstructive causes
• Fluid resuscitation
• Maintain blood pressure with inotrope or vasopressor
• Avoid nephrotoxic medications
• Trial loop diuretics after optimal restoration of intravascular volume
• Dopamine infusion does not affect the likelihood of progression to acute tubular necrosis.

23. Answer B

Alpha-1-adrenergic receptor antagonists such as tamsulosin can promote the chances of stone passage (Bultitude and Rees, 2012). Alpha-1 receptors are located in the human ureter, especially the distal ureter, and alpha-blockers have been demonstrated to increase expulsion rates of distal ureteral stones, decrease time to expulsion and decrease need for analgesia during stone passage. Up to 98% of small stone of less than 5 mm may pass spontaneously. No benefits have been seen with diuretics or intravenous fluids, though calcium channel antagonists may also promote expulsion.

 Bultitude, M. and Rees, J. (2012). Management of renal colic. *BMJ* 345, e5499.
http://www.bmj.com/content/345/bmj.e5499

24. Answer B
Post-transplantation lymphoproliferative disease (PTLD) carries a high mortality (Carbone et al., 2008). Most cases of PTLD are induced by Epstein–Barr virus (EBV). A seronegative renal transplant recipient who receives a seropositive kidney is at high risk of developing PTLD.

The initial treatment for PTLD will depend on the patient's medical conditions, balancing the immediate risk for death with possible rejection of the allograft. The reduction of immunosuppression forms the cornerstone of all treatment and may be sufficient by itself, with a complete remission rate of 63% in some reports. This man has had a localised PTLD. The initial approach would be to reduce his overall immunosuppression and monitor his response. Withdrawal of immunosuppression would likely result in acute rejection and the risk of dying from PTLD is low in this patient. Rituximab has been shown to induce remission in PTLD but there is no evidence to support maintaining current levels of immunosuppression and treating with rituximab at the same time. Anti-viral treatment with valganciclovir or acyclovir has not been shown to have benefit in the treatment of PTLD.

 Carbone, A., Gloghini, A., and Dotti, G. (2008). EBV-associated lymphoproliferative disorders: classification and treatment. *Oncologist* 13, 577–585.
http://theoncologist.alphamedpress.org/content/13/5/577.full

25. Answer D
The prognosis for patients with cirrhosis and renal failure is poor. Patients with type 1 hepatorenal syndrome have a median survival of 1 month compared to patients with type 2 hepatorenal syndrome who have a median survival of 6 months. The great majority of patients with hepatorenal syndrome have a poor short-term outcome unless they undergo liver transplantation. Patients who respond to terlipressin live longer than those with no response. However, vasoconstrictor therapy has not been shown to improve survival in the long-term. Continuous renal replacement therapy improves short-term survival in patients with severe acute kidney injury with a reversible decompensation and can be beneficial in bridging patients to transplant. However, the long-term outcome in patients with type 1 hepatorenal syndrome is very poor. The Hepatorenal Syndrome: The 8th International Consensus Conference of the Acute Dialysis Quality Initiative (ADQI) Group recommended withholding renal replacement therapy in patients with decompensation of cirrhosis who are not candidates for liver transplantation. Transjugular intrahepatic portosystemic shunts may be effective in

selected patients. However, there are limited data on long-term survival. There are also limited data on the use of norepinephrine (noradrenaline) in patients with hepatorenal syndrome.

Ginès, P. and Schrier, R. (2009). Renal failure in cirrhosis. *N Engl J Med* 361, 1279–1290.
http://www.ncbi.nlm.nih.gov/pubmed/19776409

26. Answer C

The patient in the vignette has tubulointerstitial nephritis and uveitis (TINU) syndrome (Li et al., 2008). The proposed diagnostic criteria for definite TINU specifies that affected patients' renal biopsy should be consistent with acute tubulointerstitial nephritis (ATIN) and the onset of bilateral uveitis 2 months or less before or less than 12 months after ATIN.

Most patients with TINU are adolescents and young women. Renal disease in these patients is usually self-limited but some may develop progressive renal failure. Histocompatibility leucocyte antigen (HLA) haplotype DQA1*01/DQB1*05/DRB1*01 may be of importance in TINU susceptibility.

ATIN in this syndrome is typically treated with prednisolone and good results have been reported. Topical and systemic corticosteroids have been used for uveitis with success. Recurrences of uveitis are common.

Li, J.Y., Yong, T.Y., Bennett, G., Barbara, J.A., and Coates, P.T. (2008). Human leucocyte antigen DQ alpha heterodimers and human leucocyte antigen DR alleles in tubulointerstitial nephritis and uveitis syndrome. *Nephrology (Carlton)* 13, 755–757.
http://www.ncbi.nlm.nih.gov/pubmed/19154326

27. Answer G

Primary focal segmental glomerulosclerosis (FSGS) may recur rapidly in the renal allograft (Ponticelli, 2010). The rapidity of recurrence in some cases strongly suggests the presence in primary FSGS of a circulating factor in plasma, with resulting toxicity to the glomerular capillary wall, glomerular basement membrane (GBM) and podocytes. The reported recurrence rate averages about 20%. There are two clinical presentations of FSGS after transplantation: an early recurrence, the most frequent, characterised by a massive proteinuria within hours to days after implantation of the new kidney; and a late recurrence which develops insidiously several months or years after transplantation.

The management of patients with recurrent FSGS is difficult and not well established. The administration of high-dose angiotensin converting enzyme (ACE) inhibitors, angiotensin receptor blockers and statins is recommended in order to exploit their anti-proteinuric and anti-lipaemic effects. Increased doses of steroids and calcineurin inhibitors may protect from FSGS recurrence, but may increase the risk of over-immunosuppression. The most commonly used therapeutic approach is the use of plasmapheresis or immunoadsorption with protein A. In the absence of contraindication, a course with rituximab may be attempted if there is no response to plasmapheresis.

In spite of the risk of recurrence, patients with primary FSGS should not be excluded from transplantation. In the case of living donation, the possibility of recurrence and its consequences should be clearly expressed to and discussed with the donor and the recipient, and pre-emptive plasmapheresis should be planned.

Ponticelli, C. (2010). Recurrence of focal segmental glomerular sclerosis (FSGS) after renal transplantation. *Nephrol Dial Transplant* 25, 25–31. http://ndt.oxfordjournals.org/content/25/1/25.full.pdf

28. Answer C

Patients with the nephrotic syndrome (NS) are at increased risk for venous thrombosis, particularly deep vein and renal vein thrombosis (DVT and RVT) (Radhakrishnan, 2012). Pulmonary embolisation (mostly asymptomatic) is relatively common. Arterial thromboses (e.g. limb and cerebral) also occur with higher frequency than in the general population. The absolute risks of venous thromboembolism (VTE) (rate of 1.02% per year) and arterial thromboembolism (ATE) (rate of 1.48% per year) are each eight times higher than the estimated age- and sex-weighted annual incidences in the general population. Risks of both VTE and ATE are particularly high within the first 6 months of NS. The annual incidence for thromboembolism in idiopathic membranous nephropathy (MN) is 1.4%. The risk of thrombosis seems to be related to the severity and duration of the nephrotic state and is particularly increased with serum albumin concentrations of less than 20 g/L. Furthermore, among the causes of NS, the risk is highest with idiopathic MN, followed by membranoproliferative glomerulonephritis and minimal change disease. The cause of the hypercoagulable state in patients with NS is not well understood. A variety of haemostatic abnormalities have been described, including decreased levels of anti-thrombin and plasminogen (due to urinary losses), increased platelet activation, hyperfibrinogenaemia, inhibition of plasminogen activation and the presence of high molecular weight fibrinogen in the circulation. There is no prospective, controlled study comparing the risks associated with undiagnosed venous thrombosis with the risk of long-term anticoagulation in patients with NS.

Radhakrishnan, J. (2012). Venous thromboembolism and membranous nephropathy: so what's new? *Clin J Am Soc Nephrol* 7, 3–4. http://cjasn.asnjournals.org/content/7/1/3.full

29. Answer F

Most cases of minimal change disease (MCD) are idiopathic and not clearly associated with an underlying disease or event (Waldman et al., 2007). With secondary MCD, the onset of nephrotic syndrome occurs concurrently or following an extraglomerular or glomerular disease process. MCD can be associated with the following:

• Drugs
• Neoplasms

- Infections
- Allergy.
Non-steroidal anti-inflammatory drugs (NSAIDs) and selective COX-2 inhibitors are the most common cause of secondary MCD.

Waldman, M., Crew, R.J., Valeri, A., et al. (2007). Adult minimal-change disease: clinical characteristics, treatment, and outcomes. *Clin J Am Soc Nephrol* 2, 445–453.
http://cjasn.asnjournals.org/content/2/3/445.long

30. Answer C

The M-type phospholipase A2 receptor (PLA2R), a transmembrane receptor that is highly expressed in glomerular podocytes, has been identified as a major antigen in human idiopathic membranous nephropathy (MN) (Beck and Salant, 2010; Beck et al., 2009). Anti-PLA2R antibodies have been identified in 70–80% of patients with idiopathic MN. In contrast, there was no evidence of PLA2R antibodies in serum from patients with secondary MN due to lupus or hepatitis B or from patients with nephrotic syndrome other than MN (such as diabetic nephropathy or focal segmental glomerulosclerosis). In one study, anti-PLA2R strongly correlated with clinical status and in another study, a decline in anti-PLA2R predicted the clinical response to immunosuppressive therapy. The association of these anti-PLA2R autoantibodies with disease activity might suggest a causal role, but it has not yet been demonstrated that these antibodies cause MN.

Beck, L.H., Jr., Bonegio, R.G., Lambeau, G., et al. (2009). M-type phospholipase A2 receptor as target antigen in idiopathic membranous nephropathy. *N Engl J Med* 361, 11–21.
http://www.ncbi.nlm.nih.gov/pubmed/19571279

Beck, L.H., Jr. and Salant, D.J. (2010). Membranous nephropathy: recent travels and new roads ahead. *Kidney Int* 77, 765–770.
http://www.ncbi.nlm.nih.gov/pubmed/20182413

31. Answer E

The renal biopsy shows the characteristic histological features of type I MPGN (Sethi and Fervenza, 2012). There is global and diffuse thickening of the capillary walls, caused by mesangial interposition into the subendothelial zone of the capillary loops. There is also mesangial proliferation and hypercellularity. There is lobular accentuation, meaning that the segments or lobules are discernible because of cleft-like spaces between adjacent lobules. Immunofluorescence staining shows a coarse granular pattern along the glomerular capillaries. Electron microscopy shows a segment of a glomerular capillary with large, discrete, electron-dense deposits in the subendothelial space.

Sethi, S. and Fervenza, F.C. (2012). Membranoproliferative glomerulonephritis – a new look at an old entity. *N Engl J Med* 366, 1119–1131.
http://www.ncbi.nlm.nih.gov/pubmed/22435371

5 Endocrinology

Questions

BASIC SCIENCE

Answers can be found in the Endocrinology Answers section at the end of this chapter.

1. Parathyroid hormone (PTH) plays a central role in the regulation of calcium and phosphate through its action on the bone, kidney and intestine. Which is the primary target cell of PTH in bone?
- **A.** Osteoclast
- **B.** Osteoblast
- **C.** Osteocyte
- **D.** Mesenchymal stem cell
- **E.** Adipocyte

2. Which one of the following hormones leads to decreased food intake?
- **A.** Ghrelin
- **B.** Glucagon
- **C.** Neuropeptide Y
- **D.** Leptin
- **E.** Cortisol

3. Diuretics can alter calcium homeostasis. Which one of the following effects is most likely?
- **A.** Thiazide diuretics increase gastrointestinal calcium absorption
- **B.** Thiazide diuretics reduce urinary calcium excretion
- **C.** Thiazide diuretics reduce serum calcium concentration
- **D.** Loop diuretics reduce urinary calcium excretion
- **E.** Loop diuretics increase serum calcium concentration

4. Which protein is involved in glucose reabsorption at the brush border membrane of the tubular epithelial cells in the kidney?
- **A.** Glucose transporter type 1 (GLUT1)
- **B.** Glucose transporter type 2 (GLUT2)

Passing the FRACP Written Examination: Questions and Answers, First Edition. Jonathan Gleadle, Tuck Yong, Jordan Li, Surjit Tarafdar, and Danielle Wu.
© 2013 John Wiley & Sons, Ltd. Published 2013 by John Wiley & Sons, Ltd.

    C. Sodium-dependent glucose co-transporter (SGLT)
    D. Peroxisome proliferator-activated receptor γ (PPARγ)
    E. Hepatocyte nuclear factor (HNF)

5. Which one of the following inhibits the formation of 1, 25-dihydroxy-vitamin D?
    A. Circulating fibroblast growth factor-23
    B. Parathyroid hormone
    C. Low serum phosphate level
    D. Pregnancy
    E. Sun exposure

6. Which one of the followings best describes the biological action of glucagon-like peptide 1 (GLP-1)?
    A. Glucose-dependent inhibition of insulin secretion
    B. Suppression of glucagon secretion
    C. Decreased synthesis of proinsulin
    D. Acceleration of gastric emptying
    E. Stimulation of appetite

7. What is the first physiological response to hypoglycaemia in an individual without diabetes mellitus?
    A. Increased epinephrine (adrenaline)
    B. Increased glucagon
    C. Decreased insulin
    D. Increased growth hormone
    E. Increased cortisol

8. In addition to its effects on glucose homeostasis, which one of the following is an effect of increased glucagon level?
    A. Decreased energy expenditure
    B. Decreased ketogenesis
    C. Decreased bile acid synthesis
    D. Decreased thermogenesis
    E. Decreased food intake

9. Hyponatraemia is a frequent manifestation of primary adrenal insufficiency. Which one of the following hormone changes explains this manifestation?
    A. Increase in corticotrophin-releasing hormone
    B. Increase in prolactin
    C. Increase in thyroid-stimulating hormone
    D. Reduction in anti-diuretic hormone release
    E. Reduction in adrenocorticotropin hormone

10. Which one of the following is an effect of amiodarone on thyroid function?
- **A.** Decreased sensitivity of the pituitary to thyroxine (T_4) and tri-iodothyronine (T_3)
- **B.** Inhibition of conversion of thyroxine (T_4) to tri-iodothyronine (T_3)
- **C.** Inhibition of thyroid stimulating hormone (TSH) release
- **D.** Stimulation of tri-iodothyronine (T_3) synthesis
- **E.** Inhibition of thyrotropin-releasing hormone (TRH) secretion

Theme: Thyroid physiology (for Questions 11–14)
- **A.** Thyroid-stimulating hormone
- **B.** Thyroid-stimulating hormone receptor antibody
- **C.** Thyroxine-binding globulin
- **D.** Thyroglobulin
- **E.** Thyroperoxidase antibody
- **F.** Reverse tri-iodothyronine (T_3)
- **G.** Thyrotropin-releasing hormone
- **H.** Thyroxine (T_4)

For each of the following conditions, select the most likely hormone, antibody or protein to be altered.

11. An increase in which one of the above occurs in normal maternal thyroid physiology during pregnancy as a result of reduced hepatic clearance and increased synthesis?

12. Which one of the above is produced only by normal or neoplastic thyroid follicular cells and is helpful in monitoring for thyroid cancer recurrence?

13. Which one of the above is metabolised by de-iodinase to generate tri-iodothyronine (T_3)?

14. Which one of the above is a tripeptide hormone released by the hypothalamus?

CLINICAL

15. A 36-year-old woman has an abdominal computed tomography (CT) performed because of abdominal pain. A 1.9-cm mass in her right adrenal gland with an attenuation value of less than 10 Hounsfield units was the only abnormality found. She has no significant past medical history. She is normotensive and overnight dexamethasone suppression test, urinary fractionated metanephrines, plasma aldosterone/plasma renin activity and electrolytes are all normal. What should be the further management plan?
   A. Magnetic resonance imaging of the adrenal glands
   B. Selective adrenal venous sampling for aldosterone
   C. Arrange for surgical resection of the mass
   D. Repeat CT at 6, 12 and 24 months
   E. 24-h urinary cortisol levels

16. A 30-year-old woman with Cushing syndrome returns for her recent investigation results which are shown below. Magnetic resonance imaging of the pituitary did not reveal any mass. What is the next appropriate step to take?

	Value	Reference range
8 am plasma cortisol (nmol/L)	800	200–650
8 am plasma adrenocorticotrophic hormone (ACTH) (ng/L)	68	<50
Urine free cortisol (nmol/24 h)	850	100–300
Low-dose dexamethasone suppression test (2 mg/day): urine free cortisol (nmol/24 h)	575	
High-dose dexamethasone suppression test (8 mg/day): urine free cortisol (nmol/24 h)	400	

   A. Bilateral adrenal vein sampling
   B. Inferior petrosal sinus sampling
   C. Midnight salivary free cortisol
   D. Computed tomography of the abdomen
   E. Refer the patient to a neurosurgeon

17. Which one of the following observations is correct regarding type 2 diabetes in the Australian indigenous population compared to the non-indigenous population?
   A. Age of onset of type 2 diabetes in the indigenous and non-indigenous population is the same
   B. There is an earlier average age of onset of macrovascular complications in the indigenous population
   C. There is a later age of onset of microvascular complications in the indigenous population
   D. Body mass index is not a predictor of the development of type 2 diabetes in the indigenous population

E. The prevalence of type 2 diabetes is higher in the non-indigenous population

18. Which one of the following statements is true concerning subclinical hypothyroidism?

A. Thyroid stimulating hormone (TSH) levels are suppressed but thyroxine levels are normal

B. TSH levels are increased but thyroxine levels are normal

C. It does not progress to overt hypothyroidism

D. Thyroxine replacement should be initiated if TSH is elevated

E. Population screening for subclinical hypothyroidism is of proven benefit

19. A 34-year-old man has been concerned about a change in facial appearance, headaches, hypertension and excessive sweating. Which one of the following tests should be undertaken to investigate possible acromegaly?

A. Growth hormone-releasing hormone levels following a 75-g oral glucose load

B. 24-h urinary insulin-like growth factor 1 (IGF-1) levels

C. Growth hormone-releasing hormone suppression test

D. Growth hormone (GH) levels following insulin stimulation test

E. Insulin-like growth factor I (IGF-1) and growth hormone (GH) levels during a 2-h period after a 75-g oral glucose load

20. Which one of the following is the most important reason to measure thyroid stimulating hormone receptor antibodies during pregnancy in a woman with Graves disease?

A. To detect fetal goitre

B. To predict the risk of thyrotoxic storm

C. To titrate dose of anti-thyroid therapy

D. To predict the risk of neonatal thyrotoxicosis

E. To predict the risk of post-partum hypothyroidism

21. An 18-year-old man presents for investigation of delayed puberty. On examination, his height is 1.85 m and weight is 80 kg. He has a complete loss of the sense of smell and small testes. The results of investigations are shown below. What is the likely diagnosis?

	Value	Reference ranges
Prolactin (mU/L)	350	50–450
Testosterone (nmol/L)	4	11–36
Luteinising hormone (LH) (IU/L)	<0.1	0.5–9.0
Follicular stimulating hormone (FSH) (IU/L)	0.5	1.0–8.0
Serum cortisol at 9.00 am (nmol/L)	165	200–700

A. Hypopituitarism
B. Kallman syndrome
C. Klinefelter syndrome
D. Noonan syndrome
E. Turner syndrome

22. A 28-year-old woman with type 1 diabetes is 13 weeks' pregnant. She is on a basal-bolus insulin treatment. She is seen in the high-risk pregnancy clinic for the first time. Her blood pressure (BP) is 120/70 mmHg. Her most recent HbA$_{1c}$ is 8.3%. Which one of the following should be included in her management plan?

A. HbA$_{1c}$ level should be monitored every 3 months
B. Intensify her insulin treatment to achieve a pre-prandial glucose level of 5.6–6.5 mmol/L
C. Intensify her insulin treatment to achieve a post-prandial glucose level at 1 h of less than 8 mmol/L
D. Intensify her insulin treatment to lower her HbA$_{1c}$ level to a target of 7.5%
E. Commence angiotensin converting enzyme (ACE) inhibitor

23. A 50-year-old woman presents with a sudden onset of severe headache associated with vomiting for the preceding 24 h. She has previously been healthy and does not take any medications. On examination, her temperature is 37°C, pulse is 100 beats/min and blood pressure is 85/50 mmHg. There is also a partial right-sided third nerve palsy present. The results of her investigations are shown below. What is the most likely diagnosis?

	Value	Reference ranges
Haemoglobin (g/L)	120	115–155
White cell count (cells/L)	14.5×10^9	$4.0–11.0 \times 10^9$
Platelet count (cells/L)	240×10^9	$150–450 \times 10^9$
C-reactive protein (g/L)	32	0–10
Sodium (mmol/L)	126	137–145
Potassium (mmol/L	4.3	3.2–4.3
Urea (μmol/L)	6.8	2.7–8.0
Creatinine (μmol/L)	110	60–100
Thyroid-stimulating hormone (mIU/L)	1.3	0.4–4.5
Free thyroxine (T4) (pmol/L)	7	10–22
Serum cortisol at 9.00 am (nmol/L)	165	200–700

A. Brainstem ischaemic stroke
B. Encephalitis
C. Meningitis
D. Pituitary apoplexy
E. Subarachnoid haemorrhage

24. You are referred a 19-year-old woman with newly diagnosed diabetes. She has no symptoms, but had a random glucose of 17 mmol/L. A subsequent fasting glucose was 5.8 mmol/L and HbA$_{1c}$ was 6.8%.

Her medical history is significant for cystic fibrosis diagnosed as an infant. She has had numerous hospitalisations over the years for pulmonary infections. Her current medications include salbutamol inhaler 200 µg four times a day, pancreatic enzymes of variable dose three times a day, ciprofloxacin 500 mg twice a day, and one multi-vitamin tablet daily. Her weight is 55 kg (BMI 17.5 kg/m^2).

You arrange for her to be taught home blood glucose monitoring by a diabetic educator. What is the best therapeutic option at this point?

- **A.** Acarbose three times a day with meals
- **B.** Metformin twice daily with meals
- **C.** Gliclazide slow release once daily
- **D.** Once-daily basal insulin
- **E.** Rapid-acting insulin with meals

25. Regarding diagnosis and management of prolactinoma, which one of the following is INCORRECT?

- **A.** There is an increased risk of cardiac valve regurgitation with the use of cabergoline in patients with Parkinson disease
- **B.** Patients with bitemporal hemianopia and severe headache should have transphenoidal surgery
- **C.** Elevated prolactin levels can be observed in patient with hepatic or renal failure
- **D.** Anti-depressants and anti-psychotic medications are associated with elevated prolactin levels
- **E.** In patients with a pituitary macroadenoma, prolactin level can be greatly underestimated with immunoradiometric assays

26. A 45-year-old man was diagnosed to have hypergastrinaemia due to Zollinger–Ellison syndrome associated with multiple endocrine neoplasia syndrome type 1. Which one the following findings can be observed?

- **A.** Decrease in lower oesophageal sphincter (LES) pressure
- **B.** Decrease in pepsinogen secretion
- **C.** Increase in gastric motility
- **D.** Increase in ileo-caecal sphincter pressure
- **E.** Inhibition of gastric mucosa growth

27. A 65-year-old woman has had a total thyroidectomy and radioactive iodine for treatment of papillary thyroid carcinoma. She is on an appropriate dose of thyroxine therapy. Six months later she has a neck ultrasound which shows no residual thyroid disease. What other test should be considered at this time?

- **A.** Anti-thyroperoxidase antibody
- **B.** Thyroid-stimulating hormone
- **C.** Free thyroxine (free T$_4$)

D. Thyroglobulin

E. Anti-thyroid stimulating hormone receptor antibody

28. A 39-year-old woman with a history of primary hyperparathyroidism treated with subtotal parathyroidectomy presents with episodic headaches and palpitations. She is found to be hypertensive. Further investigations reveal that her 24-h urinary norepinephrine (noradrenaline) and epinephrine (adrenaline) are 600 nmol/L (0–450) and 752 nmol/L (0–100), respectively. In addition her serum calcitonin is also elevated at 1355 ng/L (0–5.5). Which one of the following genes should be considered for mutational analyses?

A. Adenomatous polyposis coli (APC) gene

B. Breast cancer type 1 (BRCA1) gene

C. K-ras oncogene

D. RET oncogene

E. Von Hippel–Lindau (VHL) gene

29. A 27-year-old woman presented with amenorrhoea since stopping her oral contraceptive pill 4 months ago. She has no significant past medical problems. The results of investigations are shown below. What is the most likely cause of her amenorrhoea?

	Value	Reference range
Prolactin (ng/mL)	24	5–20
Oestrogen (pmol/L)	28676	100–2400
Testosterone (nmol/L)	2.9	0.5–2.5
Luteinising hormone (LH) (IU/L)	<1.0	3.0–12.0
Follicle stimulating hormone (FSH) (IU/L)	<1.0	2.0–10.0

A. Prolactinoma

B. Pregnancy

C. Congenital adrenal hyperplasia (CAH)

D. Premature ovarian failure

E. Polycystic ovary syndrome (PCOS)

30. A 59-year-old man has chronic kidney disease secondary to diabetic nephropathy. His estimated glomerular filtration rate is 45 mL/min/1.73 m^2. Which one of the following glucose-lowering agents poses the highest risk of hypoglycaemia in the setting of the renal impairment?

A. Acarbose

B. Exenatide

C. Glimepiride

D. Metformin

E. Sitagliptin

Theme: Endocrine investigations (for Questions 31–34)

A. 24-h urinary catecholamines and metanephrines
B. Plasma catecholamines
C. Blood renin-to-aldosterone ratio
D. Insulin-like growth factor-I
E. Saline suppression test
F. Thyroid function test
G. Urinary sodium and osmolality
H. Water deprivation test

31. The hypertension in a 40-year-old woman is known to be difficult to control. She is currently taking three anti-hypertensive medications. She also complains of recurrent anxiety attacks and episodes of palpitations. Which one of the above is the next most appropriate investigation?

32. A 76-year-old woman presents with confusion. Her family reports her being constipated and gaining weight in recent months. On examination, she is alert but disoriented in time and place. Her heart rate is 52 beats/min and blood pressure is 138/95 mmHg. There is non-pitting oedema in both legs. The chest X-ray reveals cardiomegaly and bilateral small pleural effusions. Apart from mild hyponatraemia (serum sodium level 133 mmol/L), other biochemistry results are unremarkable. What is the next most appropriate investigation?

33. A 40-year-old man presents with recent changes in his vision and headaches. He reports that he has had two near-miss traffic accidents because he failed to spot cars approaching him at a T-junction. His medical history is unremarkable though his wife reports the recent onset of severe snoring and he recently had bilateral carpal tunnel release. On examination, he is hypertensive with a blood pressure of 160/95 mmHg and he is tanned from a recent holiday. The rest of his cardiovascular, respiratory and abdominal examination is normal. What is the next investigation to undertake?

34. A 68-year-old woman presents after a 2-day history of vomiting. She is found to have hypernatraemia but her elevated serum sodium concentration did not improve despite adequate fluid replacement. She has a history of bipolar disorder and has been taking lithium for the past 8 years. What is the appropriate investigation after stabilising this patient clinically?

Answers

BASIC SCIENCE

1. Answer B

The primary function of parathyroid hormone (PTH) is to maintain the extracellular fluid calcium concentration within a narrow normal range. The hormone acts directly on bone and the kidney and indirectly on the intestine through its effects on synthesis of 1, 25-dihydroxy-vitamin D to increase serum calcium concentration (Kousteni and Bilezikian, 2008).

Osteoblasts (or stromal cell precursors), which have PTH receptors, are crucial to the bone-forming effect of PTH; osteoclasts, which appear to lack PTH receptors, mediate bone breakdown. PTH-mediated stimulation of osteoclasts is thought to be indirect, acting in part through cytokines released from osteoblasts to activate osteoclasts. In in vitro experiments, osteoblasts must be present for PTH to activate osteoclasts to reabsorb bone. Intermittent PTH treatment increases osteoblast numbers, induces differentiation of committed osteoblast precursors and prolongs osteoblast survival. Understanding the cell biology of PTH is important in appreciating the mechanism of action of PTH analogues in the treatment of osteoporosis (Kraenzlin and Meier, 2011). Continuous exposure to elevated levels of PTH for days leads to increased osteoclast-mediated bone reabsorption, but intermittent administration leads to a net stimulation of bone formation rather than bone breakdown.

Kousteni, S. and Bilezikian, J.P. (2008). The cell biology of parathyroid hormone in osteoblasts. *Curr Osteoporos Rep* 6, 72–76.
http://www.ncbi.nlm.nih.gov/pubmed/18778567

Kraenzlin, M.E. and Meier, C. (2011). Parathyroid hormone analogues in the treatment of osteoporosis. *Nat Rev Endocrinol* 7, 647–656.
http://www.ncbi.nlm.nih.gov/pubmed/21750510

2. Answer D

Leptin is a circulating peptide hormone that is produced primarily in adipose tissue and leads to suppression of appetite.

Leptin acts on receptors in the hypothalamus where it inhibits appetite by counteracting the effects of neuropeptide Y (a potent appetite stimulant) and promotes the synthesis of α-melanocyte-stimulating hormone, an appetite suppressant. Genetic deficiency of leptin or the leptin receptor leads to severe obesity.

Ghrelin is an appetite-stimulating hormone that is produced mainly by the stomach and pancreas. Its secretion increase with starvation or reduced food intake and it stimulates secretion of growth hormone, increases appetite and leads to weight gain. Reduced ghrelin production may partially account for the effectiveness of some bariatric surgery.

Glucagon is a counter-regulatory hormone to hypoglycaemia and it increases glucose production in the liver by increasing both gluconeogenesis and glycogenolysis.

3. Answer B
Thiazide diuretics tend to lead to a reduction in urinary calcium excretion. This effect can be therapeutically helpful in the treatment of recurrent stone formers with hypercalciuria. The fall in calcium excretion also tends to induce positive calcium balance or to minimise the degree of negative calcium balance that is commonly seen in older patients. This may be manifested clinically by an increase in bone density, possibly by a reduction in the incidence of hip fracture. Chronic use of a loop diuretic may have the opposite effect as it tends to promote calcium loss and negative calcium balance may enhance the risk of hip fracture. Thiazide diuretics can be associated with hypercalcaemia, but usually in the presence of co-existing hyperparathyroidism.

4. Answer C
The kidney contributes to glucose homeostasis through gluconeogenesis, glucose filtration, reabsorption and consumption. Under normal circumstances, up to 180 g/day of glucose is filtered by the renal glomerulus and virtually all of it is reabsorbed in the proximal convoluted tubule. This reabsorption is carried out by two sodium-dependent glucose co-transporter (SGLT) proteins, SGLT1 and SGLT2, which are present on the brush border membrane of epithelial tubular cells. SGLT1, situated in the S3 segment, is a high-affinity low-capacity transporter reabsorbing about 10% of filtered glucose. SGLT2, situated in the S1 segment, is a low-affinity high-capacity transporter reabsorbing the other 90%. In patients with type 2 diabetes mellitus, renal absorptive capacity is maladaptively increased. Once glucose has been reabsorbed and concentrated in the tubular epithelial cells, it diffuses into the interstitium across specific facilitative glucose transporters (GLUTs) located on the basolateral membrane of cells (Mather and Pollock, 2011).

SGLT2 inhibitors have been examined as a novel drug for treating diabetes. SGLT2 inhibitors enhance renal glucose excretion by inhibiting renal glucose reabsorption. Consequently, SGLT2 inhibitors reduce plasma glucose and improve insulin resistance in diabetes. To date, various SGLT2 inhibitors have been developed and evaluated in clinical studies.

Peroxisome proliferator-activated receptor γ (PPARγ) is expressed most abundantly in adipose tissue, but is also found in pancreatic beta cells, vascular endothelium and macrophages. PPARγ is essential for normal adipocyte differentiation and proliferation as well as fatty acid uptake and storage.

Hepatocyte nuclear factors (HNFs) are transcription factors found in the liver, pancreatic islets, the kidneys and genital tissues. In pancreatic beta cells, these transcription factors regulate the expression of the insulin gene and the expression of genes encoding proteins involved in glucose transport, metabolism and mitochondrial metabolism – all of which are linked to protein secretion. Mutation of HNFs is found in patients with mature-onset diabetes of the young (MODY).

Patients with mutation of HNF-1β are associated with MODY 5, which is characterised by both diabetes mellitus and renal cysts. However, the role of HNF-1β in glucose transport is not known.

Mather, A. and Pollock, C. (2011). Glucose handling by the kidney. *Kidney Int* 79 (Suppl 120), S1–S6.
http://www.ncbi.nlm.nih.gov/pubmed/21358696

Isaji, M. (2011). SGLT2 inhibitors: molecular design and potential differences in effect. *Kidney Int* 79 (Suppl 120), S14–S19.
http://www.ncbi.nlm.nih.gov/pubmed/21358697

5. Answer A

1, 25-dihydroxy [(OH)$_2$] vitamin D is formed from 25-hydroxy (OH) vitamin D, facilitated by 1-α hydroxylase found in the inner mitochondrial membrane of cells in the proximal tubule of the kidneys. Serum 1, 25-(OH)$_2$ vitamin D stimulates the uptake of calcium and phosphate across the upper gastrointestinal tract and also stimulates absorption of phosphate by renal tubular cells (Bowyer et al., 2009).

The formation of 1, 25-(OH)$_2$ vitamin D is stimulated by circulating parathyroid hormone (PTH) and low serum phosphate levels, and is inhibited by circulating fibroblast growth factor (FGF)-23. The receptor for FGF-23 is FGF receptor-1 and it requires the membrane-bound protein klotho as a co-factor for its action. 1, 25-(OH)$_2$ vitamin D, acting through its vitamin D receptor, up-regulates both FGF-23 mRNA and klotho mRNA. 1, 25-(OH)$_2$ vitamin D also inhibits the secretion of PTH so that serum 1, 25-(OH)$_2$ vitamin D is involved in a complex homeostatic mechanism whereby reducing serum PTH levels reduces renal phosphate loss and increasing serum FGF-23 increases renal phosphate loss.

Serum 1, 25-(OH)$_2$ vitamin D levels increase during pregnancy and are correlated with levels of serum 25-OH vitamin D. The increase in serum 1, 25-(OH)$_2$ vitamin D levels is probably due to increased 1-α hydroxylase acting on the placenta. By the end of the first trimester, the serum 1, 25-(OH)$_2$ vitamin D level is about three times higher than the average value in non-pregnant women and may be responsible for the increased calcium absorption in pregnant women.

Bowyer, L., Catling-Paull, C., Diamond, T., Horner, C., Davis, G., and Craig, M.E. (2009). Vitamin D, PTH and calcium levels in pregnant women and their neonates. *Clin Endocrinol* 70, 372–377.
http://www.ncbi.nlm.nih.gov/pubmed/18573121

6. Answer B

Glucagon-like peptide 1 (GLP-1) is a gut-derived incretin hormone that stimulates insulin and suppresses glucagon secretion, inhibits gastric emptying and reduces appetite and food intake (Drucker and Nauck, 2006). Therapeutic approaches to enhancing incretin action include incretin mimetics (egexenatide and liraglutide) and inhibitors of dipeptidyl peptidase-4 (DPP-4), which is responsible for the degradation of incretins (egsitagliptin and vildagliptin). These agents have been shown to be efficacious in lowering haemoglobin A_{1c} in clinical trials, but long-term studies are still needed to determine their benefits for the treatment of type 2 diabetes.

Drucker, D.J. and Nauck, M.A. (2006). The incretin system: glucagon-like peptide-1 receptor agonists and dipeptidyl peptidase-4 inhibitors in type 2 diabetes. *Lancet* 368, 1696–1705.
http://www.ncbi.nlm.nih.gov/pubmed/17098089

7. Answer C

Insulin secretion begins to decrease as blood glucose approaches the lower limit of normal levels and it is the body's first defence mechanism against hypoglycaemia (Cryer et al., 2009). This reverses the normal effects of insulin, which are to increase the peripheral uptake of glucose and decrease its hepatic production. This response is lost in patients with absolute beta-cell failure, as in type 1 diabetics or long-standing type 2 diabetics.

The second defence against hypoglycaemia is an increase in glucagon secretion, which leads to increased hepatic production of glucose by increasing both gluconeogenesis and glycogenolysis. The third mechanism is an increase in epinephrine (adrenaline) secretion, which, acting via the beta-2-adrenergic receptors, increases the hepatic production of glucose and impairs peripheral uptake of glucose. Epinephrine (adrenaline) also decreases insulin secretion via its alpha-2-adrenergic receptors effects.

Growth hormone and cortisol begin to rise if hypoglycaemia persists for hours. They enhance hepatic glucose production and limit peripheral utilisation of glucose.

Cryer, P.E., Axelrod, L., Grossman, A.B., et al (2009). Evaluation and management of adult Hypoglycemic Disorders: An Endocrine Society Clinical Practice Guideline. *J Clin Endocrinol Metab* 94, 709–728.
http://jcem.endojournals.org/content/94/3/709.long

8. Answer E

In addition to its well-known effects on glucose metabolism, glucagon has the following effects:
- Increases lipolysis
- Increases fatty acid oxidation and ketogenesis
- Increases satiety and decreases food intake
- Increases thermogenesis and energy expenditure
- Increases bile acid synthesis.

The ability of glucagon to stimulate energy expenditure, along with its hypolipidaemic and satiating effects, make it an attractive pharmaceutical agent for the treatment of metabolic syndrome (Habegger et al., 2010).

Habegger, K.M., Heppner, K.M., Geary, N., et al. (2010). The metabolic actions of glucagon revisited. *Nat Rev Endocrinol* 6, 689–697.
http://www.ncbi.nlm.nih.gov/pubmed/20957001

9. Answer A

Hyponatraemia was present in 78% of 50 patients with primary adrenal insufficiency in one study. Cortisol deficiency causes hyponatraemia because it increases corticotrophin-releasing hormone (CRH), which stimulates anti-diuretic hormone (ADH) release, whereas aldosterone deficiency causes hyponatraemia because of renal sodium loss, hypovolaemia and baroreceptor-mediated ADH release (Bornstein, 2009). When cortisol concentration is low, its feedback to the hypothalamus is lost. Consequently, CRH is no longer inhibited. High CRH concentrations stimulate the secretion of ADH. Hydrocortisone replacement therapy leads to rapid normalisation of serum sodium levels.

Bornstein, S.R. (2009). Predisposing factors for adrenal insufficiency. *N Engl J Med* 360, 2328–2339.
http://www.ncbi.nlm.nih.gov/pubmed/19474430

10. Answer B

In 14–18% of amiodarone-treated patients, there is overt thyroid dysfunction, either amiodarone-induced thyrotoxicosis (AIT) or amiodarone-induced hypothyroidism (AIH) (Ursella et al., 2005). Amiodarone is extremely rich in iodine and, being highly lipophilic, is avidly bound to adipose, thyroid and skeletal muscle tissue with a half-life of about 100 days. With excess intra-thyroidal iodine, iodine transport and thyroid hormone synthesis are transiently inhibited (Wolff–Chaikoff effect). Amiodarone inhibits conversion of thyroxine (T_4) to tri-iodothyronine (T_3). Amiodarone also has a direct toxic effect on thyroid cells. AIH results from the thyroid gland's inability to escape from the transient Wolff–Chaikoff effect in the presence of amiodarone. There may be a background of unrecognised Hashimoto thyroiditis.

There are two types of AIT. Type I is caused by an excess of iodine-induced thyroid hormone synthesis (Jod–Basedow effect) and usually occurs on a background of pre-existing multinodular goitre or latent Graves disease. Type II AIT is a destructive thyroiditis that results in excess release of pre-formed T_4 and T_3 without increased hormone synthesis. In type I AIT the main medical treatment consists of the administration of thionamides and potassium perchlorate, while in type II AIT, glucocorticoid is the most useful therapeutic option.

Ursella, S., Testa, A., Mazzone, M., and Silveri, N.G. (2005) Amiodarone-induced thyroid dysfunction in clinical practice. *Eur Rev Med Pharmacol Sci* 10, 269–278.
http://www.ncbi.nlm.nih.gov/pubmed/17121321

11. Answer C

Several alterations in thyroid physiology occur during normal pregnancy (Stagnaro-Green and Pearce, 2012). These changes occur at different times of gestation, are reversible post-partum and collectively stimulate the maternal thyroid gland.

The best recognised alteration in maternal thyroid physiology is the increase in thyroxine-binding globulin (TBG). This increase begins early in the first trimester, plateaus during mid-gestation and persists until shortly after delivery. The increased concentration of TBG expands the extrathyroidal pool, triggering a concomitant increase in maternal thyroid hormone synthesis and elevation of total thyroxine (T_4) and tri-iodothyronine (T_3) levels. The increase in concentration of TBG is a result of reduced hepatic clearance and increased synthesis stimulated by oestrogen. The concentration plateaus at 20 weeks' gestation and falls again post-partum.

Other changes in thyroid physiology during pregnancy include a fall in iodide store because of increased renal clearance and transplacental transfer to the fetus, a rise in thyroglobulin that corresponds to the increase in thyroid size, and a decrease in thyroid-stimulating hormone (TSH) receptor antibody titre with progression of the pregnancy.

 Stagnaro-Green, A. and Pearce, E. (2012). Thyroid disorders in pregnancy. *Nat Rev Endocrinol* 8, 650–658.
http://www.ncbi.nlm.nih.gov/pubmed/23007317

12. Answer D

Thyroglobulin is a glycoprotein that is produced only by normal or neoplastic thyroid follicular cells (Spencer and Lopresti, 2008). Therefore it should not be detectable in patients who have undergone total thyroid ablation, and its detection in such patients signifies the presence of persistent or recurrent thyroid carcinoma.

Good thyroglobulin assays can detect concentrations as low as 1 ng/mL or lower. However, the results can be altered artefactually by the presence of serum anti-thyroglobulin antibodies, which are found in about 15% of patients with thyroid carcinoma. Tests for these antibodies should always be performed when serum thyroglobulin is measured. The extent to which serum thyroglobulin assays are altered by the presence of antibodies depends on whether a radioimmunoassay or an immunoradiometric assay is performed.

The production of thyroglobulin by both normal and neoplastic thyroid tissue is also in part dependent on thyroid-stimulating hormone (TSH). Therefore when interpreting the serum thyroglobulin value, one should take into account the serum TSH value and the presence or absence of thyroid remnants. If serum thyroglobulin is detectable during thyroxine treatment, it will increase after thyroxine is withdrawn. Serum thyroglobulin is a good prognostic indicator for follicular and papillary thyroid carcinoma.

Spencer, C.A. and Lopresti, J.S. (2008). Measuring thyroglobulin and thyroglobulin autoantibody in patients with differentiated thyroid cancer. *Nat Clin Pract Endocrinol Metab* 4, 223–233.
http://www.ncbi.nlm.nih.gov/pubmed/18268520

13. Answer H

Thyroxine (T_4) is converted to the active T_3 (which is three to four times more potent than T_4) within cells by selenium-containing de-iodinase (5'-iodinase) enzyme.

14. Answer G

Thyrotropin-releasing hormone (TRH) is produced by the hypothalamus and initially synthesised as a 242-amino acid precursor polypeptide. Through proteolysis this is then processed to form the mature tripeptide TRH molecule. It travels across the median eminence to the anterior pituitary via the hypophyseal portal system where it stimulates the release of thyroid-stimulating hormone from thyrotrope cells. It is used in the TRH test to help diagnose secondary (or central) hypothyroidism.

CLINICAL

15. Answer D
An adrenal 'incidentaloma', which on computed tomographic (CT) scanning has benign characteristics and which is not cortisol secreting, aldosterone secreting or a phaeochromocytoma, needs regular follow-up with repeat imaging (Young, 2007).

Unsuspected adrenal masses are discovered in 4–7% of imaging studies or at post-mortem and incidence increases with age. Although the majority are hormonally silent and have no malignant potential, 15% are cortisol-secreting adenomas, phaeochromocytomas, adrenal carcinomas, metastatic disease or aldosterone-producing adenomas. After a complete history and physical examination, the hormonal activity of the incidentaloma should be determined with an overnight dexamethasone suppression test, urinary fractionated metanephrines and plasma aldosterone/plasma renin activity.

On imaging, a diameter of greater than 4 cm has 90% sensitivity for adrenocortical carcinoma. An attenuation of less than 10 Hounsfield units suggests a high lipid content and hence is more likely an adenoma. Adenomas have regular margins and take up less contrast in contrast studies. Non-hormonal secreting adenomas less than 4 cm should be followed up radiologically at 6, 12 and 24 months, while for larger ones surgical resection is advised.

Young, W.F., Jr. (2007). Clinical practice. The incidentally discovered adrenal mass. *N Engl J Med* 356, 601–610.
http://www.ncbi.nlm.nih.gov/pubmed/17287480

16. Answer B
There are many ways to evaluate a patient with Cushing syndrome with the aim of:
- Establishing the presence of hypercortisolism
- Determining whether the hypercortisolism is adrenocorticotrophic hormone (ACTH) dependent or independent
- If ACTH dependent, whether it is a consequence of Cushing disease or ectopic production of ACTH (Newell-Price et al., 2006).

Increased excretion of cortisol in a 24-h urine collection occurs with primary or secondary adrenocortical hyperfunction, although increased levels may also be seen in obesity, stress, depression and alcoholism.

In dexamethasone suppression tests, suppression is defined as a reduction of cortisol to less than 50% of the basal value. Suppression of cortisol levels on low-dose dexamethasone 2 mg/day excludes Cushing syndrome. Failure to suppress cortisol after 2 mg/day, with suppression on 8 mg/day, indicates pituitary Cushing syndrome (Cushing disease). Failure to suppress cortisol on 8 mg/day indicates adrenal neoplasm or ectopic ACTH syndrome. In Cushing disease, ACTH is suppressed by high-dose dexamethasone; in the ectopic ACTH syndrome, ACTH is not suppressed; in adrenal neoplasia, ACTH levels are low in the baseline specimen.

If there is suppression of urine cortisol with the high-dose dexamethasone and an obvious pituitary neoplasm on magnetic resonance imaging (MRI), surgery is indicated. If, however, after the high-dose test there is suppression (as in this case), but no visible lesion in the sella, inferior petrosal sinus sampling should be pursued. A basal central-to-peripheral ratio of more than 2:1 or a ratio after stimulation with corticotropin-releasing hormone of more than 3:1 is consistent with Cushing disease. Petrosal sinus sampling has no role in the evaluation of ectopic ACTH syndrome and would needlessly place the patient at risk of morbidity, such as bleeding, dissection and stroke.

 Newell-Price, J., Bertagna, X., Grossman, A.B., and Nieman, L.K. (2006). Cushing's syndrome. *Lancet* 367, 1605–1617. http://www.ncbi.nlm.nih.gov/pubmed/16698415

17. Answer B

Type 2 diabetes represents a serious public health problem for indigenous Australians, occurring at a higher prevalence than in the non-indigenous population, and with an earlier age of onset of the disease and of its micro- and macro-vascular complications (Azzopardi et al., 2012; O'Dea et al., 2007). It is likely that diabetes is an important contributor to the considerably higher cardiovascular mortality rate among indigenous Australians at young ages (9–10 times higher in indigenous men aged 25–44 years and 12–13 times higher in indigenous women aged 35–54 years). Body mass index and age are the two strongest predictors of diabetes for indigenous Australians, while leanness is protective.

Like the general population, preventing and managing the complications of diabetes in indigenous Australians involves lifestyle modification. Through changes in food supply, increased physical activity and health promotion, some indigenous communities have been able to achieve amelioration of dyslipidaemia, improved insulin action (even in the absence of weight loss), increased red cell folate and reduced homocysteine levels.

 Azzopardi, P., Brown, A.D., Zimmet, P., et al. (2012). Type 2 diabetes in young Indigenous Australians in rural and remote areas: diagnosis, screening, management and prevention. *Med J Aust* 197, 32–36. https://www.mja.com.au/journal/2012/197/1/type-2-diabetes-young-indigenous-australians-rural-and-remote-areas-diagnosis

 O'Dea, K., Rowley, K.G., and Brown, A. (2007). Diabetes in Indigenous Australians: possible ways forward. *Med J Aust* 186, 494–495. https://www.mja.com.au/journal/2007/186/10/diabetes-indigenous-australians-possible-ways-forward

18. Answer B

Subclinical hypothyroidism should be distinguished from other causes of physiological, artefactual or transiently increased serum thyroid-stimulating hormone

(TSH) (Cooper and Biondi, 2012). Subclinical hypothyroidism is defined as a persistently elevated serum TSH with thyroid hormone levels within the reference range. Subclinical hypothyroidism is detected in 4–8% of the general population and in up to 15–18% of women aged older than 60 years. Approximately 4–18% of patients will progress to overt hypothyroidism each year. A recent Cochrane review found that thyroxine versus no treatment for subclinical hypothyroidism did not improve overall survival, cardiovascular morbidity, health-related quality of life or symptoms ascribed to subclinical hypothyroidism. However, there was some evidence to suggest that thyroxine replacement improved surrogate markers for cardiovascular disease, such as lipid profile, vascular compliance and left ventricular function. Most experts advocate treatment with thyroxine only when TSH is greater than 10 mIU/L.

Serum TSH concentrations are raised in overweight and obese individuals, which might falsely suggest subclinical hypothyroidism. The mild increase is usually associated with serum concentration of free tri-iodothyronine (T_3) at the upper limit of the normal range, which might be caused by increased de-iodinase activity as a compensatory mechanism for fat accumulation to raise energy expenditure. This altered thyroid hormone pattern is reversible with weight loss.

Cooper, D.S, and Biondi, B. (2012). Subclinical thyroid disease. *Lancet* 379, 1142–1154.
http://www.ncbi.nlm.nih.gov/pubmed/22273398

19. Answer E

Diagnosis of acromegaly is based on biochemistry tests, such as serum insulin-like growth factor I (IGF-I) and growth hormone (GH) levels during a 2-h period after a standard 75-g oral glucose load (oral glucose-tolerance test). If there is inadequate growth hormone suppression, pituitary MRI is used to assess for the presence of a pituitary mass. However, in cases with no obvious pituitary masses, a CT chest and abdomen is performed to search for extrapituitary masses that may cause acromegaly. Transphenoidal surgery is the mainstay of treatment for microadenomas, with surgical cure achieved in more than 80% of patients. Surgical cure rate is only 50% in patients with macroadenomas and even lower in patients with invasive macroadenomas (Melmed, 2006).

Medical treatment with somatostatin analogues (e.g. octreotide or lanreotide) has been used as adjuvant therapy after unsuccessful surgery. Emerging data have shown somatostatin analogues used as first-line therapy in patients with invasive macroadenomas can achieve biochemical control of acromegaly and tumour shrinkage. Patients resistant to medical therapy are often referred for radiotherapy. Dopamine agonists can be used in conjunction with somatostatin analogues in patients whose biochemical cure is not achieved by somatostatin alone to provide an additive suppressive effect.

Pegvisomant is a pegylated recombinant analogue of human growth hormone that acts as a growth hormone receptor antagonist. Pegvisomant can be used in patients with acromegaly not cured by surgery and not responding to somatostatin analogues. Pegvisomant is currently not available in Australia and may elevate transaminases.

Melmed, S. (2006). Medical progress: Acromegaly. *N Engl J Med* 355, 2558–2573.
http://www.ncbi.nlm.nih.gov/pubmed/17167139

20. Answer D

Measurement of maternal serum thyroid-stimulating hormone (TSH) receptor antibodies (TRAb) during the third trimester (24–28 weeks) in pregnant women with Graves disease helps to identify those infants who are at higher risk for the development of fetal and neonatal Graves hyperthyroidism. A high maternal thyroid-stimulating immunoglobulin predicts neonatal thyrotoxicosis with a sensitivity of 100%, specificity of 76.0%, positive predictive value of 40.0% and negative predictive value of 100% (De Groot et al., 2012).

Because thyroid receptor antibodies freely cross the placenta and can stimulate the fetal thyroid, these antibodies should be measured by 22 weeks in mothers with:

- Current Graves disease
- A history of Graves disease and treatment with ^{131}I or thyroidectomy before pregnancy
- A previous neonate with Graves disease
- Previously elevated TRAb.

Women who have a negative TRAb and do not require anti-thyroid drug treatment (ATD) have a very low risk of fetal or neonatal thyroid dysfunction.

In women with TRAb elevated at least two- to three-fold above the normal level and in women treated with ATD, maternal free T_4 and fetal thyroid dysfunction should be screened during the fetal anatomy ultrasound done in the 18th–22nd week and repeated every 4–6 weeks or as clinically indicated. Evidence of fetal thyroid dysfunction can include thyroid enlargement, growth restriction, hydrops, goitre, advanced bone age, tachycardia or cardiac failure. If fetal hyperthyroidism is diagnosed and thought to endanger the pregnancy, treatment using propylthiouracil should be given with frequent clinical, laboratory and ultrasound monitoring.

De Groot, L., Abalovich, M., Alexander, E.K., et al. (2012). Management of Thyroid Dysfunction during Pregnancy and Postpartum: An Endocrine Society Clinical Practice Guideline. *J Clin Endocrinol Metab* 97, 2543–2565.
http://www.ncbi.nlm.nih.gov/pubmed/22869843

21. Answer B

Kallman syndrome (KS) describes the occurrence of hypothalamic gonadotrophin-releasing hormone deficiency (hence low testosterone and sex hormones) and deficient olfactory sense (anosmia). It is usually inherited as an X-linked or autosomal recessive disorder with greater penetrance in the male (Dode and Hardelin, 2009).

Most cases are diagnosed at puberty because of the lack of sexual development, identified by small testes and absent virilisation in males or the lack of breast development and primary amenorrhea in females. KS is diagnosed when low serum gonadotropins and gonadal steroids are coupled with a compromised sense of smell. The latter should be ascertained by means of detailed questioning and olfactory screening tests, because it is rarely mentioned spontaneously. Magnetic resonance imaging (MRI) of the forebrain can be carried out to show the hypoplasia or aplasia of the olfactory bulbs and tracts. MRI is also useful to exclude hypothalamic or pituitary lesions as the cause of hypogonadotropic hypogonadism (HH). The gonadotrophin-releasing hormone (GnRH) deficiency can be indirectly assessed by means of endocrinological tests.

The treatment of hypogonadism in KS aims first to initiate virilisation or breast development, and second to develop fertility. Hormone replacement therapy, usually with testosterone for males and combined oestrogen and progesterone for females, is the treatment to stimulate the development of secondary sexual characteristics. For those desiring fertility, either gonadotropins or pulsatile GnRH can be used to obtain testicular growth and sperm production in males or ovulation in females. Both treatments restore fertility in the vast majority of affected individuals.

Dode, C. and Hardelin, J.P. (2009). Kallmann syndrome. *Eur J Hum Genet* 17, 139–146.
http://www.nature.com/ejhg/journal/v17/n2/full/ejhg2008206a.html

22. Answer C

Pregnancy in women with type 1 or type 2 diabetes is associated with a two- to four-fold increased risk of pre-eclampsia, preterm delivery and perinatal mortality compared with the background population (Mathiesen et al., 2012). Strict glycaemic control during pregnancy is important but may be difficult because pregnant women with type 1 diabetes have an increased risk of severe hypoglycaemia. Development of pre-eclampsia is more frequent in women with higher levels of HbA_{1c} in early pregnancy.

Self-monitoring of blood glucose is mandatory. It is recommended that tests be performed before meals and 1–2 h after meals. The blood glucose targets are: fasting and pre-prandial 4.0–5.5 mmol/L, and post-prandial less than 8.0 mmol/L at 1 h or less than 7 mmol/L at 2 h. A basal-bolus regimen of insulin generally provides the best opportunity for good glycaemic control. Insulin pump therapy is a suitable alternative where there is local experience. The HbA_{1c} level should be monitored every 4–8 weeks and kept within the normal range. It is important to note that the HbA_{1c} level is normally lower in pregnancy, but most laboratories do not report a reference range specific to pregnancy. Pregnant women with type 1 diabetes are more prone than usual to ketoacidosis.

Women should be monitored for signs or progression of diabetic complications, particularly retinopathy and proteinuria. Formal eye review should be at least 3 monthly if baseline retinopathy is present, if there is a rapid improvement in glycaemic control, or if there has been a long duration of pre-existing diabetes. Proteinuria should be assessed by dipstick at regular intervals and quantitated where appropriate.

McElduff, A, Cheung, N.W., McIntyre, H.D., et al. (2005). The Australasian Diabetes in Pregnancy Society consensus guidelines for the management of type 1 and type 2 diabetes in relation to pregnancy. *Med J Aust* 183, 373–377. https://www.mja.com.au/journal/2005/183/7/australasian-diabetes-pregnancy-society-consensus-guidelines-management-type-1

23. Answer D

Pituitary apoplexy is characterised by sudden onset of headache, visual symptoms, altered mental status and hormonal dysfunction due to acute haemorrhage or infarction of a pituitary gland (Kearney and Dang, 2007). Lateral extension of haemorrhage and necrosis can cause third, fourth or fifth (first and second divisions) or sixth cranial nerve palsies. The third cranial nerve is most commonly affected in isolation or combined with other nerve palsies.

Hypopituitarism with variably decreased levels of all or multiple pituitary hormones is evident on presentation in the majority of patients presenting with apoplexy. In this vignette, there is evidence of hypocortisolism and secondary hypothyroidism.

Pituitary apoplexy is usually caused by an acute expansion of a pituitary adenoma or, less commonly, in a non-adenomatous gland, from infarction or haemorrhage. The anterior pituitary gland is perfused by its portal venous system, which passes down the hypophyseal stalk. This unusual vascular supply probably contributes to the frequency of pituitary apoplexy. Apoplexy has been reported after cardiac bypass surgery, during induction chemotherapy for acute myeloid leukaemia and in patients with dengue fever or thrombocytopenia.

Pituitary apoplexy during pregnancy may be due to temporary enlargement of a pituitary adenoma, which compromises the blood supply. Sheehan syndrome refers to post-partum hypopituitarism caused by ischaemic necrosis of the pituitary in association with massive blood loss and hypovolaemic shock during labour or post-partum.

Kearney, T. and Dang, C. (2007). Diabetic and endocrine emergencies. *Postgrad Med J 83*, 79–86. http://www.ncbi.nlm.nih.gov/pmc/articles/PMC2805944/

24. Answer E

Cystic fibrosis-related diabetes (CFRD) is a common complication in adults with cystic fibrosis (CF) (O'Sullivan and Freedman, 2009). One report noted that 50% of adults with CF had abnormal glucose tolerance. CFRD is not the same as typical type 1 or type 2 diabetes mellitus. Several factors unique to CF affect glucose metabolism, including raised energy expenditure, acute and chronic infection, glucagon deficiency, liver dysfunction, decreased intestinal transit time and increased work of breathing, as well as islet fibrosis leading to insulin deficiency. Because of the association between CFRD and more severe pulmonary disease, more frequent pulmonary exacerbations and poorer nutritional status, any patient, irrespective of age, who has unexplained weight loss or a decrease in pulmonary function should be assessed for CFRD.

Periodic screening with a random glucose concentration should be done in all CF patients; a yearly oral glucose-tolerance test is thought to be the best screening method for those aged 10 years and older.

These patients tend to be quite sensitive to insulin due to pancreatic glucagon deficiency. Because the basic problem is predominantly deficiency of insulin rather than resistance to its action, insulin sensitisers such as metformin and thiazolidinediones (rosiglitazone), which act largely by enhancing insulin sensitivity, are unlikely to be effective.

Acarbose also is an inappropriate choice. The process of carbohydrate digestion requires the pancreas to release into the intestine alpha-amylase enzymes which digest the large carbohydrates into smaller carbohydrates called oligosaccharides. The small intestine then releases alpha-glucosidase enzymes that further digest the oligosaccharides into glucose. Acarbose is a man-made oligosaccharide designed to slow down the actions of alpha-amylase and alpha-glucosidase enzymes, thereby slowing the absorption of sugar after the meal. In a patient receiving pancreatic enzyme supplement due to fat malabsorption caused by pancreatic insufficiency, inducing a delay in carbohydrate absorption with its concomitant gastrointestinal side effects seems a poor choice.

The use of an insulin secretagogue may have short-term benefit, but is not the best choice. Patients with CFRD do not usually have a good response to sulphonylureas. CFRD patients generally have a progressive loss of insulin secretion, which explains why those who do respond only derive short-term benefit from sulfonylureas. In patients with pancreatic diabetes of any aetiology, the treatment is usually replacement of the deficient hormone: insulin. Most patients need supplemental insulin for post-prandial hyperglycaemia and require minimal insulin during the night unless they are receiving continuous nocturnal nasogastric or gastrostomy feeding. Therefore, multiple rapid-acting insulin injections before meals with dose adjustment to match the carbohydrate content of each meal is the most appropriate choice.

 O'Sullivan, B.P. and Freedman, S.D. (2009). Cystic fibrosis. *Lancet* 373, 1891–1904.
http://www.ncbi.nlm.nih.gov/pubmed/19403164

25. Answer B

Dopamine agonists are recommended as the first-line therapy for patients with prolactin-secreting microadenomas or macroadenomas. Medications currently available in Australia are bromocriptine, cabergoline and quinagolide. Tumour shrinkage happens within 1–2 weeks after the start of treatment and may continue for months to years. It is reasonable to switch to another dopamine agonist if there is no response to the first dopamine agonist prescribed. There are extensive safety data on bromocriptine in pregnancy. The use of cabergoline may also be safe in early pregnancy. Insufficient safety data on quinagolide preclude its use during pregnancy.

Elevated prolactin levels are associated with many other causes, such as pregnancy, stress, primary hypothyroidism, chest wall injury (due to nerve stimulation), nipple stimulation (transient elevation of prolactin level), reduced clearance of prolactin secondary to renal failure and hepatic failure, and medications, such as anti-depressants, anti-psychotic agents (in particular, risperidone), dopaminergic blockers (e.g. metoclopramide), some anti-hypertensive agents, opiates and H_2-receptor blockers. These causes need to be ruled out before considering further investigation for prolactinomas.

The diagnosis of prolactinoma rests on the prolactin level and a pituitary MRI scan. When there is a significant discrepancy between the very large size of the prolactinoma and a mildly elevated prolactin level, serial dilution of serum samples is recommended to eliminate the artefact of a falsely low prolactin level that occurs with some immunoradiometric assays when excess antigen (e.g. prolactin) is present during testing (the 'hook effect'). The lower dose of cabergoline required for treatment of hyperprolactinaemia has not been found to be associated with clinically significant valvular heart disease.

Klibanski, A. (2010). Clinical practice. Prolactinomas. N Engl J Med 362, 1219–1226.
http://www.ncbi.nlm.nih.gov/pubmed/20357284

26. Answer C
The main functions of gastrin are:
- Increases hydrochloric acid secretion (via parietal cells)
- Simulates growth of gastric mucosa
- Increases gastric motility
- Increases lower oesophageal sphincter pressure (preventing reflux)
- Lowers ileo-caecal sphincter pressure
- Increases pepsinogen secretion.

Neuroendocrine tumours of the gastrointestinal system are rare, and are either functional, secreting one of a variety of neuropeptides, or non-functioning, where elevated levels of neuropeptides are not detected. Of the functional tumours, the commonest hormone secreted is gastrin, accounting for up to 30% of such neoplasms. The majority of gastrinomas are sporadic; however, 12–20% are associated with the multiple endocrine neoplasia syndrome type 1 (MEN1), in association with functional adenomas of the parathyroid (90%), pituitary [e.g. prolactinomas (17%)] and pancreas [e.g. insulinomas (10%)].

Burkitt, M.D., Varro, A., and Pritchard, D.M. (2009). Importance of gastrin in the pathogenesis and treatment of gastric tumors. *World J Gastroenterol* 7, 1–16.
http://www.ncbi.nlm.nih.gov/pmc/articles/PMC2653300/

27. Answer D

Measurement of the serum thyroglobulin level with anti-thyroglobulin antibody to validate accuracy of the thyroglobulin assay could be considered at this time (Sherman, 2003). In the absence of residual normal thyroid tissue (after surgical and radioiodine ablation), thyroglobulin is a marker of residual or recurrent papillary or follicular thyroid carcinoma.

Sherman, S.I. (2003). Thyroid carcinoma. *Lancet* 361, 501–511.
http://www.ncbi.nlm.nih.gov/pubmed/12583960

28. Answer D

RET is an abbreviation for 'rearranged during transfection', as the DNA sequence of this gene was originally found to be rearranged within a 3T3 fibroblast cell line following its transfection with DNA taken from human lymphoma cells. The human gene RET is localised to chromosome 10 (10q11.2) and contains 21 exons. The RET proto-oncogene encodes a receptor tyrosine kinase for members of the glial cell line-derived neurotrophic factor family of extracellular signalling molecules. RET loss of function mutations are associated with the development of Hirschsprung disease, while gain of function germline mutations are associated with the development of various types of human cancer, including medullary thyroid carcinoma, multiple endocrine neoplasia (MEN) type 2A and 2B, phaeochromocytoma and parathyroid hyperplasia.

MEN2 is an autosomal dominant syndrome that is characterised by medullary thyroid carcinoma, phaechromocytoma and primary hyperparathyroidism. If MEN2 is suspected, the underlying mutation in the RET gene should be sought. Autosomal dominant inheritance of MEN2 means that the offspring of an affected person has a 50% chance of inheriting the mutated gene. Identification of the underlying genetic mutation allows predictive testing in relatives, monitoring for early detection of disease in mutation carriers and reassurance for non-carriers.

Somatic K-ras mutations are found at high rates in leukaemias, colon cancer, pancreatic cancer and lung cancer. The breast cancer type 1 (BRCA1) gene mutation is associated with familial breast or ovarian carcinoma. The adenomatous polyposis coli (APC) gene mutation is associated with familial polyposis coli, while von Hippel–Lindau (VHL) gene mutation is associated with renal cell cancer, phaechromocytoma, retinal angioma and hemangioblastoma.

Brandi, M.L., Gagel, R.F., Angeli, A., et al. (2001). Guidelines for diagnosis and therapy of MEN type 1 and type 2. *J Clin Endocrinol Metab* 86, 5658–5671.
http://jcem.endojournals.org/content/86/12/5658.long

29. Answer B

Pregnancy leads to raised oestrogen levels. It is associated with raised human chorionic gonadotrophin (hCG; which is used as a diagnostic test), progesterone, testosterone and prolactin levels, while luteinising hormone (LH) and follicle-stimulating hormone (FSH) are suppressed (Norman et al., 2007).

Prolactinoma is usually associated with higher prolactin levels and oestrogen will not be elevated. Late-onset congenital adrenal hyperplasia (CAH) is rare and these patients will have hirsutism/acne along with menstrual irregularities. The LH level is usually raised. Whilst premature ovarian failure is a relatively common cause of secondary amenorrhoea, oestrogen is not elevated but FSH is commonly raised.

Patients with polycystic ovarian syndrome (PCOS) usually present with menstrual irregularities due to anovulation together with clinical signs of hyperandrogenism, e.g. hirsutism, acne and male-pattern balding. Along with raised androgens, they often exhibit a raised LH/FSH ratio.

Norman, R.J., Dewailly, D., Legor, R.S., and Hickey, T.E. (2007). Polycystic ovary syndrome. *Lancet* 370, 685–697.
http://www.ncbi.nlm.nih.gov/pubmed/17720020

30. Answer C

Metformin is eliminated almost entirely unchanged via the kidney, partly by filtration and partly by secretion. In order to avoid any accumulation of metformin, the product information currently advises stopping metformin when the estimated glomerular filtration rate (eGFR) falls below 60 mL/min/1.73 m^2. However, given the extensive clinical experience with this drug, national authorities such as the United Kingdom's National Institute for Health and Clinical Excellence (NICE) have sanctioned the use of metformin at lower rates of eGFR. NICE guidelines recommend a reduced dose of metformin at an eGFR of less than 45 mL/min/1.73 m^2. In addition, regular checks of renal function are important. Australian Diabetes Society and National Institute of Health and Care Excellence (NICE) guidelines advise cessation of metformin when the eGFR is 30 mL/min/1.73 m^2 or less. Patients should be advised to stop metformin if they develop diarrhoea or sepsis. Metformin monotherapy is associated with a low risk of hypoglycaemia.

The sulphonylureas vary with respect to metabolism and route of elimination. Glimepiride produces long-acting metabolites that are at the highest risk of causing hypoglycaemia in the setting of chronic kidney disease. In order to avoid drug accumulation, caution should be exercised (i.e. dose reduction or discontinuation of the agent) when these sulphonylureas are used in patients with an eGFR of less than 60 mL/min/1.73 m^2.

Acarbose is mostly degraded in the intestine. Those metabolites that are absorbed are generally inactive and mostly eliminated in the urine. Therefore, there is no need to reduce the dose in patients with chronic kidney disease.

The glucagon-like peptide 1 (GLP-1) receptor agonist, exenatide, is mostly eliminated via the kidneys; therefore, caution should be exercised when prescribing this agent to a patient with an eGFR of less than 60 mL/min/1.73 m². Liraglutide is partly degraded in the circulation, partly by the liver and partly in the kidney; however, it also should be used with caution in patients with an eGFR of less than 60 mL/min/1.73 m². When used as monotherapy, hypoglycaemia is unlikely, since GLP-1 receptor agonists stimulate the 'glucose-dependent' release of insulin. If GLP-1 receptor agonists are combined with secretagogues, hypoglycaemia is possible (Ismail-Beigi, 2012).

The dipeptidyl peptidase-4 (DPP-4) inhibitors undergo a mix of pathways of metabolism and elimination. Sitagliptin, for example, is mostly eliminated in the urine unchanged; it can be used at the various stages of moderate and severe renal impairment with a gradually reduced dosage. In clinical practice, DPP-4 inhibitors do not cause weight gain and are weight neutral, with a very low incidence of hypoglycaemia as a side effect.

Ismail-Beigi, F. (2012). Glycemic management of type 2 diabetes mellitus. *N Engl J Med* 366, 1319–1327.
http://www.ncbi.nlm.nih.gov/pubmed/22475595

31. Answer A

This patient's clinical presentation raises the suspicion of phaeochromocytoma. Plasma fractionated metanephrine level can be used as a first-line test for phaeochromocytoma (Pacak et al., 2007). The predictive value of a negative test is extremely high. Although measurement of plasma fractioned metanephrines has a sensitivity of 96–100%, the specificity is poor at 85–89% and the specificity falls to 77% in patients older than 60 years and taking multiple anti-hypertensive medications. In one study, 97% of patients with hypertension seen in a tertiary care clinic who had a positive plasma fractionated metanephrine measurements did not have a phaeochromocytoma.

The 24-h urinary fractionated catecholamines and metanephrines should be measured if a high level of plasma metanephrine is found. Specificity is highest for urinary epinephrine (adrenaline) (99.9%), followed by urinary norepinephrine (noradrenaline) and dopamine (99.5% and 99.3%, respectively), and urinary total metanephrines (97.8%). Furthermore, the clonidine suppression test can be used as a confirmatory test.

Plasma catecholamines no longer have a role in testing for phaeochromocytoma because of the poor overall accuracy of measurement of plasma catecholamines. Measurement of 24-h urinary vanillylmandelic acid (VMA) excretion has poor diagnostic sensitivity and specificity compared with measurement of 24-h urinary fractionated metanephrines. Biochemical confirmation of the diagnosis should be followed by radiological evaluation to locate the tumour.

Pacak, K., Eisenhofer, G., Ahlman, H., et al. (2007). Pheochromocytoma: recommendations for clinical practice from the First International Symposium. October 2005. *Nat Clin Pract Endocrinol Metab* 3, 92–102.
http://www.nature.com/nrendo/journal/v3/n2/full/ncpendmet0396.html

32. Answer F

Hypothyroidism may present in the elderly with very non-specific symptoms and signs. It should be considered in the differential diagnosis of anyone presenting with confusion (part of the so-called 'dementia' screen) and general deterioration with no readily identifiable cause. As one of the most common endocrine disturbances alongside diabetes mellitus, it should not be missed as a cause of a range of symptoms, from neurological signs, typically bradykinesia, reduced deep tendon reflexes and parasthaesias from nerve entrapment (especially carpal tunnel syndrome) to abdominal pain from chronic constipation to mental disturbance manifest as confusion and apparent memory impairment. Other subtle signs of hypothyroidism include loss of the outer one-third of the eyebrows with male-pattern frontal balding, hypothermia, bradycardia, non-pitting oedema (myxoedema) and dry, coarse skin.

Thyroid function tests are usually diagnostic and demonstrate a low free thyroxine (T_4) with a compensatory high thyroid-stimulating hormone (TSH) in primary hypothyroidism. Very occasionally, a low TSH and a low free T_4 may be seen in the context of pan-hypopituitarism, and assay of levels of the sex hormones, ACTH and other pituitary hormones will confirm the diagnosis.

33. Answer D

The presentation of acromegaly can often be very subtle, with those closest to the patient often bringing the changes to attention (Ribeiro-Oliveira and Barkan, 2012). It is often helpful to look at old photographs if there is a suspicion of acromegaly as coarsening of features, protrusion of the jaw (prognathism) and change in clothing or shoe size may all point to a retrospective diagnosis. Acromegaly is most often due to a pituitary adenoma (80% macroadenoma, 20% microadenoma) and visual symptoms may be a complaint alongside headache. Visual field testing may reveal a defect, commonly a bitemporal hemianopia (tunnel vision). Sausage fingers (leading to an inability to wear rings), greasy coarse skin and a thickening of the forehead are all signs of growth-hormone excess that characterise acromegaly. Hypertension, obstructive sleep apnoea, carpal tunnel syndrome, joint pains, back pain and glucose intolerance are other common features.

Acromegaly results from increased secretion of growth hormone (GH), which stimulates hepatic secretion of insulin-like growth factor-I (IGF-I) and this causes most of the clinical manifestations of acromegaly. The measurement of circulating IGF-I levels has been an important biochemical tool in the diagnosis and follow-up of acromegaly. The best single test for the diagnosis of acromegaly is measurement of serum IGF-I. Unlike growth hormone, serum IGF-I concentrations do not alter according to food intake or activity, but reflect integrated GH secretion during the preceding day or longer. Elevated serum IGF-I concentrations are highly specific and sensitive for a diagnosis of acromegaly. Trans-sphenoidal hypophysectomy is usually employed as a treatment modality, sometimes in conjunction with medical therapy, to reduce the size of a very large macroadenoma or surgically incompletely resected tumour.

Ribeiro-Oliveira, A., Jr. and Barkan, A. (2012). The changing face of acromegaly – advances in diagnosis and treatment. *Nat Rev Endocrinol* 8, 605–611.
http://www.ncbi.nlm.nih.gov/pubmed/22733271

34. Answer H

Lithium is used in the treatment of bipolar disorder. It can cause major disturbance in water balance, manifest as polyuria and secondary polydipsia (Grunfeld and Rossier, 2009). This is because of the decreasing urinary concentrating ability resulting from impaired responsiveness of the distal nephron to anti-diuretic hormone (ADH), which is known as nephrogenic diabetes insipidus. In most cases there is a correlation between impaired urinary concentrating ability and duration of lithium therapy or total lithium dose.

Nephrogenic diabetes insipidus in adults is usually partial with mild symptoms. Usually the serum sodium is normal or mildly elevated, the plasma osmolality is within normal range, the urine osmolality is low (<300 mOsm/kg) and the urine volume is between 2.5 and 6 L/day. However, when patients are fluid depleted, there is a marked rise in serum sodium, a rise in plasma osmolality and a urine osmolality that may exceed that of plasma. The water deprivation test is useful in diagnosis: the urine osmolality is usually less than 300 mosmol/kg after dehydration with no further or a minimal (<95 mOsm/kg) rise after desmopressin. In partial nephrogenic diabetes insipidus, the urine osmolality is between 300 and 750 mOsm/kg after dehydration and is less than 750 mOsm/kg after desmopressin. Lithium-induced nephrogenic diabetes insipidus is usually reversible on stopping therapy, but a few patients remain symptomatic long after lithium has been discontinued. If the urine volume exceeds 4 L/day, treatment with thiazides and amiloride has been advocated. Preventive measures include education of patients and their carers about maintaining adequate hydration. The serum lithium level should be kept between 0.5 and 0.8 mmol/L. Annual measurement of 24-h urine volume is a simple and effective screening test.

Grunfeld, J.P. and Rossier, B.C. (2009). Lithium nephrotoxicity revisited. *Nat Rev Nephrol* 5, 270–276.
http://www.ncbi.nlm.nih.gov/pubmed/19384328

6 Neurology

Questions

BASIC SCIENCE

Answers can be found in the Neurology Answers section at the end of this chapter.

1. The pathogenesis of myasthenia gravis is best explained by:
   A. Antibody-mediated decrease in the number of available acetylcholine receptors (AChR) at the postsynaptic neuromuscular junctions
   B. Antibodies against P/Q type calcium channels in motor nerve terminals
   C. Defect in acetylcholine release by the nerve terminals at the neuromuscular junctions
   D. Genetic or acquired deficiency of choline acetyltransferase leading to a deficiency of acetylcholine
   E. Autoantibodies that bind to choline acetyltransferase at the neuromuscular junctions

2. A 75-year-old woman develops sudden movements of her arm; she throws her arm outwards, and uncontrollably injures herself. Which one of the following areas in her brain could have sustained an insult?
   A. Corpus callosum
   B. Globus pallidus
   C. Hippocampus
   D. Subthalamic nucleus
   E. Thalamus

3. Partial epilepsy is most commonly associated with:
   A. Mesial temporal sclerosis
   B. Abnormal thalamocortical circuits
   C. Abnormality in the frontal cortex
   D. Stroke
   E. Head trauma

4. Which one of the following can explain the sudden onset of a right third nerve palsy and a left hemiplegia involving the face, arm and leg?
   A. Left internal capsule infarct
   B. Left medullary infarct

Passing the FRACP Written Examination: Questions and Answers, First Edition. Jonathan Gleadle, Tuck Yong, Jordan Li, Surjit Tarafdar, and Danielle Wu.
© 2013 John Wiley & Sons, Ltd. Published 2013 by John Wiley & Sons, Ltd.

    C. Right medullary infarct
    D. Right midbrain infarct
    E. Right occipital lobe infarct

5. Which one of the following is associated with a right-sided Horner syndrome?
    A. Dilated right pupil
    B. Increased sweating of the right side of the face
    C. Constricted right pupil
    D. Weakness of lateral movement of the right eye
    E. Weakness of the left orbicularis oculi muscle

6. Which one of the following is correct concerning these demyelinating diseases?
    A. Acute disseminated encephalomyelitis (ADEM) involves the grey matter of the brain and spinal cord
    B. Adrenoleucodystrophy is an autosomal recessive disorder
    C. Guillain–Barré syndrome does not involve the autonomic nervous system
    D. Multiple sclerosis is frequently hereditary
    E. Progressive multifocal leucoencephalopathy (PML) is caused by a polyomavirus

7. A 64-year-old man presents with loss of feeling in the left little toe. On examination he has difficulty standing on tiptoe on the left side and left ankle jerk is absent. This is most likely due to:
    A. Common peroneal nerve compression
    B. S1 radiculopathy
    C. L5 radiculopathy
    D. Sciatic nerve compression
    E. Posterior tibial nerve compression

Theme: Pathophysiology of neurological disorders
(for Questions 8 and 9)
    A. Wallerian degeneration
    B. Presynaptic block of the release of acetylcholine
    C. Segmental demyelination
    D. Reduced acetylcholine in presynaptic vesicles
    E. Axonal destruction
    F. Antibodies against postsynaptic receptors
    G. Loss of anterior horn cells
    H. Antibodies against presynaptic calcium channels
For each of the following disorders, select the most appropriate pathophysiological explanation.

8. What is the major pathophysiological feature of idiopathic inflammatory polyneuropathy (also known as Guillain–Barré syndrome)?

9. Which is the correct description of the pathophysiological feature of Lambert–Eaton myasthenic syndrome?

Theme: Genetic basis of neurological disorders
(for Questions 10 and 11)
- **A.** Hexosaminidase A
- **B.** KALIG-1
- **C.** Apo E4
- **D.** Retinoblastoma (Rb) protein
- **E.** Amyloid precursor protein
- **F.** Neurofibromin
- **G.** Beta-amyloid protein
- **H.** Merlin (also known as schwannomin)

For each of the following patients, select the most likely genetic abnormality that can explain the presentation.

10. A large brain tumour is seen on computed tomography (CT) in a 30-year-old man. The finding on examination is shown in the photo below. Which gene mutation will account for this clinical presentation?

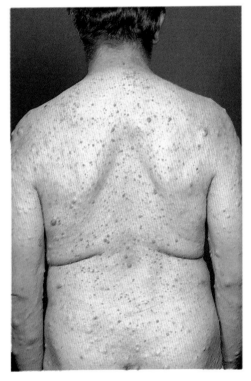

11. A 20-year-old woman presents with progressive speech and swallowing difficulties, unsteadiness of gait, spasticity, cognitive decline and psychosis. Which gene mutation might explain this clinical presentation?

CLINICAL

12. A 49-year-old man presents with sudden onset of left facial weakness. He experienced a respiratory infection 2 weeks ago and has had a dull ache behind the left ear for 2 days. This morning while shaving, he noticed a drooping of the left side of his face. Examination reveals complete paralysis of the left upper face and forehead. Hearing, taste and sensation are normal, and the other cranial nerves are functioning normally. No rash or vesicles are noted. Which one of the following clinical features would suggest a poorer prognosis and prompt early treatment with prednisolone?

    A. Abrupt onset of symptoms
    B. Age younger than 60 years
    C. Complete paralysis
    D. Previous similar episode
    E. Recent respiratory infection

13. A 37-year-old woman presents with a severe headache and new-onset ptosis of the left eye. Her pupil sizes are normal. She does not have fatigability of her eye movements, but fundoscopy shows mild bilateral papilloedema. She has a full range of eyes movements. Computed tomography of her head is normal. What is the most likely diagnosis?

    A. Cerebral venous thrombosis
    B. Herpes simplex encephalitis
    C. Cerebral abscess
    D. Glioblastoma multiforme
    E. Third nerve palsy

14. A 28-year-old woman is seen in neurology outpatients several weeks following a witnessed unprovoked grand mal convulsion. She had another episode 6 months previously that was not witnessed but involved an unexplained loss of consciousness, urinary incontinence and tongue injury. Magnetic resonance imaging (MRI), electroencephalography (EEG) and electrocardiography (ECG) are all normal. She wants to know more about epilepsy and the likelihood of further episodes. You should tell her that:

    A. With treatment, the risk of a further seizure is greater than 50% within 2 years
    B. Without treatment, the risk of a further seizure is less than 25% within 2 years
    C. Appropriate drug treatment can maintain more than 70% of patients with epilepsy seizure free
    D. Epilepsy is associated with a standardised mortality rate of 1.1
    E. Epilepsy affects 1 in 500 people in developed countries

15. A 37-year-old man has had several 30-min episodes of a severe unilateral headache over the last day following alcohol intake. He has had three previous similar episodes. His eye waters, is red and the most intense pain is felt behind the eye and the temple. Which one of the following diagnosis is most likely?

   A. Classical migraine
   B. Trigeminal neuralgia
   C. Acute closed angle glaucoma
   D. Cluster headache
   E. Temporal arteritis

16. Which one of the following features of Parkinson disease is most likely to respond to deep brain stimulation?

   A. Autonomic dysfunction
   B. Cognitive decline
   C. Loss of balance
   D. On–off fluctuations
   E. Sleep disorders

17. A 64-year-old woman presents with a rapid onset of symmetrical weakness in her legs. Magnetic resonance imaging (MRI) of her brain and spinal cord is normal and a diagnosis of Guillain–Barré syndrome is suspected. Which one of the following is correct?

   A. In the first week following onset albuminocytological dissociation [high level of protein in the cerebrospinal fluid (CSF) with normal cell count] is present in over 95% of patients
   B. The presence of knee-jerk reflexes cannot exclude the diagnosis
   C. Over 95% of patients will completely recover
   D. Sensory symptoms with distal paraesthesia excludes the diagnosis
   E. Autonomic dysfunction occurs in 50% of patients and is associated with arrhythmias

18. In a patient with features of parkinsonism and dementia, which one of the following clinical manifestations is most likely to be present in Lewy body dementia?

   A. Tremor
   B. Rigidity
   C. Visual hallucinations
   D. Improvement with neuroleptics
   E. Myoclonic jerks

19. A 25-year-old man presents with an acute right-sided weakness and slurred speech. He has had one tonic–clonic seizure prior to this presentation. He does not smoke and has no history of hypertension, diabetes mellitus or hyperlipidae-mia. On examination he has hypotonia and greater weakness in the proximal muscles than the distal muscles of the arms and legs. Laboratory investigation shows a high lactate-to-pyruvate ratio. Which is the most likely diagnosis?

   A. Dermatomyositis
   B. Inclusion body myositis

C. Mitochondrial myopathy, encephalopathy, lactic acidosis and stroke-like episodes (MELAS)
D. Motor neurone disease
E. Polymyositis

20. A 62-year-old woman presents following multiple falls, which have been increasing in frequency over the past 6 months. She says that she feels unsteady almost all the time and is frequently light-headed. On examination, she has bradykinesia, cogwheeling of both upper extremities, gait ataxia and a systolic blood pressure fall of 35 mmHg on standing with no change in pulse. Which one of the following is the most likely diagnosis for this patient?
   A. Huntington disease
   B. Multiple system atrophy
   C. Parkinson disease
   D. Progressive supranuclear palsy
   E. Primary adrenal insufficiency

21. A 65-year-old woman who is known to have myasthenia gravis for the past 4 years had been started on oral antibiotics for an upper respiratory tract infection. Two days later she is brought to the hospital with confusion and arterial blood gases reveal an elevated partial arterial carbon dioxide ($PaCO_2$) of 55 mmHg (37–45 mmHg). What is the most appropriate treatment for her presentation?
   A. Combination of high-dose prednisolone and azathioprine
   B. Plasmapheresis
   C. Intravenous pyridostigmine
   D. Urgent thymectomy
   E. Intravenous antibiotics

22. A 58-year-old man presents with a 2-month history of progressively worsening weakness of both legs. On examination, he has bilateral proximal and distal leg weakness with diminished tendon reflexes. What is the next most appropriate investigation?
   A. Magnetic resonance imaging of the cervical spine
   B. Computed tomography of the brain
   C. Nerve biopsy
   D. Muscle biopsy
   E. Nerve conduction study

23. A 35-year-old woman complains of an uncontrollable urge to move her legs at night accompanied by an aching discomfort. Which of the following features would be consistent with a diagnosis of restless legs syndrome?
   A. Improvement in symptoms with the dopaminergic agonist ropinirole
   B. Improvement in symptoms with the dopaminergic antagonist chlorpromazine
   C. Evidence of iron overload with elevated ferritin

D. Improvement during pregnancy
E. Glove and stocking peripheral sensory neuropathy

24. A 28-year-old woman presents with visual loss in her right eye and pain behind the eye with eye movement. Fundoscopy reveals optic neuritis in that eye. Magnetic resonance imaging (MRI) of the head and cerebrospinal fluid (CSF) examination are normal. Which one of the following statements is true for this patient?
   A. Optic neuritis is a distinct clinical entity unrelated to multiple sclerosis
   B. It is possible that this patient will progress to multiple sclerosis in spite of normal MRI head and CSF examination
   C. This patient has a greater than 90% chance of progress to definite multiple sclerosis within 12 months
   D. Without treatment, this patient has a high likelihood of permanent unilateral visual loss
   E. Treatment with high-dose methylprednisolone will preserve her vision at 12 months

25. A 26-year-old Thai man presents with profound weakness after a meal with friends. He reports that for several years he has had similar episodes after exercise and large meals. Which one of the following diagnostic tests should be performed immediately for this patient?
   A. Assessment of serum potassium level
   B. Blood glucose
   C. Synacthen test
   D. Electromyography
   E. Testing for acetylcholine receptor antibodies

26. An 83-year-old woman with a past history of controlled hypertension presents 3½ h following a sudden onset of left-sided weakness due to an ischaemic stroke. Which one of the following statements is true regarding thrombolysis with tissue plasminogen activator (tPA)?
   A. Patients over the age of 80 years do not benefit from thrombolysis
   B. Patients do not benefit from thrombolysis later than 3 h from stroke onset
   C. Thrombolysis is associated with an increased risk of death and intracerebral haemorrhage in the first week following treatment
   D. Aspirin should be administered in conjunction with thrombolysis
   E. Intracerebral haemorrhage occurs in less than 1% of patients treated with thrombolysis

27. A 36-year-old woman presents with a sudden onset of headache and right-sided hemiparesis. She has no history of cardiovascular or neurological disease and was well and doing yoga daily before the onset of her symptoms. She does not take alcohol or illicit drugs. Her examination reveals a blood pressure of 130/70 mmHg and pulse of 80 beats/min in sinus rhythm. Her cardiac and respiratory examinations are normal, and her neurological examination confirms a hemiparesis. Laboratory studies reveal an erythrocyte sedimentation rate of 28 mm/h, a normal haematological and biochemical profile, and a negative urinary drug screen. Anti-nuclear antibody (ANA), anti-double-stranded DNA (anti-dsDNA) antibodies and anti-neutrophil cytoplasmic antibodies (ANCAs) are negative. Computed tomography (CT) of her head reveals hypodensity of her left temporal–parietal region consistent with an ischaemic region. What is the next best step for this patient?

A. Administration of high-dose intravenous corticosteroids
B. Biopsy of the temporal artery
C. Magnetic resonance angiography
D. Cerebral spinal fluid examination for oligoclonal bands
E. Visual evoked potentials

28. The first presentation of a patient with new variant Creutzfeldt–Jakob disease (nvCJD) is likely to be with:

A. Myoclonic jerks
B. Psychiatric symptoms
C. Akinesia
D. Dementia
E. Visual loss

Theme: Neuromuscular disorders (for Questions 29–32)

A. Limb girdle dystrophy
B. Guillain–Barré syndrome
C. Myotonic dystrophy
D. Dermatomyositis
E. Facioscapulohumeral dystrophy
F. Myasthenia gravis
G. Oculopharyngeal dystrophy
H. Motor neurone disease (also known as amyotrophic lateral sclerosis)

For each of the following patients, select the most likely diagnosis.

29. A 38-year-old man presents with muscle weakness and wasting. On examination, cataracts, frontal baldness and testicular atrophy were also present.

30. A 57-year-old man presents with progressive weakness and swallowing difficulties. Examination shows muscle wasting, fasciculation in the muscles of both legs, hyperactive reflexes generally and upgoing plantar responses.

31. A 53-year-old man presents with difficulty swallowing and progressive bilateral ptosis. On examination, there is also proximal weakness and ophthalmoplegia but no evidence of fatigability. His father had the same problem in his late 50s.

32. A 48-year-old Aboriginal woman has noticed difficulty rising from a chair and climbing stairs for 2 months prior to presentation. On examination, periungual telangiectasia is observed and erythematous psoriasiform dermatitis is present on the scalp.

Answers

BASIC SCIENCE

1. Answer A

The fundamental defect in myasthenia gravis is a decrease in the number of available acetylcholine receptors (AChR) at the postsynaptic muscle membrane in the neuromuscular junctions due to an autoimmune antibody mediated mechanism (Chaudhuri and Behan, 2009).

Myasthenia gravis is a neuromuscular disorder characterised by weakness and fatigability of skeletal muscles. In the neuromuscular junction, acetylcholine is released by motor nerve endings in response to the arrival of an action potential. The acetylcholine then combines with AChRs that are densely packed on the postsynaptic muscle membrane. In myasthenia gravis, an autoimmune attack by anti-AChR antibodies both reduces the number of AChRs by endocytosis and blocks the active site of the receptors (the site that normally binds acetylcholine).

The thymus is hyperplastic in 65% of patients with myasthenia gravis while 10% have thymic tumours. Muscle-like cells on the thymus (myoid cells) bear AChRs on their surface and are postulated to serve as the source of autoantigen.

Lambert–Eaton myasthenic syndrome (LEMS), which resembles myasthenia gravis, is associated with antibodies against P/Q-type calcium channels. These antibodies interfere with the normal calcium flux needed for the release of acetylcholine. Clinically, the differentiating features of LEMS are depressed or absent reflexes and incremental responses on repetitive nerve stimulation. Patients with myasthenia gravis have normal reflexes and characteristically show rapid decrease in the amplitude of evoked responses on repetitive nerve stimulation.

Chaudhuri, A. and Behan, P.O. (2009). Myasthenic crisis. *QJM* 102, 97–107.
http://qjmed.oxfordjournals.org/content/102/2/97.long

2. Answer D

Hemiballismus is a rare movement disorder characterised by a large movement of an entire limb or limbs on one side of the body (Hawley and Weiner, 2012). The acute development of hemiballismus is often caused by focal lesions in the contralateral basal ganglia and subthalamic nucleus. Many aetiologies exist for this rare disorder, with vascular causes and non-ketotic hyperglycaemia being the most common. Prognosis is favourable for most patients with complete resolution. It is first important to treat underlying causes such as hyperglycaemia, infections or neoplastic lesions. When pharmacological treatment is necessary, anti-dopaminergic drugs, such as haloperidol and chlorpromazine, can be helpful. Other treatments include topiramate, intrathecal baclofen and botulinum injections.

Hawley, J.S. and Weiner, W.J. (2012). Hemiballismus: current concepts and review. *Parkinsonism Relat Disord* 18, 125–129.
http://www.ncbi.nlm.nih.gov/pubmed/21930415

3. Answer A

While partial epilepsy, which is the most common seizure disorder in adults, can be associated with head trauma, stroke and tumour, the strongest association is with mesial temporal sclerosis (Chang and Lowenstein, 2003). This is characterised by hippocampal neuronal loss and chronic fibrillary gliosis centred on the pyramidal cell layer. It can be imaged with Magnetic resonance imaging (MRI) and features can include reduced hippocampal volume, increased signal intensity on T2-weighted imaging and disturbed internal architecture.

Epilepsy syndromes fall into two general groups – generalized and partial syndromes. In generalised epilepsy, the seizures begin with simultaneous involvement of both cerebral hemispheres. In partial epilepsy, in contrast, seizures originate in one or more local foci, although they can spread to involve the whole brain.

Most of the partial epilepsies arise from abnormality in the mesial temporal lobe. Recordings from intracranial electrodes demonstrate an ictal onset in mesial temporal structures, such as the hippocampus, amygdala and adjacent parahippocampal cortex; surgical resection of these areas in suitable patients can abolish the seizures.

Chang, B.S. and Lowenstein, D.H. (2003). Epilepsy. *N Engl J Med* 349, 1257–1266.
http://www.ncbi.nlm.nih.gov/pubmed/14507951

4. Answer D

The involvement of the right third cranial nerve and the right pyramidal tract would suggest the lesion is at the level of the third cranial nerve nucleus in the midbrain. A midbrain infarct is most commonly a consequence of hypertensive cerebral vascular disease and may arise from an embolus with a cardiac origin or proximal atherosclerotic lesion. It is also sometimes known as Weber syndrome and due to occlusion of paramedian branches of the posterior cerebral artery or of basilar bifurcation perforating arteries. The involvement of the third nerve excludes a lesion in the internal capsule, medulla, cervical cord and occipital lobe. Sometimes contralateral parkinsonism may develop due to involvement of the basal ganglia projections. On rare occasions, hemiparesis with contralateral third cranial nerve palsy can result from a hemispheric space-occupying lesion, which compresses the contralateral third cranial nerve and the cerebral peduncle against the clinoid process.

5. Answer C

Horner syndrome results from interruption of the sympathetic supply to the head and is characterised by enophthalmos, miosis, ptosis and a warm dry skin (anhydrosis) on the affected side of the face. The loss of sympathetic tone causes vasodilatation of the cutaneous vessels of the cheek and nasal mucosa with absence of sweating and a feeling of nasal obstruction. There is also narrowing of the palpebral fissure where the ptosis is due to weakness of the superior tarsal muscle or Muller's muscle. There is also a contraction of the pupil due to the unopposed action of the autonomic parasympathetic inflow via the oculomotor nerve. The movement of the eyeball is unaffected.

The sympathetic pathway may be interrupted in the cervical spinal cord, from the sympathetic trunk, the brachial plexus, over the lung apex in the superior cervical ganglion, within the adventitia of the internal carotid artery or through the cavernous sinus. Conditions that can produce a Horner syndrome include anything that might destroy the cervical sympathetic chain, such as invading malignancy at the lung apex. Brainstem stroke can also cause Horner syndrome and other neurological symptoms may then co-exist such as diplopia, vertigo and ataxia, whilst the presence of neck pain should point towards the possibility of a carotid dissection.

6. Answer E

Adrenoleucodystrophy (ALD) is a hereditary demyelinating disease (X-linked disorder). ALD is the most common peroxisomal disorder of beta-oxidation that results in accumulation of very long chain fatty acids (VLCFA) in all tissues. ALD consists of a spectrum of phenotypes, including childhood cerebral forms, adrenomyeloneuropathy and Addison disease. These disorders vary in the age at and severity of clinical presentation. ALD is caused by mutations in the ATP-binding cassette, Subfamily D, Member 1 gene (ABCD1 gene), located at Xq28, which encodes an ATP-binding cassette (ABC) transporter, similar to the cystic fibrosis transmembrane conductance regulator (CFTR). ALD is characterised by inflammatory demyelination, resulting in symmetric loss of myelin in the cerebral and cerebellar white matter. The parieto-occipital regions are usually affected first, with asymmetric progression of the lesions toward the frontal or temporal lobes.

Acute disseminated encephalomyelitis (ADEM) is an immune-mediated inflammatory disorder of the central nervous system (CNS) characterised by a widespread demyelination that predominantly involves the white matter of the brain and spinal cord (Tenembaum et al., 2007). The condition is usually precipitated by a viral infection or vaccination. The presenting features include an acute encephalopathy with multifocal neurological signs and deficits. Children are preferentially affected. In the absence of specific biological markers, the diagnosis of ADEM is still based on the clinical and radiological features. Although ADEM usually has a monophasic course, recurrent or multiphasic forms have been reported, raising diagnostic difficulties in distinguishing these cases from multiple sclerosis (MS).

Progressive multifocal leucoencephalopathy (PML) is a severe inflammatory demyelinating disease of the central nervous system that is caused by reactivation of the polyomavirus JC.

Guillain–Barré syndrome is an acute polyneuropathy. Some subtypes cause change in sensation or pain as well as dysfunction of the autonomic nervous system.

MS is an acquired inflammatory demyelinating disease which rarely shows familial aggregation, though there has been an increasing interest in associations of the disease with HLA DR and other genetic loci.

 Tenembaum, S., Chitnis, T., Ness, J., and Hahn, J.S. (2007). Acute disseminated encephalomyelitis. *Neurology* 68, S23–36. http://www.ncbi.nlm.nih.gov/pubmed/17438235

7. Answer B

S1 innervates skin over the little toe and S1 radiculopathy is associated with loss of ankle jerk. Other findings of S1 radiculopathy can be decreased plantar and toe flexion.

L5 radiculopathy is associated with decreased foot dorsiflexion and toe extension with normal ankle jerk.

Common peroneal nerve compression leads to foot drop with weakness on foot dorsiflexion and eversion. It can be seen with prolonged immobilisation such as following general anaesthesia or from a plaster cast. Reflexes are preserved.

Sciatic nerve compression may be associated with hip fracture, dislocation, repair or other trauma. There is sensory loss over the posterior aspect of the thigh, gluteal regions and entire lower leg (the medial calf and arch of the foot may be spared). The ankle jerk is lost while knee jerk is preserved.

Posterior tibial nerve compression leads to sensory symptoms, such as aching or burning over the sole of the foot, with positive Tinel's sign over the nerve posterior to the medial malleolus and sensory loss over the sole of the foot.

8. Answer C

Guillain–Barré syndrome (GBS) is an acute inflammatory demyelinating polyradiculoneuropathy (van Doorn et al., 2008). The inflammatory response in GBS strips myelin between the nodes of Ranvier in peripheral nerves. Axons are destroyed only in extensively involved areas as a secondary phenomenon. The dominant features are rapidly progressive symmetrical muscle weakness with sensory loss and widespread hyporeflexia or areflexia. It has been called the 'ascending paralysis' because in about two-thirds of patients it begins in the lower limbs and later affects the upper limbs, trunk and cranial nerves. It can affect the facial muscles (50% of cases) and respiratory muscles, with 25% of patients needing artificial ventilation. Both proximal and distal muscles tend to be affected simultaneously because demyelination occurs in the nerve roots and in nerves more peripherally.

Nerve conduction studies show features of segmental demyelination, including partial motor conduction block, prolonged distal motor and F wave latencies, temporal dispersion of motor responses and reduced maximum motor conduction velocity, although these can be normal for the first 1–2 weeks. Nerve conduction studies distinguish classical demyelinating GBS from axonal forms (acute motor axonal neuropathy), which may follow *Campylobacter jejuni* infection, although this infection may also precipitate either type of GBS.

van Doorn, P.A., Ruts, L., and Jacobs, B.C. (2008). Clinical features, pathogenesis, and treatment of Guillain–Barré syndrome. *Lancet Neurol* 7, 939–950.
http://www.ncbi.nlm.nih.gov/pubmed/18848313

9. Answer H

Lambert–Eaton myasthenic syndrome is an autoimmune disease in which antibodies are directed against the presynaptic voltage-gated calcium channels (VGCCs) (Titulaer et al., 2011). It can occur sporadically or as a paraneoplastic syndrome, most often in association with small cell lung cancer, which also expresses functional VGCCs.

The syndrome usually presents with proximal weakness, which is greater in the legs than the arms. Like myasthenia gravis, weakness is exacerbated by exercise and heat. Autonomic dysfunction occurs in 75% of patients, manifesting as dry mouth, blurred vision, constipation and orthostatic hypotension. Calcium entry into the presynaptic terminal is initially blocked, resulting in reduced release of acetylcholine and reduced muscle contraction. However, on exercise, continuous influx of calcium results in accumulation of calcium in the presynaptic nerve terminal, because its removal by mitochondria does not keep pace with its influx. This results in release of normal or near-normal amounts of acetylcholine on muscle contraction for a short time, and muscle strength may improve with repeated testing. Indeed, grip may become more powerful over several seconds of strength testing. Because of similarities in clinical presentation, Lambert–Eaton myasthenic syndrome can be mistaken for myasthenia gravis. However, ocular and bulbar muscles are affected more prominently in myasthenia gravis than in Lambert–Eaton myasthenic syndrome. Moreover, the legs are less commonly affected in patients with myasthenia gravis.

Electrophysiological studies are useful to differentiate Lambert–Eaton myasthenic syndrome from myasthenia gravis. Compound muscle action potential amplitudes are reduced in myasthenia gravis and are not increased after repetitive stimulation.

Titulaer, M.J., Lang, B., and Verschuuren, J.J. (2011). Lambert-Eaton myasthenic syndrome: from clinical characteristics to therapeutic strategies. *Lancet Neurol* 10, 1098–1107.
http://www.ncbi.nlm.nih.gov/pubmed/22094130

10. Answer F

This patient has neurofibromatosis type 1 (NF1), also known as von Recklinghausen disease (Ferner, 2007). NF1 is an autosomal dominant genetic disorder with an incidence of approximately 1 in 3000 individuals. Approximately one-half of cases are familial; the remainder are new mutations. The NF1 gene has been mapped to chromosome 17q11.2.

Neurofibromin, the cytoplasmic protein product encoded by the NF1 gene, acts as a tumour suppressor and is widely expressed, with high concentrations in the nervous system. Neurofibromin reduces cell proliferation by accelerating the inactivation of a cellular proto-oncogene, p21 ras, which is important in promoting tumour formation. Neurofibromin controls mammalian target of rapamycin (mTOR) via a common biochemical pathway with tuberin, the TSC2 gene product. The major disease features involve the nervous system, the skin, and bone, and the resulting complications are numerous, unpredictable and vary even within families. However, many patients will not have substantial problems other than cutaneous neurofibromas and mild cognitive impairment.

The neurofibromatosis type 2 (NF2) gene is located on chromosome 22q 11.2 and encodes a 595 amino acid protein known as merlin (or schwannomin). Merlin is structurally related to the moesin/ezrin/radixin proteins, which link the actin cytoskeleton to cell-surface glycoproteins that control growth and cellular remodelling. Merlin is widely expressed in Schwann cells, meningeal cells, peripheral nerves and the lens. Adults with NF2 usually present with symptoms associated with vestibular schwannoma.

Ferner, R.E. (2007). Neurofibromatosis 1 and neurofibromatosis 2: a twenty first century perspective. *Lancet Neurol* 6, 340–351.
http://www.ncbi.nlm.nih.gov/pubmed/17362838

11. Answer A

Tay–Sachs disease (also known as GM2 gangliosidosis or hexosaminidase A deficiency) is an autosomal recessive genetic disorder. In its most common variant (known as infantile Tay–Sachs disease), it causes a progressive deterioration of mental and physical abilities that commences around 6 months of age and usually results in death by the age of 4 years. A rare form of this disease, known as adult-onset or late-onset Tay–Sachs disease, usually has its first symptoms during the 30s or 40s. In contrast to the other forms, late-onset Tay–Sachs disease is usually not fatal as the effects may not progress. The disease occurs when harmful quantities of gangliosides accumulate in the lysosome of neurones, eventually leading to their death (Rucker et al., 2004).

Tay–Sachs results from mutations in the HEXA gene on human chromosome 15, which encodes the alpha-subunit of beta-N-acetylhexosaminidase A, a lysosomalenzyme. Hexosaminidase A is a vital lysosomal hydrolytic enzyme that breaks down phospholipids. When hexosaminidase A is dysfunctional, the lipids accumulate in the brain and interfere with normal biological processes. Hexosaminidase A specifically breaks down fatty acid derivatives called gangliosides; these are made and biodegraded rapidly in early life as the brain develops. Patients with and carriers of Tay–Sachs can be identified by a simple test that measures hexosaminidase A activity. In patients with a clinical suspicion of Tay–Sachs disease, at any age of onset, the initial testing involves an enzyme assay to measure the activity of hexosaminidase in serum, fibroblasts or leucocytes. Total hexosaminidase enzyme activity is decreased in individuals with Tay–Sachs, as is the percentage of hexosaminidase A. After confirmation of decreased enzyme activity in an individual, confirmation by genetic analysis can be pursued.

 Rucker, J.C., Shapiro, B.E., Han, Y.H., et al. (2004). Neuro-ophthalmology of late-onset Tay-Sachs disease (LOTS). *Neurology* 63, 1918–1926.
http://www.ncbi.nlm.nih.gov/pubmed/15557512

CLINICAL

12. Answer C

This patient has an acute, idiopathic, facial neuropathy (Bell's palsy). The abrupt onset of unilateral facial weakness with lower motor neurone (forehead) involvement preceded by pain behind the ear is classical. Over 80% of patients eventually make a full recovery. Early treatment with prednisolone significantly improves the chances of complete recovery at 3 and 9 months and is appropriate for patients with clinical features indicating a poorer prognosis. Such features include severe (complete) paralysis, older age, hyperacusis, altered taste and electromyographic evidence of axonal degeneration. Recent evidence implicates herpes simplex virus (HSV) type 1 infection in many patients. Trials of facial nerve decompression have not demonstrated efficacy (Gilden, 2004; Gilden and Tyler, 2007).

Gilden, D.H. (2004). Clinical practice. Bell's palsy. *N Engl J Med* 351, 1323–1331.
http://www.ncbi.nlm.nih.gov/pubmed/15385659

Gilden, D.H. and Tyler, K.L. (2007). Bell's palsy – is glucocorticoid treatment enough? *N Engl J Med* 357, 1653–1655.
http://www.ncbi.nlm.nih.gov/pubmed/17942879

13. Answer A

Cerebral venous thrombosis, including thrombosis of cerebral veins and major dural sinuses, is rare (Piazza, 2012), but it has a higher frequency among patients younger than 40 years of age, patients with thrombophilia and women who are pregnant or receiving hormonal contraceptive therapy. Cerebral venous thrombosis should be considered in patients who present with acute, subacute, or chronic headache with unusual features, signs of intracranial hypertension, focal neurological abnormalities in the absence of vascular risk factors, new seizure disorders, or haemorrhagic infarcts especially if multiple or in non-arterial vascular territories. Focal or generalised seizures, including status epilepticus, are observed more commonly than in other causes of stroke and are seen in 30–40% of patients with cerebral venous thrombosis. Because of variability in clinical presentation, delays in diagnosis are common.

Magnetic resonance (MR) imaging of the head combined with MR venography is the most sensitive study for detection of cerebral venous thrombosis in the acute, subacute and chronic phases. Non-contrast computed tomogram (CT) head has a poor sensitivity and shows direct signs of cerebral venous thrombosis in only one-third of patients.

Acute therapy for cerebral venous thrombosis focuses on anti-coagulation, management of sequelae, such as seizures, increased intracranial pressure and venous infarction, and prevention of cerebral herniation.

Piazza, G. (2012). Cerebral venous thrombosis. *Circulation* 125, 1704–1709.
http://circ.ahajournals.org/content/125/13/1704.long

14. Answer C

The risk of a second seizure occurring within 2 years of the first is approximately 50% (Rugg-Gunn and Sander, 2012). Early treatment with anti-epileptic drugs after the first seizure does not affect the long-term prognosis, with 75% of patients achieving remission at 5 years, regardless of whether treatment began after the first seizure or only after a recurrence. Treatment is therefore typically reserved for people who have had at least two seizures and in whom the risk of a third seizure is over 70%. The prevalence of epilepsy in developed countries is about 0.5%, whilst, the lifetime risk of a person having a non-febrile epileptic seizure is much higher at 2–5%.

The majority of people with epilepsy eventually become free of seizures on anti-epileptic drugs. However, about a quarter of patients continue to have seizures despite treatment. Epilepsy carries an increased risk of premature mortality with standardised mortality rates two- to three-fold higher than those for the general population. This increased risk is partly due to the underlying diseases associated with epilepsy, but is also a direct result of seizures, such as an increased risk of accidents such as drowning and sudden unexpected death in epilepsy (SUDEP), so seizure remission, wherever possible, is an important aim.

Rugg-Gunn, F.J. and Sander, J.W. (2012). Management of chronic epilepsy. *BMJ* 345, e4576.
http://www.bmj.com/content/345/bmj.e4576?view=long&pmid=22807075

15. Answer D

Cluster headache is an extremely painful and distressing headache disorder (Nesbitt and Goadsby, 2012). Attacks are unilateral, generally last 15 min to 3 h and have a characteristic set of ipsilateral cranial autonomic features (lacrimation, nasal congestion or rhinorrhoea, ptosis, oedema of the eyelid or the face, sweating of the forehead or the face and miosis), which are often accompanied by agitation. Attacks occur from once every other day to eight times daily, in bouts that last several weeks, usually with complete remission between bouts. Acute attacks should be treated with high flow oxygen and/or parenteral triptans. Verapamil can be helpful as prophylactic treatment. There is a marked male predominance, an association with smoking and in many people a precipitation by alcohol and occurrence during the night.

Attacks of migraine tend to be less severe and to last longer; cranial autonomic features are unusual, whilst nausea, vomiting, and bilateral photophobia are more common. Migraine lacks the striking clustering of attacks and most patients prefer not to move during a migrainous episode, in contrast to the agitation and restlessness experienced by many patients during a cluster attack.

Trigeminal neuralgia tends to affect people over the age of 50 years and consists of sudden, short stabs of pain, affecting the second and third divisions of the trigeminal nerve. It is not associated with cranial autonomic features. Acute glaucoma might mimic, but is not usually associated with, the clustering pattern, recurrence or precipitation by alcohol. Temporal arteritis affects an older population and the headaches are usually not so severe or clustering in pattern.

Nesbitt, A.D., and Goadsby, P.J. (2012). Cluster headache. *BMJ* 344, e2407.
http://www.bmj.com/content/344/bmj.e2407

16. Answer D

Typically, patients with Parkinson disease have a robust response to one or more medications. However, after 5 years of therapy, medication-related complications develop in a majority. Such complications include dyskinesia and 'on–off' fluctuations in which a sudden, often unpredictable loss of benefit from medication occurs, characterised by reduced mobility, tremor, rigidity, and other motor and non-motor manifestations. Some symptoms (difficulties with gait, balance, speech, swallowing or cognition) may become progressively resistant to pharmacological therapies. Patients with symptoms that are responsive to levodopa and selected other symptoms are appropriate potential candidates for deep-brain stimulation (Fasano et al., 2012; Okun, 2012).

Deep brain stimulation is a surgical technique in which electrodes attached to leads are implanted in specific regions of the brain. The electrodes are connected to a device called an impulse generator, which delivers electrical stimuli to brain tissue in order to modulate or disrupt patterns of neural signalling within a targeted region. Two sites in the brain have been targeted for deep brain stimulation in Parkinson disease, where much of the degenerative change occurs: the subthalamic nucleus and the internal segment of the globus pallidus. Deep brain stimulation acts on the cells and fibres closest to the implanted electrode, in most cases inhibiting cells and exciting fibres. It changes the firing rate and pattern of individual neurones in the basal ganglia. However, it remains unclear exactly how these influences lead to changes in the symptoms of Parkinson disease.

Typically, levodopa-responsive symptoms, tremor, on–off fluctuations and dyskinesia are most likely to improve with deep brain stimulation, whereas impairments in gait, balance and speech are less likely to improve and may in some cases worsen. Patients should be considered for deep brain stimulation only if adequate trials of multiple medications for Parkinson disease (carbidopa–levodopa, dopamine agonists, monoamine oxidase inhibitors and amantadine) have been unsuccessful.

Fasano, A., Daniele, A., and Albanese, A. (2012). Treatment of motor and non-motor features of Parkinson's disease with deep brain stimulation. *Lancet Neurol* 11, 429–442.
http://www.ncbi.nlm.nih.gov/pubmed/22516078

Okun, M.S. (2012). Deep-brain stimulation for Parkinson's disease. *N Engl J Med* 367, 1529–1538.
http://www.ncbi.nlm.nih.gov/pubmed/23075179

17. Answer B

Albuminocytological dissociation is seen in about 50% of cases of Guillain–Barré syndrome in the first week of presentation, with the number reaching 75% by the third week (Yuki and Hartung, 2012). Pleocytosis in a patient with typical features of Guillain–Barré syndrome may be suggestive of human immunodeficiency virus (HIV) infection.

Guillain–Barré syndrome patients present with bilateral symmetric paralysis of the limbs with arefexia/hyporeflexia, although up to 10% may have normal or brisk reflexes. The presence of distal paraesthesia is common. It is the commonest cause of flaccid paralysis worldwide. Serious and potentially fatal autonomic dysfunction, such as arrhythmias and extreme hypertension or hypotension, occurs in 20% of patients. Marked bradycardia may warrant a cardiac pacemaker and can be preceded by wide swings in systolic blood pressure. Two-thirds of cases are preceded by diarrhoea or upper respiratory infection, with *Campylobacter jejuni* identified in up to 30% of cases.

Lumbar puncture may help in diagnosis but equally importantly helps to rule out infectious conditions such as Lyme disease and malignant conditions such as lymphoma. Although nerve conduction studies help to confirm the presence, pattern and severity of the disease, they are not obligatory for diagnosis.

Up to 20% of patients remain severely disabled and, despite immunotherapy, there is a 5% mortality rate.

Yuki, N. and Hartung, H.P. (2012). Guillain-Barré syndrome. *N Engl J Med* 366, 2294–2304.
http://www.ncbi.nlm.nih.gov/pubmed/22694000

18. Answer C

Lewy body dementia (LBD) is a form of dementia that shares characteristics with both Alzheimer and Parkinson disease. It is characteristically associated with visual hallucinations (Lees et al., 2009).

LBD is caused by deposition of Lewy bodies, which are round, eosinophilic, intracytoplasmic inclusion bodies in the nuclei of neurones. Although many of the symptoms of the disorder bear a striking resemblance to Alzheimer or Parkinson disease, it is characterised by fluctuations in level of alertness, visual hallucinations, repeated falls, autonomic instability and rapid eye movement (REM) sleep behaviour disorder causing dream-enacting behaviour. Patients may display severe sensitivity to neuroleptics with acute worsening of symptoms.

Lees, A.J., Hardy, J., and Revesz, T. (2009). Parkinson's disease. *Lancet* 373, 2055–2066.
http://www.ncbi.nlm.nih.gov/pubmed/19524782

19. Answer C

This patient most likely has mitochondrial myopathy, encephalopathy, lactic acidosis and stroke syndrome (MELAS) (Goodfellow et al., 2012). It is a progressive neurodegenerative disorder. Patients may present sporadically or as members of maternal pedigrees with a wide variety of clinical presentations. Onset of the disorder may be myopathic with weakness, easy fatigability and exercise intolerance. Other features include seizures, diabetes mellitus, hearing loss, cardiac disease, short stature, endocrinopathies and neuropsychiatric dysfunction. Patients have a myopathy causing proximal muscle weakness and hypotonia, seizures and stroke-like episodes.

Lactic acidosis is an important feature of the disorder, as measured by a high lactate-to-pyruvate ratio. However, in general, lactic acidosis does not lead to systemic metabolic acidosis, and it may be absent in patients with impressive involvement of the central nervous system. The levels of serum creatine kinase are increased in some patients with MELAS syndrome.

Individuals with more severe clinical manifestations of MELAS syndrome generally have greater than 80% mutant mtDNA in stable tissues such as muscle. A skeletal muscle biopsy is required to confirm the diagnosis of MELAS.

Goodfellow, J.A., Dani, K., Stewart, W., et al. (2012). Mitochondrial myopathy, encephalopathy, lactic acidosis and stroke-like episodes: an important cause of stroke in young people. *Postgrad Med J* 88, 326–334.
http://www.ncbi.nlm.nih.gov/pubmed/22328278

20. Answer B

Multiple system atrophy (MSA) is a degenerative neurological disorder (Stefanova et al., 2009). The cause of MSA is unknown and no specific risk factors have been identified. The aggregation, deposition and dysfunction of alpha-synuclein (aSyn) in Lewy bodies and glial cytoplasmic inclusions are common events in neurodegenerative disorders known as synucleinopathies, which include Parkinson disease, dementia with Lewy bodies and multiple system atrophy. Approximately 55% of cases of MSA occur in men, with the typical age of onset in the 50s to 60s. Patients with MSA present with a heterogeneous combination of autonomic failure, urogenital dysfunction, cerebellar ataxia, parkinsonian and pyramidal signs. The diagnosis of probable MSA requires the presence of urinary dysfunction or orthostatic hypotension with a decrease in blood pressure of at least 30 mmHg systolic and 15 mmHg diastolic within 3 min after standing up, as well as a motor syndrome that includes parkinsonism with a poor response to levodopa or a cerebellar syndrome. Use of bladder function assessment often detects early abnormalities consistent with neurogenic disturbance with detrusor hyper-reflexia and abnormal urethral sphincter function followed later in disease progression by increased residual urine volume. Cardiovascular autonomic dysfunction in MSA can be investigated with a standing blood pressure test, if the patient is ambulatory, or by tilt-table testing.

Supporting features of MSA include:
- Orofacial dystonia
- Disproportionate antecollis

- Camptocormia (severe anterior flexion of the spine) with or without Pisa syndrome (severe lateral flexion of the spine)
- Contractures of the hands or feet
- Inspiratory sighs
- Severe dysphonia
- Severe dysarthria
- New or increased snoring
- Cold hands and feet
- Pathological laughter or crying.
  Features not consistent with MSA include:
- Classical pill-rolling rest tremor
- Significant neuropathy
- Onset after age 75 years
- Family history of ataxia or parkinsonism
- Dementia
- White matter lesions that suggest multiple sclerosis
- Hallucinations not induced by drugs.

Stefanova, N., Bucke, P., Duerr, S., and Wenning, G.K. (2009). Multiple system atrophy: an update. *Lancet Neurol* 8, 1172–1178.
http://www.ncbi.nlm.nih.gov/pubmed/19909915

21. Answer B

This patient has myasthenic crisis and should receive urgent ventilatory support that could include intubation and ventilation. The myasthenia gravis should be urgently treated with plasmapheresis (Chaudhuri and Behan, 2009). Myasthenic crisis is a life-threatening medical emergency requiring early diagnosis and respiratory assistance. It can affect between one-fifth and one-third of all patients with myasthenia gravis.

Myasthenic crisis is caused by severe weakness of the respiratory muscles, upper airway muscles (bulbar myasthenia) or both. It is typically precipitated by poor control of generalised disease, medical treatment for bulbar myasthenia (steroids and anti-cholinesterases); concomitant use of certain antibiotics (aminoglycosides, quinolones and macrolides), muscle relaxants, benzodiazepines, beta-blockers and iodinated radiocontrast agents. Patients must be offered elective ventilation on clinical diagnosis without waiting for blood gas changes to show hypoxaemia. Careful observation and bedside measurements (vital capacity, peak flow measurement, pulse rate and blood pressure) are more important than repeated monitoring of blood gases.

Both plasma exchange and intravenous immunoglobulin (IVIg) are comparable in terms of treatment efficacy. There is no significant advantage of an initial pulse of intravenous methylprednisolone over regular prednisolone, which is given by nasogastric tube at a pharmacological dose (1 mg/kg) and must be continued for several months after recovery from the crisis until alternative immunosuppressive or steroid-sparing agents (such as azathioprine or ciclosporin) become effective.

Intravenous pyridostigmine in a patient with myasthenic crisis is controversial as it can cause coronary vasospasm leading to myocardial infarction. Besides, large doses of anti-cholinesterases promote excessive salivary and gastric secretions, which may increase the risk of aspiration pneumonia.

 Chaudhuri, A. and Behan, P.O. (2009). Myasthenic crisis. *QJM* 102, 97–107.
http://qjmed.oxfordjournals.org/content/102/2/97.long

22. Answer E

The clinical scenario is suggestive of chronic inflammatory demyelinating neuropathy (CIDP) whose diagnosis is based mainly on the clinical presentation and nerve-conduction findings that are suggestive of demyelination (Koller et al., 2005).

CIDP is characterised by symmetrical weakness in both proximal and distal muscles that progressively increases for more than 2 months (distinguishing this condition from Guillain–Barré syndrome which is self-limited). The condition is associated with impaired sensation, absent or diminished tendon reflexes, an elevated cerebrospinal fluid protein level (with normal cell count), demyelinating nerve conduction studies, and signs of demyelination in nerve biopsy specimens. The course can be relapsing or chronic and progressive, the former being much more common in young adults.

The diagnosis of CIDP is based mainly on the clinical presentation and on nerve conduction findings that are consistent with demyelination. The electrophysiological features suggesting demyelination are the presence of three of the following four criteria: partial motor nerve conduction block, reduced motor nerve conduction velocity, prolonged distal motor latencies, and prolonged F-wave latencies.

Elevation of the protein content of the cerebrospinal fluid without pleocytosis and histological proof of demyelination and remyelination, often with inflammation, in nerve biopsy specimens can provide additional supporting evidence for the diagnosis.

 Koller, H., Kieseier, B.C., Jander, S., and Hartung, H.P. (2005). Chronic inflammatory demyelinating polyneuropathy. *N Engl J Med* 352, 1343–1356.
http://www.ncbi.nlm.nih.gov/pubmed/15800230

23. Answer A

Restless legs syndrome (RLS) is a common cause of distress and sleep disturbance (Leschziner and Gringras, 2012). It may be idiopathic or secondary to other disease, such as renal failure, diabetes or iron deficiency.

Because of its varied presentations, it is often missed or misdiagnosed. There is no specific test for RLS. The diagnosis is a clinical one. There is an urge to move the legs, usually accompanied or caused by uncomfortable sensations in the legs. It is worsened during inactivity, tends to be worse during the evening or night, and the sensations and urge to move can be partially alleviated by movement. It can lead to insomnia and sleep deprivation. It can occur or be exacerbated during pregnancy and there may be a positive family history.

Patients should be screened for iron deficiency and if deficient treated with replacement. Not all patients need treatment and non-drug-based measures include avoidance of alcohol, caffeine and smoking; good sleep hygiene; moderate regular exercise; hot baths, or leg massage before bedtime. Dopamine agonists (e.g. pramipexole and ropinirole) can be helpful but may be associated with impulse control disorders.

Leschziner, G. and Gringras, P. (2012). Restless legs syndrome. *BMJ* 344, e3056. http://www.bmj.com/content/344/bmj.e3056?view=long&pmid=22623643

24. Answer B

Typically, patients with first presentation of acute demyelinating optic neuritis are healthy young adults (Shams and Plant, 2009). A history of preceding viral illness may be present. There is a female preponderance (ratio of about 3:1) and most patients present at 20–45 years of age. The classical triad of inflammatory optic neuritis consists of loss of vision, periocular pain and dyschromatopsia, and is unilateral in 70% of adults. The typical clinical course is that of retro-orbital pain usually exacerbated by eye movement, and loss of central vision. Visual loss varies from mild reduction to no perception of light and progresses over 7–10 days before reaching a nadir.

Investigations should be guided by the clinical presentation. The diagnosis of optic neuritis is usually made on clinical grounds. Neuro-ophthalmic assessments can improve diagnostic accuracy, and early review is essential to ensure visual recovery has begun and the diagnosis reconsidered if it has not recovered.

Although more than half of all patients with multiple sclerosis (MS) have optic neuritis at some time, patients with optic neuritis who have completely normal results on magnetic resonance imaging (MRI) scanning and comprehensive cerebrospinal fluid examination may not progress to MS. It has been reported that the risk of development of MS after an episode of isolated unilateral optic neuritis is 38% at 10 years and 50% at 15 years. Another study has reported that 54% of patients with optic neuritis go on to develop MS after 30 years. Whether optic neuritis is a distinct clinical entity or part of a continuum with MS is controversial. Treatment of optic neuritis may result in hastened improvement, but even without treatment, most patients begin to recover vision within 4 weeks.

Shams, P.N, and Plant, G.T. (2009). Optic neuritis: a review. *Int MS J* 16, 82–89. http://www.ncbi.nlm.nih.gov/pubmed/19878630

25. Answer A

Hyperkalaemic and hypokalaemic periodic paralysis are both characterised by an abnormal serum potassium level at the time of symptom occurrence (Venance et al., 2006). However, the potassium levels can be normal between attacks, and thus, measurement of serum potassium during symptoms is the most important next step to take in assessing and treating this patient. Hyperkalaemic periodic paralysis is caused by a defect of a sodium channel (SCN4A), precipitated by rest following exercise, stress, potassium administration and the ingesting of certain foods. Hypokalaemic periodic paralysis is caused by a defect in a calcium channel (CACNL1A3) and is precipitated by the partaking of meals high in carbohydrates, rest following exercise, and excitement. If the potassium level is found to be low during attacks, secondary causes of hypokalaemia (diuretics, hyperaldosteronism, laxatives, etc.) or thyrotoxicosis (especially in patients of Asian descent) should be sought. A serum potassium level that is elevated without apparent cause is suggestive of hyperkalaemic periodic paralysis.

Venance, S.L., Cannon, S.C., Fialho, D., et al. (2006). The primary periodic paralyses: diagnosis, pathogenesis and treatment. *Brain* 129, 8–17.
http://brain.oxfordjournals.org/content/129/1/8.long

26. Answer C

Recent studies and meta-analyses have confirmed that patients older than 80 years achieved similar benefits from thrombolysis to those aged 80 years or younger, particularly when treated early with thrombolysis (Wardlaw et al., 2012). They have also extended the potential time interval from onset of benefit from thrombolysis to 4½ h with weaker suggestions of benefit up to 6 h in some patients. Thrombolysis is associated with an increased incidence of early mortality mainly due to intracerebral haemorrhage. Aspirin should not be started within the first 24 h of thrombolytic therapy in patients with acute ischaemic stroke, but usually should be started 24–48 h after thrombolytic therapy. Intracerebral haemorrhage is seen in 3–7% of patients treated with thrombolysis.

Wardlaw, J.M., Murray, V., Berge, E., et al. (2012). Recombinant tissue plasminogen activator for acute ischaemic stroke: an updated systematic review and meta-analysis. *Lancet* 379, 2364–2372.
http://www.ncbi.nlm.nih.gov/pmc/articles/PMC3386494/

27. Answer C

This patient has a single lesion in the distribution of a major cerebral vessel (middle cerebral artery) and no other findings on her imaging study that suggest multiple independent lesions. In young adults, carotid artery dissection is a common cause of stroke (20%), but may occur at any age (Debette and Leys, 2009). Carotid artery dissection begins as a tear in one of the carotid arteries of the neck, which allows blood under arterial pressure to enter the wall of the artery and split its layers. The result is either an intramural haematoma or an aneurysmal dilatation, either of which can be a source of microemboli. Dissection of the internal carotid artery can occur intracranially or extracranially, with the latter being more frequent. Internal carotid artery dissection can be caused by major or minor trauma, or it can be spontaneous, in which case, genetic, familial or heritable disorders are likely aetiologies. In diagnosing carotid dissection, conventional angiography has been largely replaced by non-invasive approaches, particularly brain MRI with magnetic resonance angiography (MRA) or with computed tomography angiography (CTA). Dissection may be diagnosed non-invasively with ultrasonography but may miss dissection in a significant proportion of cases.

Anti-thrombotic therapy with either anti-coagulation or anti-platelet agents has been used in the treatment of ischaemic stroke caused by carotid dissection, but the roles of thrombolysis and endovascular treatments are less well established.

This is a case of an ischaemic stroke occurring in a young, otherwise healthy female. In such cases, illicit drug use should also be considered as a potential contributing factor, although is made less likely in this case because of the lack of confirmatory history or urinary drug screen. Other sources of emboli, e.g. cardiac, and the possibility of a cardiac shunt should be considered. Vasculitis and systemic lupus erythematosus are possibilities, but against these are the negative anti-nuclear antibodies (ANA), anti-double-stranded DNA (anti-dsDNA) antibodies, and anti-neutrophil cytoplasmic antibodies (ANCAs). The absence of any illness preceding the onset of her symptoms also decreases the probability of a systemic inflammatory process. Visual evoked potentials and cerebrospinal fluid analysis are recommended if multiple sclerosis were a serious possibility, but the very acute onset makes this unlikely.

Debette, S. and Leys, D. (2009). Cervical-artery dissections: predisposing factors, diagnosis, and outcome. *Lancet Neurol* 8, 668–678.
http://www.ncbi.nlm.nih.gov/pubmed/19539238

28. Answer B
Patients with new variant Creutzfeldt–Jacob Disease (nvCJD) usually present with psychiatric symptoms such as dysphoria, anxiety, irritability, apathy, loss of energy, insomnia and social withdrawal (Tyler, 2003). Patients with CJD usually present in the sixth decade with rapidly progressive dementia and death heralded by a rigid, akinetic and mute state. Patients often have myoclonic jerks involving the face and limbs, as well as 'startle myoclonus' on stimulation. In contrast, patients with nvCJD present at a mean age of 26 years, usually with psychiatric symptoms. The diagnosis is often not suspected until neurological symptoms such as cognitive impairment, pain, paraesthesias, dysarthria and gait abnormalities appear. Myoclonus is a late feature and startle myoclonus is rarely seen.

CJD is an example of the prion diseases, which are transmissible, progressive and invariably fatal neurodegenerative conditions associated with misfolding and aggregation of a host-encoded cellular prion protein, PrP(C) (Imran and Mahmood, 2011). Human prion diseases can arise sporadically, be hereditary or be acquired. Sporadic human prion diseases include CJD, fatal insomnia and variably protease-sensitive prionopathy. Genetic or familial prion diseases are caused by autosomal dominantly inherited mutations in the gene encoding for PrP(C) and include familial or genetic CJD, fatal familial insomnia and Gerstmann–Sträussler–Scheinker syndrome. Acquired human prion diseases account for only 5% of cases of human prion disease. They include kuru, iatrogenic CJD and nvCJD, the latter probably transmitted to humans from affected cattle via meat consumption.

Imran, M. and Mahmood, S. (2011). An overview of human prion diseases. *Virol J* 8, 559.
http://www.ncbi.nlm.nih.gov/pmc/articles/PMC3296552/

Tyler, K.L. (2003). Creutzfeldt–Jakob disease. *N Engl J Med* 348, 681–682.
http://www.ncbi.nlm.nih.gov/pubmed/12594311

29. Answer C

Myotonic dystrophy is the most common muscular dystrophy observed in hospitalised patients (Turner and Hilton-Jones, 2010). Myotonia, muscle wasting, cataracts, testicular atrophy and frontal baldness all characterise hereditary myotonic dystrophy. There are currently two clinically and molecularly defined forms of myotonic dystrophy: myotonic dystrophy type 1 (DM1), also known as 'Steinert disease'; and myotonic dystrophy type 2 (DM2), also known as proximal myotonic myopathy. DM1 and DM2 are progressive multisystem genetic disorders with several clinical and genetic features in common. DM1 is the most common form of adult-onset muscular dystrophy, whereas DM2 tends to have a milder phenotype with later onset of symptoms and is rarer than DM1.

Patients with DM1 can be further divided into four subtypes:

- Congenital
- Childhood-onset
- 'Classical' adult-onset
- Asymptomatic/late-onset.

The predominant symptom in classical DM1 is distal muscle weakness, leading to difficulty with performing tasks requiring fine dexterity of the hands and foot drop, particularly affecting ankle dorsiflexors. The characteristic facies is caused by weakness and wasting of the facial, levator palpebrae and masticatory muscles giving rise to ptosis and the typical myopathic appearance. The neck flexors and finger/wrist flexors are also commonly involved. Ophthalmoplegia is described but is rare. Muscle weakness progresses slowly. Hand grip myotonia and strength may improve with repeated contractions – 'warm up phenomenon'. Conduction disturbances and tachyarrhythmias are common in DM1 and contribute significantly to the morbidity and mortality of the disease. Minor intellectual deficits are present in many patients. Endocrine abnormalities include disturbances of the thyroid, pancreas, hypothalamus and gonads.

DM2 is a multisystem disorder characterised by myotonia (90%) and muscle weakness (82%). The onset of DM2 is typically in the third decade, with the most common presenting symptom being muscle weakness, although myotonia during the first decade has been reported. DM2 patients commonly have prominent muscle pain, stiffness and fatigue in contrast to DM1 patients, although muscle pain may be underestimated in DM1. The weakness typically affects proximal muscles, including the neck, elbow extension and hip flexors, in comparison with early DM1, which initially tends to affect the distal upper limb muscles. Other clinical features include cardiac conduction defects (19%), posterior subcapsular cataracts (~78%, increasing with age) and endocrine changes, including insulin insensitivity (~75%, increasing with age) and testicular failure (~65%). Diabetes mellitus type 2 may be more common in DM2 than in DM1. Cognitive manifestations in DM2 include problems with organisation, concentration and word finding, and excessive daytime sleepiness. Conduction abnormalities are more common in DM1 than DM2, but cardiac screening is still necessary as the absolute cardiac risk in DM2 is not fully understood.

 Turner, C. and Hilton-Jones, D. (2010). The myotonic dystrophies: diagnosis and management. *J Neurol Neurosurg Psychiatry* 81, 358–367.
http://jnnp.bmj.com/content/81/4/358.long

30. Answer H
The main presentations of motor neurone disease (MND), known as amyotrophic lateral sclerosis (ALS) include:
* Limb-onset MND with a combination of upper and lower motor neurone (UMN and LMN) signs in the limbs
* Bulbar-onset MND, presenting with speech and swallowing difficulties, and with limb features developing later in the course of the disease
* The less common primary lateral sclerosis with pure UMN involvement
* Progressive muscular atrophy, with pure LMN involvement (Kiernan et al., 2011).

The clinical hallmark of MND is the presence of UMN and LMN features involving the brainstem and multiple spinal cord regions of innervation. Patients can present with bulbar-onset disease (about 25%) or limb-onset disease (about 70%), or with initial trunk or respiratory involvement (5%), subsequently spreading to involve other regions. Atypical modes of presentation can include weight loss, which is an indicator of a poor prognosis, cramps and fasciculations in the absence of muscle weakness, emotional lability and frontal lobe-type cognitive dysfunction.

In terms of presentation, UMN disturbance involving the limbs leads to spasticity, weakness and brisk deep tendon reflexes. By contrast, LMN limb features include fasciculations, wasting and weakness. Bulbar UMN dysfunction results in spastic dysarthria, which is characterised by slow, laboured and distorted speech, often with a nasal quality. The gag and jaw jerk can be pathologically brisk. Bulbar LMN dysfunction can be identified by tongue wasting, weakness and fasciculations, accompanied by flaccid dysarthria and later dysphagia. Flaccid dysarthria results in nasal speech caused by palatal weakness, hoarseness and a weak cough.

MND is relentlessly progressive; about 50% of patients die within 30 months of symptom onset and about 20% of patients survive between 5 and 10 years after symptom onset. Older age at symptom onset, early respiratory muscle dysfunction and bulbar-onset disease are associated with reduced survival, whereas limb-onset disease, younger age at presentation and longer diagnostic delay are independent predictors of prolonged survival.

 Kiernan, M.C., Vucic, S., Cheah, B.C., et al.(2011). Amyotrophic lateral sclerosis. *Lancet* 377, 942–955.
http://www.ncbi.nlm.nih.gov/pubmed/21296405

31. Answer G
Oculopharyngeal muscular dystrophy (OPMD) is an inherited disease that occurs most commonly in families of French–Canadian or middle European ancestry. OPMD is inherited in either an autosomal dominant or an autosomal recessive manner. It causes late-onset progressive ptosis and difficult swallowing. It may be difficult to distinguish from myasthenia gravis, which is not a dystrophic muscle disease. The absence of family history and the fluctuation of symptoms in myasthenia gravis usually distinguish the two conditions. If in doubt, electromyography and neostigmine testing can confirm the diagnosis of myasthenia gravis, and molecular genetic testing can confirm the diagnosis of OPMD.

32. Answer D
Dermatomyositis is a multisystem disorder (Mammen, 2010). The myopathy primarily affects the proximal muscles, is generally symmetrical and is slowly progressive during a period of weeks to months. Initial symptoms include myalgias, fatigue and weakness, manifested as inability to climb stairs, raise the arms for hair-brushing or shaving, rise from a squatting or sitting position, or a combination of these features. Dysphagia or dysphonia generally signifies a rapidly progressive course and may be associated with poor prognosis.

Cutaneous manifestation may include heliotrope rash, Gottron's papules, periungal telangiectases, poikiloderma and erythematous to violaceous psoriasiform dermatitis in the scalp.

Dermatomyositis is frequently associated with malignancy in those over the age of 60 years and assessment should include evaluation for cancer. If an early neoplasm can be found and treated, the dermatomyositis may improve without the need for high-dose glucocorticoid therapy.

 Mammen, A.L. (2010). Dermatomyositis and polymyositis: Clinical presentation, autoantibodies, and pathogenesis. *Ann N Y Acad Sci* 1184, 134–153.
http://www.ncbi.nlm.nih.gov/pubmed/20146695

7 Rheumatology

Questions

BASIC SCIENCE

Answers can be found in the Rheumatology Answers section at the end of this chapter.

1. Which one of the following is true concerning methotrexate?
  A. It activates dihydrofolate reductase
  B. It inhibits the production of the active form of tetrahydrofolate (THF) from the inactive dihydrofolate (DHF)
  C. It increases folic acid excretion
  D. It induces DNA cross-linking
  E. It is not teratogenic

2. A patient with suspected vasculitis undergoes investigation for anti-neutrophil cytoplasmic antibodies (ANCAs). While the perinuclear anti-neutrophil cytoplasmic antibodies (P-ANCA) are reported as weakly positive on indirect immunofluorescence, they are reported negative on enzyme-linked immunosorbent assay (ELISA). What could be the cause of this?
  A. Laboratory error
  B. Less specificity of ELISA
  C. Interpreter error
  D. P-ANCA positivity on indirect immunofluorescence associated with anti-cathepsin G antibodies
  E. Cross reactivity of cytoplasmic anti-neutrophil cytoplasmic antibodies (C-ANCA) with P-ANCA

3. Which one of the following is associated with an increased frequency of HLA-DR1 allele?
  A. Rheumatoid arthritis negative for rheumatoid factor
  B. Rheumatoid arthritis positive for rheumatoid factor
  C. Ankylosing spondylitis
  D. Narcolepsy
  E. Porphyria

Passing the FRACP Written Examination: Questions and Answers, First Edition. Jonathan Gleadle, Tuck Yong, Jordan Li, Surjit Tarafdar, and Danielle Wu.
© 2013 John Wiley & Sons, Ltd. Published 2013 by John Wiley & Sons, Ltd.

4. Which one of the following correctly describes the synovial immunological process in rheumatoid arthritis?
   A. Expression of interleukin-1 family cytokines is suppressed
   B. JAK (Janus kinase) pathways are suppressed in cytokine signalling
   C. Macrophages in the synovial membrane release cytokines such as tumour necrosis factor alpha (TNF-α) and interleukin-1 (IL-1)
   D. Neutrophils and mast cells in the synovial fluid do not play a major role
   E. TNF-α inhibits angiogenesis and activates regulatory T cells

5. A 43-year-old woman with long-standing scleroderma comes to you and complains of worsening constipation. She has been experiencing constipation for the past several months; recently, her constipation has become associated with abdominal pain and very hard stools. On occasion she has vomited. Which one of the following might explain her symptoms?
   A. Achalasia
   B. Autonomic nerve dysfunction
   C. Bacterial overgrowth
   D. Gastric antral vascular ectasia (watermelon stomach)
   E. Prolonged gallbladder emptying time

6. Which one of the following is observed in systemic lupus erythematosus?
   A. Anti-DNA antibodies cross-react with N-methyl-D-aspartate receptors in the kidney
   B. Complement component C1q accumulation in the brain resulting in neurocognitive defects
   C. Activation of complement by immune complexes and complement consumption
   D. Anti-Ro antibodies that interfere with the coagulation system
   E. Anti-phospholipid antibodies that alter the function of the cardiac conduction system

Theme: Biological agents (for Questions 7 and 8)
   A. Abatacept
   B. Adalimumab
   C. Anakinra
   D. Etanercept
   E. Infliximab
   F. Leflunomide
   G. Rituximab
   H. Tocilizumab

For each of the descriptions below, select the most appropriate biological agent.

7. Which drug inhibits the activity of interleukin-6?

8. Which drug neutralises the activity of interleukin-1?

CLINICAL

9. A 77-year-old man presents with severe right knee pain for 8h. There is no history of trauma or constitutional symptoms. His medical problems include congestive heart failure, chronic kidney disease and hypertension. Two months ago, the patient was admitted to the hospital for upper gastrointestinal bleeding. The patient is very uncomfortable. His examination is notable for marked swelling and erythema of the right knee and the presence of an effusion. Which one of the following treatment strategies should be undertaken?
  A. Non-steroidal anti-inflammatory drugs
  B. Cyclooxygenase-2 inhibitors
  C. High-dose colchicine for 2 weeks
  D. Allopurinol
  E. Arthrocentesis followed by administration of an intra-articular steroid

10. Which one of the following is a contraindication to the use of tumour necrosis factor inhibitor?
  A. Previous treated tuberculosis
  B. Septic arthritis 4 months ago
  C. Fully resected basal cell carcinoma 5 years ago
  D. Breast carcinoma 15 years previously
  E. Presence of pyoderma gangrenosum

11. A 23-year-old woman is evaluated for recurrent episodes of fever and abdominal pain. These episodes occur approximately once every 2 months and usually last for 1–2 days. During these episodes, she may have diarrhoea. Her leucocyte count and C-reactive protein are elevated during these episodes. Between episodes, she feels well. Exacerbations of the pain are sometimes associated with menses and were less frequent 2 years ago when she began taking the oral contraceptive pill. She had a colonoscopy and computed tomography (CT) abdomen 3 months ago which were normal. Which of the following is the most appropriate treatment for this patient?
  A. Colchicine
  B. Etanercept
  C. High-dose oestrogen oral contraceptive
  D. Interferon alpha
  E. Prednisolone

12. A 35-year-old woman is reviewed in a rheumatology clinic with fever, proximal muscle weakness, Raynaud phenomenon and swollen fingers and hands. She has also had multiple joint pains and reflux symptoms. Which serological test is most useful in the diagnosis of mixed connective tissue disease?
  A. Anti-neutrophil cytoplasmic antibody (ANCA)
  B. Hypocomplementaemia
  C. Anti-U1 small nuclear anti-ribonucleoprotein (anti-RNP)

D. Anti-Jo1 antibodies

E. Anti-nuclear antibodies

13. Which one of the following statements about polyarteritis nodosa (PAN) is correct?

    A. Hepatitis C has the strongest association as a causative pathogen of this condition

    B. It is a multisystem disease affecting the large arteries

    C. All organ systems can potentially be affected by PAN, except for the pulmonary system

    D. A renal biopsy is recommended as a first choice for diagnosis

    E. Anti-neutrophil cytoplasmic antibodies (ANCAs) are usually positive

14. A 40-year-old woman presents with fatigue and weakness for the past 2 months. She has found it difficult to get up from a chair. In addition, she has developed blanching of the hands with exposure to cold, as well as stiffness of the hands, wrists and feet lasting several hours in the morning. She has noticed finger swelling and can no longer wear her wedding ring. On examination, she has evidence of proximal muscle weakness; synovitis of the metacarpophalangeal, proximal interphalangeal, wrists and metatarsophalangeal joints. Her screening anti-nuclear antibody is positive with a titre of 1:640. Which autoantibody to extractable nuclear antigens is most likely to be positive?

    A. Anti-double-stranded DNA

    B. Anti-Scl-70

    C. Anti-Smith

    D. Anti-Jo-1

    E. Anti-SSA

15. A 30-year-old man presents acutely with oligoarthritis, urethritis and conjunctivitis. His C-reactive protein is 78 g/L (<10 g/L) and the rheumatoid factor is negative. Which one of the following features is also associated with the suspected diagnosis of Reiter syndrome or reactive arthritis?

    A. Acute interstitial nephritis

    B. Aortic stenosis

    C. Keratoderma blenorrhagica

    D. Pericarditis

    E. Pulmonary fibrosis

16. A 60-year-old man is diagnosed with rheumatoid arthritis after several months of joint pain, swelling and stiffness. His disease has been progressing and involves numerous joints. Rheumatoid nodules are present. The patient tested positive for rheumatoid factor. He is concerned about his prognosis. Which of the following is associated with a favourable course for a patient with rheumatoid arthritis?

    A. Insidious onset of disease

    B. Acute onset in a few large joints

    C. Age greater than 40 years

D. Positive rheumatoid factor

E. Constitutional symptoms

17. Which one of the following joints is most commonly affected in acute attacks of pseudogout?

A. Ankle

B. Metacarpal joint

C. Metatarsophalangeal joint

D. Knee

E. Wrist

18. A 60-year-old woman with a 16-year history of rheumatoid arthritis and who is currently on methotrexate and prednisolone is evaluated in a preoperative clinic for total hysterectomy. She has had synovectomy of both wrists and silicone implants in seven metacarpophalangeal joints. She has increasing morning stiffness and fatigue. She also has mild alopecia, shooting pains in her forearms and hands with progressively weak hand grip, and mouth ulcers. On physical examination, there is no evidence of heart, lung or abdominal abnormalities. Multiple joint deformities with arthroplasty scars are present. She has weakness of hand grip, hyper-reflexia and hypertonia. There are multiple subcutaneous nodules on the extensor surfaces. She has been noted to have a high-titre rheumatoid factor and the C-reactive protein (CRP) has never been less than 20 mg/L. Which one of the following is the most appropriate action at this time?

A. Commence a tumour necrosis factor-α inhibitor

B. Test for cryoglobulins

C. Obtain X-ray of both hands

D. Obtain magnetic resonance imaging (MRI) of the cervical spine

E. Test for anti-nuclear antibody, anti-DNA titres and complement levels

19. A 32-year-old woman has a history of dry eyes and mouth. Blood tests are positive for anti-nuclear antibody, and anti-Ro and anti-La antibodies. Which one of the following is she predisposed to developing?

A. Asthma

B. Lymphoma

C. Pleural effusion

D. Primary salivary gland neoplasms

E. Small cell lung cancer

20. An 84-year-old woman presents with a 1-week history of malaise, severe right temporal headache and visual disturbance. She has a history of polymyalgia rheumatica but was weaned off prednisolone 6 months ago. A clinical diagnosis of temporal arteritis is made, C-reactive protein (CRP) is elevated at 65 mg/L and she is commenced on prednisone 60 mg daily. One day later, she undergoes a temporal artery biopsy but the histopathological examination reveals no evidence of temporal arteritis. What is the most likely explanation for the biopsy finding?

A. The biopsy was done 1 day after taking prednisolone

B. The elevated CRP excludes a diagnosis of temporal arteritis

C. The arterial lesion is segmental
D. The patient has had polymyalgia rheumatica previously
E. The prednisolone dose administered was too high

21. A 65-year-old man with a recent transurethral resection of the prostate presents with acute onset lower back pain with tenderness over the L4 and L5 vertebrae, left-sided foot drop and fever. Blood culture is positive for *Staphylococcus aureus*. He is haemodynamically stable. What is the most appropriate initial first step of investigation?
   A. Computed tomography guided biopsy of the L4 and L5 disc
   B. Prostate-specific antigen
   C. Magnetic resonance imaging of the spine
   D. Three-phase technetium-99m bone scan
   E. Indium-111–labelled leucocyte scintigraphy

22. A 60-year-old woman presents with a 3-month history of malaise, anorexia and weight loss. She also reports experiencing epistaxis in the past 3 weeks. She has no significant past medical history. Physical examination showed that she had crackles in both lung fields and a rash on her lower limbs. Her other investigation results and chest X-ray are shown below. Urine analysis was ++ for protein and urine microscopy showed many red blood cells and granular casts. Name the most likely diagnosis paired with its supportive serological test.

	Value	Reference ranges
Haemoglobin (g/L)	108	115–155
Creatinine (μmol/L)	210	60–100
C-reactive protein (mg/L)	80	<10

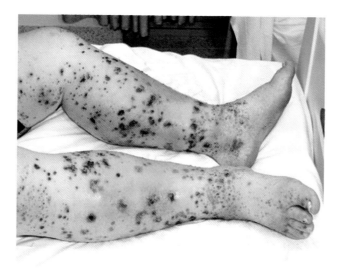

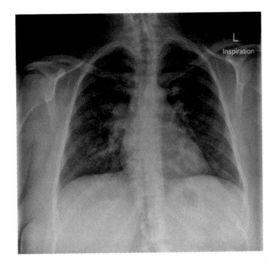

A. Systemic lupus erythematosus; anti-nuclear antibody (ANA)
B. Post-streptococcal glomerulonephritis; anti-streptolysin O titre (ASOT)
C. Goodpasture syndrome; anti-glomerular basement antibody
D. Wegener granulomatosis; anti-neutrophil cytoplasmic antibody (ANCA)
E. Cryoglobulinaemic vasculitis; cryoglobulin

23. A 46-year-old man presents with a painful and swollen left knee. He has no significant past medical history. Aspiration of the knee revealed calcium pyrophosphate crystals. The X-ray of his left knee is shown below. Which additional test should be performed?

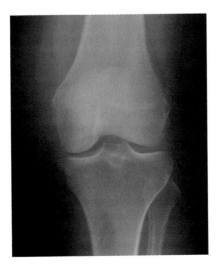

A. Skeletal survey
B. Parathyroid hormone
C. Lactate dehydrogenase
D. Serum electrophoresis
E. Serum light chain

24. A 35-year-old woman is admitted to the Intensive Care Unit because of adult respiratory distress syndrome and multiple cerebral micro-infarctions. She has a history of recurrent miscarriages but no history of thromboembolism. Her investigations reveal a creatinine of 250 μmol/L and urinalysis showing blood +++. Which one of the following investigations should be undertaken in this patient?
A. Protein C level and anti-thrombin III level
B. Protein S level and anti-thrombin III level
C. Anti-cardiolipin antibodies
D. Anti-glomerular basement membrane antibody
E. Complement levels (C3 and C4)

25. A 43-year-old man has experienced bilateral hand pain and swelling intermittently for the past 6 months. He indicates that the second and third distal interphalangeal joints on his right hand and the fourth distal interphalangeal joint on his left hand give him the most symptoms. Physical examination reveals fingers that are markedly swollen and inflamed, but are remarkably non-tender on palpation. Range of motion is preserved. Skin examination reveals no rash; however, the scalp has several small areas of silver scaling and he reports a previous scaly rash affecting his elbows. Which one of the following changes is most likely to be found on X-ray with this patient's condition?
A. Periarticular osteoporosis
B. Chondrocalcinosis in the wrist
C. Subchondral cysts
D. Periostitis at the distal phalanges
E. Subchondral bony sclerosis

26. Which one of the following is NOT included in the American College of Rheumatology (ACR) diagnostic criteria for systemic lupus erythematosus?
A. Alopecia
B. Non-erosive arthritis
C. Painless oral ulcer
D. Lymphopenia (<1.5 × 10^9 cells/L)
E. Warm antibody autoimmune haemolytic anaemia

27. A 17-year-old male with no prior medical history presented with arthralgia, abdominal pain and smoky-coloured urine. On examination a palpable rash was present on both legs (see below). Urine dipstick showed red blood cells but all other tests, including electrolytes, full blood count, liver function tests, complement levels, electrocardiography (ECG) and chest X-ray, were normal. What is the most likely diagnosis?

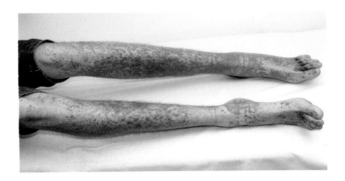

A. Erythema nodosum
B. Cryoglobulinemic vasculitis
C. Contact dermatitis
D. Erythema multiforme
E. Henoch–Schönlein purpura (HSP)

28. Amyloidosis is characterised by:
    A. Intracellular deposition of proteins which are remnants of nuclear break down
    B. Intracellular deposition of immunoglobulin light chains
    C. Extracellular tissue deposition of fibrils composed of low molecular weight subunits derived from a variety of proteins, many of which circulate as constituents of plasma
    D. Extracellular deposition of glycoproteins
    E. Extracellular deposition of antigen–antibody complexes and complement components

29. Which one of the following is a manifestation of systemic lupus erythematosus?
    A. Haemolytic anaemia
    B. Leucocytosis
    C. Lymphocytosis
    D. Eosinophilia
    E. Thrombocytosis

30. A 37-year-old woman with systemic lupus erythematosus (SLE) has been receiving glucocorticoid treatment for the past 4 years. Initially she received prednisolone 60 mg/day for 3 months, then gradually tapered down over 18 months. Her maintenance dose is 15 mg/day. She now complains of several weeks of right

groin pain and difficulty in walking; the groin pain also has occurred at rest for the past few days. She reports no falls or significant trauma. What diagnosis is likely?

A. Osteoporotic fracture of the neck of femur
B. Rheumatoid arthritis affecting the right hip joint
C. Right trochanteric bursitis
D. Gout affecting the right hip joint
E. Avascular necrosis of the right femoral head

31. A 50-year-old man who presented with Horner syndrome was found to have partial internal carotid artery dissection. He was noted to have stretchy skin and hyper-mobile joints. He has several scars, especially over his legs, and on being asked about these said that he tended to get extensive scars with minimum trauma. There was no significant family history and he had no other medical issues. What is the likely diagnosis?

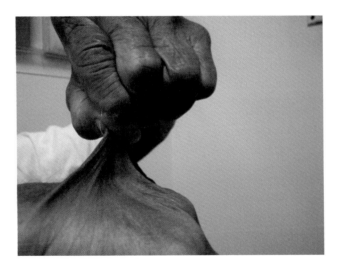

A. Marfan syndrome
B. Ehlers–Danlos syndrome
C. Tuberous sclerosis
D. Noonan syndrome
E. Klinefelter syndrome

Theme: Serological testing in rheumatological conditions (for Questions 32–35)

A. Anti-Scl-70 antibodies
B. Anti-double-stranded DNA antibodies
C. Anti-SSA or anti-Ro antibodies

    D. Antibodies to citrullinated peptides
    E. Anti-histone antibodies
    F. Anti-nuclear cytoplasmic antibodies
    G. Anti-ribosomal P protein antibodies
    H. Anti-U1 RNP antibodies

For each of the scenarios below, select the most appropriate antibody.

32. In patients with hydralazine-induced lupus, which antibody can be detected in more than 95% of cases?

33. In a woman with systemic lupus erythematosus, the presence of which antibody is associated with her children developing congenital heart block?

34. In a patient with systemic sclerosis, which antibody is associated with increased risk of interstitial lung disease?

35. In patients with rheumatoid arthritis, which antibody is associated with an increased risk of progressive joint damage?

Answers

BASIC SCIENCE

1. Answer B

Methotrexate is widely used for the treatment of rheumatoid arthritis (RA), other autoimmune conditions and in cancer chemotherapy. The mechanisms of action of methotrexate are complex. Methotrexate binds and inhibits dihydrofolate reductase. It inhibits nucleotide and DNA synthesis and cell replication by competitively inhibiting the conversion of dihydrofolate to the active tetrahydrofolate , yielding cytotoxic, immunosuppressive and anti-inflammatory action. Folinic acid rescue is usually given after methotrexate therapy to reduce myelosuppression but does not antagonise its anti-inflammatory effects.

The precise mechanism of its anti-inflammatory actions remain incompletely understood (Chan and Cronstein, 2010). There are several other pharmacological mechanisms of methotrexate action, including inhibition of purine and pyrimidine synthesis, suppression of transmethylation reactions with accumulation of polyamines, reduction of antigen-dependent T-cell proliferation, and promotion of adenosine release with adenosine-mediated suppression of inflammation. It is possible that a combination of these mechanisms is responsible for the anti-inflammatory effects of methotrexate. To date, the adenosine-mediated anti-inflammatory effect of methotrexate is the best supported by the in vitro, in vivo and clinical data. It is highly teratogenic and should be avoided in pregnancy, during breast feeding or when trying to conceive.

 Chan, E.S. and Cronstein, B.N. (2010). Methotrexate – how does it really work? *Nat Rev Rheumatol* 6, 175–178.
http://www.ncbi.nlm.nih.gov/pubmed/20197777

2. Answer D

P-ANCA-positive sera on indirect immunofluorescence, which is classically directed against the myeloperoxidase (MPO) antigen, may be associated with concomitant positivity directed against a variety of other neutrophil antigens, such as bactericidal permeability inhibitor (BPI), cathepsin G and lactoferrin (Wong et al., 2000).

In vasculitis, the two target antigens for ANCA are proteinase 3 (PR3) and myeloperoxidase (MPO). Both PR3 and MPO are located in azurophilic granules in the cytoplasm of neutrophils and peroxidase-positive lysosomes of monocytes.

Two types of ANCA assay are indirect immunofluorescence using alcohol-fixed buffy coat leucocytes and enzyme-linked immunosorbent assay (ELISA) using purified specific antigens. Of these two techniques, indirect immunofluorescence is more sensitive, while ELISA is more specific.

On indirect immunofluorescence positive for the C-ANCA pattern, staining is diffuse throughout the cytoplasm and the target antigen is PR3. This is positive in 90% of patients with granulomatosis with polyangitis (Wegener's). The P-ANCA pattern results from staining around the nucleus, which reflects an artefact of ethanol fixation. While the target antigen in this case is MPO, antibodies to a host of azurophilic granule proteins can cause a P-ANCA pattern and these include BPI, cathepsin G and lactoferrin. Approximately 70% of patients with microscopic polyangitis are positive for P-ANCA.

The optimal approach to testing for ANCA is to screen with cheaper immunofluorescence assays and to confirm positive results with ELISAs directed against vasculitis-specific target antigens.

Wong, R.C., Wilson, R, and Neil, J. (2000). M2-AMA do not directly produce ANCA indirect immunofluorescence patterns. *J Clin Pathol* 53, 643–646.
http://www.ncbi.nlm.nih.gov/pmc/articles/PMC1762931/

3. Answer B

The human leucocyte antigen (HLA)–DRB1 locus is associated with patients who are positive for rheumatoid factor or anti-citrullinated protein antibody (ACPA) (McInnes and Schett, 2011). Alleles that contain a common amino acid motif (QKRAA) in the HLA–DRB1 region, termed the shared epitope, confer particular susceptibility. These findings suggest that predisposing T-cell repertoire selection, antigen presentation, or alteration in peptide affinity plays a role in the mechanism of autoimmunity underlying rheumatoid arthritis. Other possible explanations for the link between rheumatoid arthritis and the shared epitope include molecular mimicry of the shared epitope by microbial proteins, T-cell senescence induced by shared epitope-containing HLA molecules, or a potential pro-inflammatory signalling function that is unrelated to the role of the shared epitope in antigen recognition. Smoking and exposure to silica increase the risk of rheumatoid arthritis among persons with susceptibility HLA–DR4 alleles. The HLA–DQB1*0602 genotype is associated with narcolepsy.

McInnes, I.B., and Schett, G. (2011). The pathogenesis of rheumatoid arthritis. *N Engl J Med* 365, 2205–2219.
http://www.ncbi.nlm.nih.gov/pubmed/22150039

4. Answer C

Various innate effector cells, including macrophages, mast cells and natural killer cells, are found in the synovial membrane, while neutrophils reside mainly in synovial fluid (McInnes and Schett, 2011). Macrophages are major effectors of synovitis and act through release of cytokines [e.g. tumour necrosis factor alpha (TNF-α), interleukin-1 and others], reactive oxygen intermediates and nitrogen intermediates. Neutrophils contribute to synovitis by synthesising prostaglandins, proteases and reactive oxygen intermediates. Mast cells that produce high levels of vasoactive amines, cytokines and chemokines also play a role.

Cytokine production that arises from numerous synovial cell populations is vital to the pathogenesis of rheumatoid arthritis (RA). Cytokine patterns may shift over time with early rheumatoid arthritis having a different cytokine profile to chronic disease. TNF-α plays a fundamental role through activation of cytokine and chemokine expression, expression of endothelial cell adhesion molecules, activation of synovial fibroblasts, promotion of angiogenesis and suppression of regulatory T cells. Interleukin-1 and interleukin-6 are also abundantly expressed in rheumatoid arthritis. TNF-α promotes activation of leucocytes, endothelial cells and synovial fibroblasts. Antibody-mediated suppression of interleukins, TNF-α and, more recently, JAK kinase may be of therapeutic benefit in RA (Fox, 2012).

Fox, D.A. (2012). Kinase inhibition – a new approach to the treatment of rheumatoid arthritis. *N Engl J Med* 367, 565–567.
http://www.ncbi.nlm.nih.gov/pubmed/22873537

McInnes, I.B. and Schett, G. (2011). The pathogenesis of rheumatoid arthritis. *N Engl J Med* 365, 2205–2219.
http://www.ncbi.nlm.nih.gov/pubmed/22150039

5. Answer B

Although not fully understood, gastrointestinal tract (GIT) involvement in scleroderma appears to be the result of autonomic nerve dysfunction of the GIT (Gabrielli et al., 2009; Gyger and Baron, 2012). In time, this autonomic nerve dysfunction leads to smooth muscle atrophy and eventually irreversible muscle fibrosis of the gut. As a consequence, hypomotility of the oesophagus, stomach, and small and large intestine are seen in patients with systemic sclerosis. Oesophageal dysmotility is associated with reflux and, eventually, strictures and even changes associated with Barrett oesophagus. Involvement of the stomach and small intestine is associated with gastroparesis and pseudo-obstruction, respectively. The presence of wide-mouth diverticula is pathognomonic of scleroderma. The lower two-thirds of the oesophagus show an absence of peristaltic waves and incompetence of the lower oesophageal sphincter. Achalasia is characterised by an increase, not a decrease, in activity of the lower oesophageal sphincter.

Gabrielli, A., Avvedimento, E.V., and Krieg, T. (2009). Scleroderma. *N Engl J Med* 360, 1989–2003.
http://www.ncbi.nlm.nih.gov/pubmed/19420368

Gyger, G. and Baron, M. (2012). Gastrointestinal manifestations of scleroderma: recent progress in evaluation, pathogenesis, and management. *Curr Rheumatol Rep* 14, 22–29.
http://link.springer.com/article/10.1007%2Fs11926-011-0217-3

6. Answer C

Immune complexes are central players in the tissue injury in systemic lupus erythematosus (SLE) (Tsokos, 2011). They are formed in large amounts as anti-nuclear antibodies (ANAs) bind to the abundant nuclear material in blood and tissues, and are not cleared promptly because the Fc and complement receptors are deficient. In active SLE, complement is activated and levels of C3 and C4 depressed. In the kidney, immune complexes accumulate in the subendothelial and mesangial areas first, followed by deposition in the basement membrane and subepithelial areas. Immune complexes containing cationic anti-DNA antibodies and antibodies against the collagen-like region of C1q have an increased tendency to accumulate in the kidney. Anti-DNA and anti-nucleosome antibodies contribute to lupus nephritis, and anti-chromatin–chromatin immune complexes are present in the mesangium of patients with lupus nephritis. In addition, immune complexes may accumulate in the skin and the central nervous system. Immune complexes may bind to receptors expressed by tissue-specific cells, alter their function and cause an influx of inflammatory cells by activating the complement cascade.

Anti-Ro antibodies, which may alter the function of myocytes and cells of the conduction system, have been linked to neonatal lupus and specifically to congenital heart block. The presence of anti-Ro antibodies calls for close fetal monitoring (neonatal lupus develops in only 2% of fetuses of mothers who are positive for such antibodies) and treatment. Some anti-DNA antibodies cross-react with N-methyl-D-aspartate receptors (NMDARs); these are widely distributed across the brain, with the highest density in the hippocampus and amygdala. Anti-NMDAR antibodies in the cerebrospinal fluid and brain in patients with SLE have been linked to neurocognitive defects. Some patients with SLE have antibodies against phospholipids and β_2-glycoprotein 1. The presence of such antibodies is linked to thrombotic events and fetal loss and is known as the anti-phospholipid syndrome. Anti-phospholipid antibodies interfere with the coagulation system (especially protein C) and the function of endothelial cells. These antibodies increase adhesion molecule expression on the surface of endothelial cells, induce the production of tissue factor and promote thrombosis.

Tsokos, G.C. (2011). Systemic lupus erythematosus. *N Engl J Med* 365, 2110–2121.
http://www.ncbi.nlm.nih.gov/pubmed/22129255

7. Answer H
Tocilizumab inhibits the activity of interleukin-6 (IL-6), a cytokine involved in the pathogenesis of rheumatoid arthritis (RA) and systemic juvenile idiopathic arthritis, by binding to its receptors. Elevated levels of IL-6 in the serum and synovial fluid of RA patients contribute to the chronic inflammatory process characterising RA and correlate positively with disease activity. Tocilizumab binds selectively and competitively to soluble and membrane-expressed IL-6 receptors, blocking IL-6 signal transduction. The combination therapy of tocilizumab and methotrexate was found to be more efficacious than tocilizumab monotherapy. As for its safety profile, tocilizumab was well tolerated by adult patients with early and long-standing RA.

8. Answer C
Anakinra is a recombinant form of human interleukin-1 (IL-1) receptor antagonist; it neutralises the activity of IL-1, which is involved in acute inflammatory

response. Anakinra has a half-life of 4–6 h and is administered as a 100-mg sub-cutaneous daily injection. It has been used for treating rheumatoid arthritis and may have a role in familial Mediterranean fever.

For Questions 7 and 8:

Kukar, M., Petryna, O., and Efthimiou, P. (2009). Biological targets in the treatment of rheumatoid arthritis: a comprehensive review of current and in-development biological disease modifying anti-rheumatic drugs. *Biologics* 3, 443–457.

http://www.ncbi.nlm.nih.gov/pmc/articles/PMC2763315/

CLINICAL

9. Answer E

The clinical presentation is consistent with an acute attack of gout (Neogi, 2011; Burns and Wortmann, 2011). Agents available for terminating the acute attack include colchicine, non-steroidal anti-inflammatory drugs (NSAIDs) and corticosteroids. Corticosteroids have been used more often in recent years in patients with multiple co-morbid conditions, because of the relatively low toxicity profile of these agents. Colchicine has been used for centuries to treat acute attacks of gout. However, many patients experience nausea, vomiting, abdominal cramps and diarrhoea with the dosages required to treat acute attacks of gout. Colchicine should be given more cautiously in elderly patients and in patients with renal or hepatic insufficiency. NSAIDs are useful in most patients with acute gout and remain the agents of choice for young, healthy patients without co-morbid diseases. The use of all NSAIDs is limited by the risks of gastric ulceration and gastritis, acute and chronic renal failure, fluid retention and interference with anti-hypertensive therapy. The use of intra-articular steroids after arthrocentesis is useful in providing relief, particularly in large effusions, in which the initial aspiration of fluid results in rapid relief of pain and tightness in the affected joint. Evaluation of the fluid can also provide diagnostic confirmation and exclude infection.

Burns, C.M. and Wortmann, R.L. (2011). Gout therapeutics: new drugs for an old disease. *Lancet* 377, 165–177.
http://www.sciencedirect.com/science/article/pii/S0140673610606654

Neogi, T. (2011). Clinical practice. Gout. *N Engl J Med* 364, 443–452.
http://www.ncbi.nlm.nih.gov/pubmed/21288096

10. Answer B

There are many case reports of toxicities related to tumour necrosis factor (TNF) inhibitors, including severe injection-site reactions, infection (particularly mycobacterial and opportunistic organisms), lymphoproliferative disorders, lupus-like autoimmune disease, demyelinating disease, haematological abnormalities including aplastic anaemia, and cardiac failure (Scott and Kingsley, 2006). These findings are important as infection (particularly pulmonary infection), cardiovascular disease and osteoporosis cause the greatest morbidity and mortality in rheumatoid arthritis.

Many infections can occur in patients treated with TNF inhibitors, especially in patients over 65 years of age. These include serious bacterial infections, tuberculosis, atypical mycobacterial infection, aspergillosis, histoplasmosis, listeriosis, *Pneumocystis jirovecii* pneumonia and cryptococcal infections. Reactivation of tuberculosis has been reported in association with all TNF inhibitors. This usually occurs within the first 2–5 months of commencing treatment. The majority of cases present as extra-pulmonary and disseminated tuberculosis. A recent study has shown that screening for previous pulmonary tuberculosis with chest X-ray and Mantoux testing followed by appropriate treatment before starting TNF inhibitors, significantly reduces the incidence of tuberculosis. Latent viral infections such as herpes simplex virus (including genital herpes), herpes zoster virus and cytomegalovirus may be reactivated.

The development of systemic or localised infection warrants cessation or postponement of TNF inhibitor therapy. Treatment can be continued after the infection has resolved. For patients exposed to shingles during therapy, their serological status should be obtained. Those with a negative serology will require treatment with zoster immunoglobulin to prevent disseminated infection. For major surgery, it is prudent to interrupt TNF inhibitor treatment until the risk of postoperative infection has declined. Minor surgery does not require cessation of therapy.

The current contraindications for TNF inhibitors include:
- Previous untreated tuberculosis
- Recurrent chest infections/bronchiectasis
- Septic arthritis within 12 months
- Infected prosthesis
- Indwelling urinary catheter
- Multiple sclerosis/demyelinating illness
- Malignancy within 10 years (apart from fully resected basal cell carcinoma more than 5 years before)
- Pregnancy and lactation
- Congestive heart failure
- Chronic cutaneous ulceration (but not pyoderma gangrenosum).

 Scott, D.L. and Kingsley, G.H. (2006). Tumor necrosis factor inhibitors for rheumatoid arthritis. *N Engl J Med* 355, 704–712.
http://www.ncbi.nlm.nih.gov/pubmed/16914706

11. Answer A

The patient's presentation is highly consistent with familial Mediterranean fever (FMF), which is a hereditary autoinflammatory disease characterised by recurrent and short duration (1–3 days) of fever, and serositis (peritonitis or pleuritis, arthritis, myalgia or erysipelas-like skin lesions) (Onen, 2006). It is usually inherited as an autosomal recessive condition due to mutations in the gene encoding pyrin. The continuous inflammation in FMF is associated with increased serum amyloid A (SAA) protein, which may lead to secondary amyloidosis and deposition of this insoluble protein in the kidney, gut, spleen, liver, heart, etc. Therefore, treatment of patients with FMF is beneficial not only for the prevention of the acute attacks but also for improving their prognosis.

Colchicine is the main therapeutic option in FMF. It is effective in various manifestations of the disease, such as fever, peritonitis and pleuritis. It prevents the development of amyloidosis. It is less effective in arthritis or myalgia, requiring additional treatment with NSAIDs and steroids. In the few cases where FMF is resistant to colchicine, other measures, including corticosteroids, non-biological and biological disease-modifying anti-rheumatic drugs (DMARDs), interferon-alpha and thalidomide should be employed. Because colchicine crosses the placenta, considerable concern exists about the potential mutagenic and teratogenic effects of this medication. In some reports, colchicine therapy during conception and the first trimester of pregnancy had no adverse effects on the offspring.

There are several other periodic fever syndromes, Muckle–Wells syndrome, the familial cold autoinflammatory syndrome and neonatal-onset multisystem inflammatory disease, which are due to mutations in cryopyrin whose function is central to innate immunity and the function of the inflammasome (Drenth and van der Meer, 2006).

Drenth, J.P. and van der Meer, J.W. (2006). The inflammasome – a linebacker of innate defense. *N Engl J Med* 355, 730–732.
http://www.ncbi.nlm.nih.gov/pubmed/16914711

Onen, F. (2006). Familial Mediterranean fever. *Rheumatol Int* 26, 489–496.
http://link.springer.com/article/10.1007%2Fs00296-005-0074-3

12. Answer C

This woman shows overlapping symptoms of connective tissue diseases. The most specific serological test for mixed connective tissue disease (MTCD) is anti-RNP. MCTD is a well-defined entity with mixed clinical features of rheumatoid arthritis (RA), systemic lupus erythematosus (SLE), systemic sclerosis (SSc), and polymyositis (PM)/dermatomyositis (DM) (Ortega-Hernandez and Shoenfeld, 2012). MCTD is more prevalent in women in the third decade; however, it has also been reported in children and in patients over 80 years of age. The most common clinical features at the onset of disease are Raynaud phenomenon, polyarthralgias, swollen hands, sausage-like fingers and muscle weakness. Fatigue and myalgias are also frequently observed. MCTD was once thought to be a benign disease with good prognosis. However, some patients may have mild self-limited disease, whereas others may have major life-threatening organ involvement. MCTD has systemic manifestations and patients can develop pulmonary arterial hypertension, glomerulonephritis, vasculitis, oesophageal dysfunction, gastrointestinal bleeding and severe central nervous involvement. Patients with pulmonary arterial hypertension have the highest mortality rate and the worst prognosis. Currently there is no consensus about the treatment of MCTD. In general, corticosteroids, hydroxychloroquine and cyclophosphamide are the most commonly used immunosuppressants.

Ortega-Hernandez, O.D. and Shoenfeld, Y. (2012). Mixed connective tissue disease: an overview of clinical manifestations, diagnosis and treatment. *Best Pract Res Clin Rheumatol* 26, 61–72.
http://www.ncbi.nlm.nih.gov/pubmed/22424193

13. Answer C

Polyarteritis nodosa (PAN) is a rare systemic vasculitis causing necrotising inflammation of medium-sized (muscular) or small arteries without glomerulonephritis or vasculitis in arterioles, capillaries, or venules (Colmegna and Maldonado-Cocco, 2005). PAN should be suspected in patients with constitutional symptoms and multisystem involvement. PAN may be 'idiopathic' where no identifiable associated pathogen is found or 'secondary' to a known cause (most frequently associated with hepatitis B infection). Association with other pathogens, including Group A streptococcus, hepatitis C virus, human T-cell leukaemia virus-1, cytomegalovirus, Epstein–Barr virus and parvovirus B19, have been found. Other diseases, such as hairy cell leukaemia, Sjögren syndrome and rheumatoid arthritis, have also been linked to PAN.

Clinical features suggestive of vasculitis include skip lesions of varying chronological ages not corresponding to a single vascular supply, ischaemic regions in skin, kidneys, gastrointestinal tract and testes (causing orchitis from testicular artery ischaemia). The 'gold standard' for the diagnosis of PAN is the demonstration of focal, segmental pan-mural necrotising inflammation of medium-sized arteries with a predilection for bifurcations and branch points of muscular arteries. Multiple aneurysms and less often stenosis, luminal irregularities and occlusions can be observed in segmental branches of renal arteries and can cause perirenal haematomas, renal infarctions and renin-mediated hypertension.

PAN affects all organ systems other than the pulmonary system for unknown reasons. In patients with systemic vasculitis the findings of orchitis, anti-neutrophil cytoplasmic antibodies negativity and abnormal renal or mesenteric angiography in the absence of glomerulonephritis are highly suggestive of PAN. Treatment for idiopathic PAN includes corticosteroids and cyclophosphamide, whereas hepatitis-related PAN is treated with plasmapheresis and anti-viral agents.

Colmegna, I. and Maldonado-Cocco, J.A. (2005). Polyarteritis nodosa revisited. *Curr Rheumatol Rep* 7, 288–296.
http://www.ncbi.nlm.nih.gov/pubmed/16045832

14. Answer D

This patient's presentation is most compatible with polymyositis (Mammen, 2010). Extramuscular manifestations are frequently seen in patients with polymyositis. The joints, skin, cardiac and pulmonary systems, and the gastrointestinal tract are affected. One of the most common finding is interstitial lung disease (ILD). Cardiac manifestations include arrhythmia, conduction abnormalities, cardiac arrest, congestive heart failure, myocarditis, pericarditis, angina and secondary fibrosis. Joint involvement is characterised by arthralgia and arthritis. It is usually noted early in the course of disease, involving the wrists, knees and small joints of the hands. Joint involvement is classically non-erosive and frequently responsive to the treatment of the underlying inflammatory myopathy. Extramuscular organ involvement, such as cardiac involvement and ILD, is associated with a worse prognosis.

Autoantibodies to nuclear RNAs and certain cytoplasmic antigens involved in protein synthesis are observed in up to 55% of patients with polymyositis. Anti-Jo-1 is one of the anti-synthetase antibodies currently found only in patients with myositis (about 20–30%). Besides pulmonary fibrosis, the anti-synthetase syndrome includes Raynaud phenomenon, polyarthritis and, in some cases, so-called mechanic's hands. The last condition causes cracked and fissured skin on the hands.

Anti-dsDNA and anti-Sm are autoantibodies found only in systemic lupus erythematosus, anti-Scl-70 is seen in patients with scleroderma, and anti-SSA is found in patients with either systemic lupus erythematosus or Sjögren syndrome.

Mammen, A.L. (2010). Dermatomyositis and polymyositis: Clinical presentation, autoantibodies, and pathogenesis. *Ann N Y Acad Sci* 1184, 134–153.
http://www.ncbi.nlm.nih.gov/pubmed/20146695

15. Answer C
Reiter syndrome or reactive arthritis usually manifests with urethritis, conjunctivitis and seronegative arthritis (Carter and Hudson, 2009). The typical patient is a young male with a recent history of urethritis or dysentery, and joint symptoms commonly occur 1–4 weeks after the initial infection. The associated infective agents include urethritis due to chlamydia trachomatis and enteric infections due to campylobacter, shigella, yersinia and salmonellae. The seronegative arthritis is usually either a mono- or oligo-arthritis, particularly in the legs. The arthritis may relapse or remain chronic in 15% of patients.

Other features may include conjunctivitis, anterior uveitis, keratoderma blenorrhagica (a hyperkeratotic brownish rash on the palms and soles), mouth ulcers, plantar fasciitis and Achilles tendinitis (enthesopathy), circinate balanitis and aortic incompetence. There is an increased prevalence of HLA-B27 in affected individuals (50%). The disease is self-limiting in the majority of patients and management includes treatment of the underlying infection and non-steroidal anti-inflammatory drugs. Glucocorticoid injection of severely affected joints can be helpful and in severe cases, systemic treatment with glucocorticoids, sulphasalazine, methotrexate or even tumour necrosis factor (TNF) inhibitors can be considered.

Carter, J.D. and Hudson, A.P. (2009). Reactive arthritis: clinical aspects and medical management. *Rheum Dis Clin North Am* 35, 21–44.
http://www.ncbi.nlm.nih.gov/pubmed/19480995

16. Answer B
In approximately 75% of patients with rheumatoid arthritis (RA), the disease waxes and wanes in severity over a number of years. A favourable course and long remissions are associated with acute onset restricted to a few large joints, disease duration of less than 1 year, and negative test results for rheumatoid factor (RF) (da Mota et al., 2010; Scott et al., 2010).

Factors that suggest a worse joint and functional prognosis include early (before age 20 years) or late (after age 60 years) onset of the disease, a greater number of involved joints (>20), persistently changing inflammatory indicators, high titres of RF, positivity for anti-cyclic citrullinated peptide (CCP) antibodies, and early development of radiological erosion. Patients with the most aggressive form of the disease experience a significant loss in quality of life and a shortened life expectancy. Early aggressive management with disease-modifying agents is clearly indicated for patients with an unfavourable prognosis.

da Mota, L.M., Laurindo, I.M., de Carvalho, J.F., and dos Santos-Neto, L.L. (2010). Prognostic evaluation of early rheumatoid arthritis. *Swiss Med Wkly* 140, w13100.
http://www.smw.ch/content/smw-2010-13100/

Scott, D.L., Wolfe, F., and Huizinga, T.W. (2010). Rheumatoid arthritis. *Lancet* 376, 1094–1108.
http://www.ncbi.nlm.nih.gov/pubmed/20870100

17. Answer D

The knee is affected in over 50% of acute attacks of pseudogout, whereas the first metatarsophalangeal joint is most frequently involved in gout. Pseudogout describes acute attacks of calcium pyrophosphate dihydrate (CPPD) crystal-induced synovitis, which clinically often resembles urate gout. However, the majority of individuals with CPPD crystal deposition remain asymptomatic.

The term chondrocalcinosis refers to CPPD crystal deposits typically appearing as punctate and linear radiodensities in fibrocartilage, hyaline or articular cartilage. While commonly present in patients with pseudogout, this radiological finding is neither absolutely specific for CPPD nor universally present among affected patients. Although most cases of CPPD deposition are idiopathic, association is seen with joint trauma, familial chondrocalcinosis (autosomal dominant inheritance), haemochromatosis, hyperparathyroidism, hypomagnesaemia, and hypophosphatasia.

During an acute attack, synovial fluid analysis by polarised light microscopy shows positively birefringent CPPD crystals within polymorphonuclear leucocytes. In contrast, negatively birefringent monosodium urate crystals are seen in acute gouty arthritis.

Treatment consists of joint aspiration (both for diagnosis and for treatment) combined with intra-articular glucocorticoid injection. When more than two joints are inflamed, medical therapy using an oral non-steroidal anti-inflammatory drug or colchicine is preferred.

18. Answer D

The shooting pains in her arms, hyper-reflexia and hypertonia suggest that this patient may have atlantoaxial subluxation (AAS) secondary to erosion or stretching of the transverse ligament that holds the odontoid process in place anterior to the spinal cord. Impingement or compression of the cervical cord can result, especially when the neck is flexed forward. It is essential to document the presence or absence of subluxation, particularly when general anaesthesia is planned for total hysterectomy (Fombon and Thompson, 2006). The mortality rate of patients with AAS is eight times higher than that of unaffected patients. The magnitude of AAS can appear smaller when measured by functional magnetic resonance imaging (MRI) rather than by functional radiography; for this reason, MRI is the modality of choice for detecting possible spinal cord compression in severe rheumatoid arthritis.

Although the combination of alopecia and oral ulcers may suggest that the patient also has systemic lupus erythematosus, methotrexate can cause alopecia and oral ulcers. Autoantibody testing is not a high priority. Cryoglobulins are rarely present in rheumatoid arthritis. Addition of a tumour necrosis factor-α (TNF-α) inhibitor may be appropriate if serious cervical spine disease does not preclude hysterectomy. In this case it would be appropriate to defer TNF-α inhibition therapy until she is stable after surgery. It is also important to ensure that there are no contraindications to anti-TNF-α therapy, such as evidence of infection or previous tuberculosis (Scott et al., 2010).

Scott, D.L., Wolfe, F., and Huizinga, T.W. (2010). Rheumatoid arthritis. *Lancet* 376, 1094–1108.
http://www.ncbi.nlm.nih.gov/pubmed/20870100

Fombon, F.N. and Thompson, J.P. (2006). Anaesthesia for the adult patient with rheumatoid arthritis. *Contin Educ Anaesth Crit Care Pain* 6, 235–239.
http://ceaccp.oxfordjournals.org/content/6/6/235.full

19. Answer B

The patient has primary Sjögren syndrome and this predisposes to lymphoma (Kokosi et al., 2010). The risk of lymphoma in patients with Sjögren syndrome is 44 times higher than the incidence in an age-matched healthy population. It has been estimated by several studies that 4–8% of patients with Sjögren syndrome will develop lymphoma in the course of their disease. The most common type is non-Hodgkin lymphoma. Multiple histological types of non-Hodgkin lymphoma have been described in patients with Sjögren syndrome, such as follicular, lymphoplasmacytoid and diffuse large B-cell lymphoma, with mucosa-associated lymphoid tissue (MALT) lymphoma, a subtype of marginal zone B-cell lymphoma, being the most frequent. The presence of severe involvement of the exocrine glands, vasculitis, hypocomplementaemia, and cryoglobulinaemia at diagnosis increases the risk of developing lymphoma among patients with Sjögren syndrome. The prevalence of primary pulmonary lymphoma is estimated to be 1–2% in patients with Sjögren syndrome.

Kokosi, M., Riemer, E.C., and Highland, K.B. (2010). Pulmonary involvement in Sjogren syndrome. *Clin Chest Med* 31, 489–500.
http://www.ncbi.nlm.nih.gov/pubmed/20692541

20. Answer C

This patient's clinical presentation is typical for temporal arteritis. Temporal artery biopsy should be performed as soon as possible, but should not delay the commencement of oral corticosteroid treatment. The major risk is the rapid development of irreversible visual loss. Although corticosteroid treatment will reduce the chance of a positive biopsy result, this is unlikely with just 1 day of therapy. Diagnostic results have been reported up to a week and even 3–6 months after starting corticosteroids (Salvarani et al., 2008). C-reactive protein (CRP) and erythrocyte sedimentation rate (ESR) are commonly elevated in temporal arteritis.

The biopsy should be taken from the clinically affected side. The sensitivity of the biopsy depends on its quality, particularly its length and its preparation for histological examination. The artery lesions can be segmental. If the biopsy is negative and the diagnosis of temporal arteritis is highly suspected clinically, the other superficial temporal artery should be biopsied. If both biopsies are negative, the diagnosis is clinical. The corticosteroid should not be discontinued suddenly for the purpose of obtaining a biopsy.

Salvarani, C., Cantini, F., and Hunder, G.G. (2008). Polymyalgia rheumatica and giant-cell arteritis. *Lancet* 372, 234–245.
http://www.ncbi.nlm.nih.gov/pubmed/18640460

21. Answer C

This patient has neurological impairment and clinical features of vertebral osteomyelitis. magnetic resonance imaging (MRI) should be the first diagnostic step to rule out nerve compression from a herniated disc and to look for an epidural, a paravertebral or a disc-space abscess (Zimmerli, 2010). MRI has a high accuracy (90%) for diagnosing spinal osteomyelitis. It shows high-signal intensity within the disc on T2-weighted sequences and loss of the intranuclear cleft in patients with vertebral osteomyelitis. MRI also shows rapidly-destroyed vertebral endplates and high-signal-intensity marrow oedema. The blood culture is positive for the likely causative organism so a biopsy is unlikely to add information. If blood culture is negative and MRI shows evidence of vertebral osteomyelitis, a CT-guided or an open biopsy is required to identify microorganisms to guide antibiotic selection. Bone scans are positive a few days after the onset of symptoms. However, the findings are not specific for vertebral osteomyelitis, with a reported accuracy of 67%. Indium-111-labelled leucocyte scintigraphy and anti-granulocyte scintigraphy are more specific for the diagnosis of an epidural abscess but have a low sensitivity for vertebral osteomyelitis (<20%).

Staphylococcus aureus is the most common organism involved, followed by *Escherichia coli*. In patients with recent spinal surgery, coagulase-negative staphylococci and *Propionibacterium acnes* are most commonly identified to cause vertebral osteomyelitis, particularly if fixation devices are used. However, in patients with prolonged bacteraemia (e.g. infection associated with pacemaker electrodes), a low-virulence microorganism, such as coagulase-negative staphylococci, has been described to cause haematogenous vertebral osteomyelitis. A source of bacteraemia such as endocarditis should be considered.

Although clinical trials are lacking, it is generally recommended to treat vertebral osteomyelitis with organism-specific antibiotics for 6 weeks.

Zimmerli, W. (2010). Clinical practice. Vertebral osteomyelitis. *N Engl J Med* 362, 1022–1029.
http://www.ncbi.nlm.nih.gov/pubmed/20237348

22. Answer D

The clinical presentation and initial investigation results are suggestive of Wegener granulomatosis because of pulmonary and renal involvement. In Wegener granulomatosis there is often pulmonary haemorrhage, haemoptysis, epistaxis, infiltrates on chest X-ray, as well as possible cavitation. It is also associated with rapidly progressive segmental necrotising glomerulonephritis (in about 75% of patients) that may lead to renal insufficiency.

A diffuse, cytoplasmic pattern of staining results from binding of anti-neutrophil cytoplasmic antibody (ANCA) to antigen targets throughout the neutrophil cytoplasm, the most common protein target being proteinase 3 (PR3) (Bosch et al., 2006).

Bosch, X., Guilabert, A., and Font, J. (2006). Antineutrophil cytoplasmic antibodies. *Lancet* 368, 404–418.
http://www.ncbi.nlm.nih.gov/pubmed/16876669

23. Answer B

Definite diagnosis of calcium pyrophosphate dihydrate (CPPD) deposition is based on the demonstration of CPPD crystals in the synovial fluid. Acute crystal-induced synovitis due to CPPD crystals is possibly the most common cause of acute mono-arthritis in the elderly. Any joint may be involved, but the knees and wrists are the commonest sites. As with gout, the attack is self-limiting. Several provoking factors are recognised, the most common being stress response to intercurrent illness or surgery, including lavage of the affected joint.

The knee X-ray reveals chondrocalcinosis (radiographic calcification in hyaline and/or fibrocartilage). It is commonly present in patients with CPPD crystal deposition disease but is neither absolutely specific for CPPD nor universal among affected patients. Haemochromatosis is associated with the full spectrum of CPPD crystal-related joint disease (i.e. pseudogout, chondrocalcinosis and chronic arthropathy). A variety of metabolic and endocrine disorders other than haemochromatosis are associated with CPPD crystal deposition. Clinical or radiographic evidence for CPPD crystal deposition disease, therefore, warrants exclusion of these disorders, particularly among younger individuals. The following have been associated with CPPD:

- Hyperparathyroidism, hypomagnesemia and hypophosphatasia
- Gitelman syndrome

- Hypothyroidism
- X-linked hypophosphataemic rickets
- Familial hypocalciuric hypercalcaemia.

 Richette, P., Bardin, T., and Doherty, M. (2009). An update on the epidemiology of calcium pyrophosphate dihydrate crystal deposition disease. *Rheumatology (Oxf)* 48, 711–715.
http://rheumatology.oxfordjournals.org/content/48/7/711.long

24. Answer C

The constellation of recurrent miscarriages, lung and renal disease with cerebral micro-infarctions suggests the patient may have anti-phospholipid syndrome ('Hughes syndrome'). A patient with the anti-phospholipid syndrome (APS) must meet at least one of two clinical criteria (vascular thrombosis or complications of pregnancy) and at least one of the laboratory criteria [lupus anti-coagulant, anti-cardiolipin (aCL) antibody and/or anti-β2 glycoprotein-I (anti-β2GPI) antibody present on two or more occasions, at least 12 weeks apart) (Lim, 2009). In general, lupus anti-coagulant antibodies are more specific for the anti-phospholipid syndrome, whereas anti-cardiolipin antibodies are more sensitive. The specificity of anti-cardiolipin antibodies for APS increases with titre and is higher for the IgG than for the IgM isotope. However, there is no definitive association between specific clinical manifestations and particular subgroups of anti-phospholipid antibodies. There are a variety of other clinical and laboratory manifestations that may be present including heart valve disease, livedo reticularis, thrombocytopenia, nephropathy, neurological manifestations, IgA aCL, IgA anti-β2GPI, anti-phosphatidylserine antibodies (aPS), anti-phosphatidyl ethanolamine(aPE) antibodies, antibodies against prothrombin alone (aPT-A), and antibodies to the phosphatidylserine–prothrombin (aPS/PT) complex.

'Catastrophic' APS is defined by the clinical involvement of at least three different organ systems over a period of days or weeks with histopathological evidence of multiple occlusions of large or small vessels. Venous or arterial thrombosis of large vessels is less common in patients with catastrophic APS, who tend to present with an acute thrombotic microangiopathy affecting small vessels of multiple organs. The kidney is the organ most commonly affected (in 78%) followed by the lungs (66%), the central nervous system (56%), the heart (50%) and the skin (50%).

 Lim, W. (2009). Antiphospholipid antibody syndrome. *Hematology Am Soc Hematol Educ Program*, 233–239.
http://asheducationbook.hematologylibrary.org/content/2009/1/233.long

25. Answer D

The patient in the vignette is suspected to have psoriatic arthritis. A characteristic change is the whittling of the distal ends of phalanges, giving the joints a so-called pencil-in-cup appearance, which is radiographically distinctive for psoriatic arthritis. Periostitis, bony erosions and joint effusions are also common. Subchondral cysts and bony sclerosis are seen in X-ray changes of osteoarthritis. Soft tissue swelling, periarticular osteoporosis and marginal erosions of the bone are seen in the early stage of rheumatoid arthritis. Chondrocalcinosis in the wrist, knee and symphysis pubis is typically seen with calcium pyrophosphate deposition disease.

Psoriatic arthritis is an inflammatory arthritis occurring in patients with psoriasis. The Classification Criteria for Psoriatic Arthritis study group has recently developed a set of classification criteria for psoriatic arthritis with a sensitivity of 91.4% and a specificity of 98.7%. Three main clinical patterns have been identified: oligoarticular (four or fewer involved joints) or polyarticular (five or more involved joints) peripheral disease and axial disease with or without associated peripheral arthritis. Recurrent episodes of enthesitis and dactylitis are also seen in psoriatic arthritis. The severity of psoriatic arthritis is not correlated with the extent of skin disease. Psoriasis appears to precede the onset of psoriatic arthritis in 60–80% of patients. However, in as many as 15–20% of patients, arthritis appears before the psoriasis.

Although used previously, hydroxychloroquine is no longer recommended for use in the treatment of psoriatic arthritis (Gossec et al., 2012). Use of oral glucocorticoids in patients with psoriatic arthritis should be avoided, since there is a chance of developing pustular psoriasis. Care should be taken in patients who require intra-articular glucocorticoid injections to avoid injection through psoriatic plaques. Methotrexate is commonly used in the treatment of psoriatic arthritis and there is an increasing use of anti-tumour necrosis factor (TNF) agents.

Gossec, L., Smolen, J.S., Gaujoux-Viala, C., et al. (2012). European League Against Rheumatism recommendations for the management of psoriatic arthritis with pharmacological therapies. *Ann Rheum Dis* 71, 4–12.
http://ard.bmj.com/content/71/1/4.full

26. Answer A
Systemic lupus erythematosus (SLE) is an autoimmune disease that has protean manifestations and follows a relapsing and remitting course. It is characterised by an autoantibody response to nuclear and cytoplasmic antigens. SLE can affect any organ system, but mainly involves the skin, joints, kidneys, haematological and nervous system. American College of Rheumatology (ACR) criteria summarise features necessary for diagnosis:

- Serositis: Pleurisy, pericarditis on examination or diagnostic electrocardiogram (ECG) or imaging
- Oral ulcers: Oral or nasopharyngeal, usually painless; palate is most specific
- Arthritis: Non-erosive, two or more peripheral joints with tenderness or swelling
- Photosensitivity: Unusual skin reaction to light exposure
- Blood disorders: Leukopenia ($<4 \times 10^9$ cells/L on more than one occasion), lymphopenia ($<1.5 \times 10^9$ cells/L on more than one occasion), thrombocytopenia

($<100 \times 10^9$ cells/L in the absence of offending medications), haemolytic anaemia

- Renal involvement: Proteinuria (>0.5 g/day or 3+ positive on dipstick testing) or cellular casts
- Anti-nuclear antibodies (ANAs): Higher titres generally more specific ($>1:160$); must be in the absence of medications associated with drug-induced lupus
- Immunological phenomena: dsDNA; anti-Smith (Sm) antibodies; anti-phospholipid antibodies [anti-cardiolipin immunoglobulin G (IgG) or immunoglobulin M (IgM) or lupus anti-coagulant]; biological false-positive serological test results for syphilis, lupus erythematosus (LE) cells (omitted in 1997 revised criteria)
- Neurological disorder: Seizures or psychosis in the absence of other causes
- Malar rash: Fixed erythema over the cheeks and nasal bridge, flat or raised
- Discoid rash: Erythematous raised-rimmed lesions with keratotic scaling and follicular plugging, often scarring.

Although alopecia is common in SLE, it is not include in the ACR diagnostic criteria in SLE.

27. Answer E

The combination of palpable purpura, arthritis/arthralgia, abdominal pain and haematuria in a young person is highly suggestive of Henoch–Schönlein purpura (HSP). HSP is an immune-mediated vasculitis associated with immunoglobulin A (IgA) deposition. Skin biopsy shows leucocytoclastic vasculitis with IgA staining of superficial dermal vessels. Some degree of renal involvement is seen in 20–54% of children with higher degrees of involvement in adults. Renal biopsy primarily shows IgA deposition in the mesangium in both HSP and IgA nephropathy, suggesting a similar pathogenesis.

Erythema nodosum usually presents as tender nodules of 1–10 cm in diameter on the lower limbs; these tend to coalesce and turn bluish purple, brownish or green over days to weeks.

Patients with cryoglobulinemic vasculitis will present with palpable purpura and may have arthralgia and nephritis. However, they usually have low complement levels.

Erythema multiform varies from a mild, self-limited rash to a severe, life-threatening condition that also involves mucous membranes. The commoner mild form usually presents with mildly itchy, pink–red papules, symmetrically arranged and starting on the extremities, which often take on the classical 'target lesion' appearance (central erosion on an erythematous base, surrounded by a pale oedematous rim and a peripheral erythematous halo).

 Roberts, P.F., Waller, T.A., Brinker, T.M., et al (2007). Henoch-Schönlein purpura. *South Med J* 100, 821–824.
http://www.ncbi.nlm.nih.gov/pubmed/17713309

28. Answer C

Amyloidosis is a generic term that refers to the extracellular tissue deposition of fibrils composed of low molecular weight subunits derived from a variety of proteins, many of which circulate as constituents of plasma. The generation of these fibrils is the result of misfolding of extracellular protein, often in parallel with or as an alternative to physiological folding, generating insoluble, toxic protein aggregates that are deposited in tissues in bundles of β-sheet fibrillar protein (Merlini et al., 2003).

While several types of amyloidosis are hereditary with clinical disease linked to missense mutations of the precursor proteins, mostly it arises sporadically. The commonest are AL amyloidosis and AA amyloidosis. While the former is due to deposition of protein derived from immunoglobulin light chain fragments, the latter condition is seen in chronic diseases where there is ongoing or recurring inflammation, such as rheumatoid arthritis, spondyloarthropathy, or inflammatory bowel disease with the fibrils being composed of fragments of the acute phase reactant serum amyloid A (SAA).

All amyloid deposits contain serum amyloid P (SAP), a glycoprotein that binds amyloid independently of the protein of origin. It has a specific binding motif for the common conformation of amyloid fibrils and this property makes radiolabelled SAP a diagnostic tool for the imaging of amyloid deposits.

Merlini, G. and Bellotti, V. (2003). Molecular mechanisms of amyloidosis. *N Engl J Med* 349, 583–596.
http://www.ncbi.nlm.nih.gov/pubmed/12904524

29. Answer A

Haematological abnormalities are present at some stage in the majority of systemic lupus erythematosus (SLE) patients. Normochromic normocytic anaemia occurs in 75% and warm-type autoimmune haemolytic anaemia in 10–20%. Low total white cell count is an important clinical feature in SLE and lymphopenia is the commonest, occurring in 65%. Neutropenia (<1.0 × 10⁹ cells/L) occurs in 10–20%. Mild thrombocytopenia is common, but more severe thrombocytopenia is unusual (<10%) and many precede the diagnosis by years. SLE is also associated with anti-phospholipid antibodies, which predisposes to thrombosis.

30. Answer E

Osteonecrosis, also known as avascular necrosis or aseptic necrosis, is a pathological process that is associated most notably with corticosteroid use and excessive alcohol intake. The overall incidence of osteonecrosis as a consequence of steroid therapy is about 4–25%. Patients treated with prolonged high doses of corticosteroids appear to be at the greatest risk of developing osteonecrosis; however, these patients often have other risk factors. A high index of suspicion is necessary for those with known or probable risk factors, particularly high-dose steroid use. Magnetic resonance imaging (MRI) is far more sensitive than plain radiographs or bone scanning in making the diagnosis, with a sensitivity approaching 100%.

Therefore, MRI is effective in the evaluation of suspected osteonecrosis when plain X-ray or bone scintigraphy is negative or equivocal.

31. Answer B

Ehlers–Danlos syndrome (EDS) is a heterogeneous group of inherited connective tissue disorders characterised by hyperelasticity and fragility of the skin and hypermobilty of the joints. It is caused by a genetic defect in collagen and connective tissue synthesis and structure.

The underlying defect in collagen synthesis has been identified in most but not all of the 11 types of EDS. EDS type IV, which is characterised by a decreased amount of type III collagen, can lead to arterial aneurysms and rupture, valvular prolapse, intestinal perforation and spontaneous pneumothorax. Pregnancy can increase the likelihood of a uterine or vascular rupture in women suffering from EDS type IV.

Individuals with Marfan syndrome present with characteristic skeletal findings, including long bones and arachnodactyly, joint laxity and aortic root disease leading to aortic regurgitation and dissection.

Individuals with tuberous sclerosis present with characteristic skin lesions (hypopigmented macules, angiofibromas, shagreen patches), central nervous system lesions (cortical glioneural hamartomas and subependymal nodules), seizures, cognitive defects, renal angiomyolipomas and benign renal cysts, and characteristic pulmonary disease known as lymphangioleiomyomatosis.

The cardinal features of Noonan syndrome include unusual facies (i.e. hypertelorism, down-slanting eyes, webbed neck), congenital heart disease (in 50%), short stature and chest deformity.

32. Answer E

Anti-histone antibodies are present in more than 95% of cases of drug-induced lupus; this percentage is representative for those taking procainamide, hydralazine, chlorpromazine and quinidine; however, anti-histone antibodies have been found in a smaller proportion of patients with drug-induced lupus associated with other medications, including minocycline, propylthiouracil and statins. Other autoantibodies are uncommon in this disorder. Anti-histone antibodies are also seen in up to 80% of patients with idiopathic lupus; however, patients with idiopathic systemic lupus erythematosus (SLE) also form a variety of other autoantibodies, including those directed against DNA and small ribonucleoproteins.

The anti-histone antibodies in drug-induced lupus are primarily formed against a complex of the histone dimer H2A–H2B and DNA. DNA is required either to stabilise the complex or perhaps to contribute part of the antigenic epitope. Although the drugs that can cause drug-induced lupus are heterogeneous, there may be a common pathway for disease induction since the autoantibodies produced in patients receiving procainamide, hydralazine, quinidine, acebutolol, penicillamine, isoniazide and chlorpromazine are in most cases nearly identical. In contrast, the anti-histone antibodies in idiopathic lupus are primarily directed against the H1 and H2B histone subunits.

Anti-double-stranded DNA antibodies are typically absent in drug-induced lupus due to procainamide, hydralazine and isoniazid; instead such antibodies are associated with drug-induced disease with other agents, particularly interferon-alpha and anti-tumour necrosis factor (TNF) agents.

Borchers, A.T., Keen, C.L., and Gershwin, M.E. (2007). Drug-induced lupus. *Ann N Y Acad Sci* 1108, 166–182.
http://onlinelibrary.wiley.com/doi/10.1196/annals.1422.019/abstract

33. Answer C

These anti-nuclear antibodies recognise cellular proteins with molecular weights of approximately 52 and 60 kDa. The 60-kDa protein is complexed with the hy1– 5 species of small nuclear RNAs. Anti-Ro/SSA antibodies are primarily found in patients with systemic lupus erythematosus (SLE) and Sjögren syndrome. They are infrequently seen in other connective tissue diseases such as scleroderma, polymyositis, mixed connective tissue disease and rheumatoid arthritis. Anti-Ro/SSA antibodies are found in approximately 10–60% of patients with SLE; the prevalence depends upon the methodology employed as well as the race of those tested and other factors. Anti-Ro/SSA antibodies have been associated with photosensitivity, a rash known as subacute cutaneous lupus, cutaneous vasculitis (palpable purpura), interstitial lung disease, neonatal lupus and congenital heart block (CHB).

A major concern among women with anti-Ro/SSA and anti-La/SSB antibodies is the development of congenital heart block (CHB), most often occurring in the offspring of mothers with SLE. These antibodies cross the placenta beginning at 16 weeks of gestation and reach the fetal tissues, where they can induce a *myocarditis* or be *arrhythmogenic*. The immune-mediated damage of the cardiac conduction system ultimately ends with its substitution with fibrotic tissue. The incidence of CHB in the offspring of anti-Ro-positive women is about 1–2%, and the risk of recurrence is 10 times higher in the following pregnancies. Non-fluorinated steroids (prednisone, prednisolone and methylprednisolone) are recommended only for maternal indications, not for prevention of CHB in anti-Ro/SSA-positive women.

34. Answer A

Anti-DNA topoisomerase I (Scl-70) antibodies are associated with diffuse cutaneous SSc (DcSSc) and a higher risk of severe interstitial lung disease and digital ulcers. Scl-70 levels have been shown to correlate positively with disease severity and disease activity in DcSSc. Patients in whom Scl-70 disappear during follow-up have been reported to have milder disease and better survival.

Nihtyanova, S.I. and Denton, C.P. (2010) Autoantibodies as predictive tools in systemic sclerosis. *Nat Rev Rheumatol* 6, 112–116.
http://www.ncbi.nlm.nih.gov/pubmed/20125179

35. Answer D

Patients positive for antibodies to citrullinated peptides (anti-CCP) with early rheumatoid arthritis (RA) are at increased risk of progressive joint damage. Anti-CCP testing may predict erosive disease more effectively than rheumatoid factor (RF). Positive anti-CCP testing also appears to predict an increased risk for radiographic progression in patients with early oligo- or poly-arthritis who are IgM-RF negative. Patients with an established diagnosis of RA who have a positive test for RF, anti-CCP or both are at a higher risk of developing erosive joint damage and functional impairment. As a result, such patients should receive disease-modifying anti-rheumatic drug (DMARDs) therapy that suppresses disease activity early in the course of their disease.

 Avouac, J., Gossec, L., and Dougados, M. (2006). Diagnostic and predictive value of anti-cyclic citrullinated protein antibodies in rheumatoid arthritis: a systematic literature review. *Ann Rheum Dis* 65, 845–851.
http://ard.bmj.com/content/65/7/845.abstract

8 Dermatology

Questions

BASIC SCIENCE

Answers can be found in the Dermatology Answers section at the end of this chapter.

1. Which one of the following is frequently altered in melanoma, resulting in dysregulation of the mitogen-activated protein kinase (MAPK) pathway?
  A. B-raf
  B. Vascular endothelial growth factor (VEGF)
  C. K-ras
  D. Epidermal growth factor receptor (EGFR)
  E. p53

2. A patient enquires about sun protection. Which of the following is correct about sun protection and the use of sunscreen?
  A. Regular use of sunscreens reduces the development of pre-cancerous actinic keratosis
  B. Sunburn is caused by ultraviolet A radiation
  C. Sun protection factor (SPF) of a sunscreen product is based on how effectively it blocks ultraviolet A rays
  D. Sunscreens only block ultraviolet A radiation
  E. Ultraviolet B rays can penetrate below the dermis

Passing the FRACP Written Examination: Questions and Answers, First Edition. Jonathan Gleadle, Tuck Yong, Jordan Li, Surjit Tarafdar, and Danielle Wu.
© 2013 John Wiley & Sons, Ltd. Published 2013 by John Wiley & Sons, Ltd.

CLINICAL

3. Which one of the following features can be found in patients with Stevens–Johnson syndrome?
   A. Cutaneous lesions are usually found on the limbs
   B. Eosinophilia is seen on complete blood examination
   C. Full thickness loss of epidermis
   D. Minimal inflammatory cells in skin biopsy
   E. Mucosal involvement is infrequent

4. A 50-year-old construction worker has noticed several rough-surfaced, irregularly shaped lesions on his face, scalp and backs of his hands. On examination, they appear hyperkeratotic and have a small rim of surrounding erythema. These lesions are not painful, do not itch and have been appearing over several years. Which one of the following statements regarding this patient's risk of skin cancer is true?
   A. This patient's risk of developing a cutaneous malignancy in relation to the lesions is less than 1%
   B. The lesions are precursors to melanoma and should be removed
   C. Treatment of the lesions by cryotherapy or curettage has been found to be effective in preventing the progression of such lesions to carcinoma
   D. The most important risk factor in the development of these lesions is family history
   E. Small squamous cell carcinomas arising in sun-exposed areas are more likely to metastasise

5. A 51-year-old man presents with a 4-month history of gradually worsening rash on the backs of his hands. He noticed a few small blisters developing initially but the rash has worsened, especially when exposed to sun. He is concerned about the scarring marks left on his hands. He is a non-smoker but drinks two to three standard drinks of alcohol per day. He has no history of previous skin disease or other medical problems. He does not take any medication. His hands are shown below. The full skin examination reveals similar small lesions and scars on his face. The biochemistry results and full blood count are unremarkable, except for elevated serum alanine aminotransferase (ALT) and aspartate aminotransferase (AST). What is the most likely diagnosis?

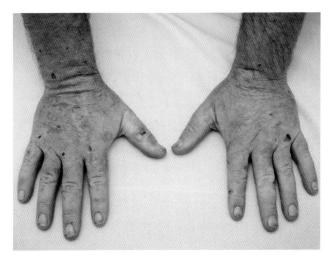

A. Bullous pemphigoid
B. Cutaneous lichen planus
C. Dermatitis herpetiforms
D. Eczema
E. Porphyria cutanea tarda

6. Which one of the following factors is most important in determining the prognosis for a patient diagnosed with malignant melanoma?
A. Depth of invasion in the skin and cutaneous tissue
B. History of pigmented naevus
C. Absence of pigmentation
D. Number of mitotic figures in the microscopic specimen
E. Ulceration of the primary melanoma

7. A 58-year-old woman with a long-standing history of type 2 diabetes and hypertension presents with a rash on her leg that in the past few months has progressively worsened. Her most recent HbA1c is 9.2% and she also has both chronic kidney disease and retinopathy. On physical examination, the rash shown below is observed on her shin. What is the most likely diagnosis in this patient?

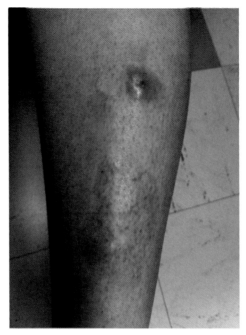

A. Acanthosis nigricans
B. Necrobiosis lipoidica
C. Erythrasma
D. Contact dermatitis
E. Plaque-type psoriasis

8. A 27-year-old man develops a reddish brown macule on his face soon after taking a trimethoprim–sulphamethoxazole tablet for urinary infection. The lesion heals over the next few weeks with hyperpigmentation. He had a similar lesion on his face 3 years ago after exposure to trimethoprim–sulphamethoxazole. What is the most likely diagnosis?
   A. Discoid lupus
   B. Fixed drug reaction
   C. Pemphigus vulgaris
   D. Atopic dermatitis
   E. Pityriasis rosea

9. A 36-year-old woman has redness and itching of the hands with tiny vesicles, scaling and fissuring, accompanied by itching on the palms. A diagnosis of hand eczema has been made, but simple emollients have not improved matters. Which one of the following agents is NOT used for the treatment of severe hand eczema?
   A. Topical glucocorticoids
   B. Topical tacrolimus

C. Oral retinoids
D. Oral ciclosporin
E. Hydroxychloroquine

10. A 56-year-old woman who had received a kidney transplant 5 years ago presents with a 4-day history of painful lesions on the anterior surface of both legs, as shown below. On examination the lesions are firm and tender. A biopsy shows panniculitis involving inflammation of septa in the subcutaneous fat tissue without any evidence of vasculitis. What is the most likely diagnosis?

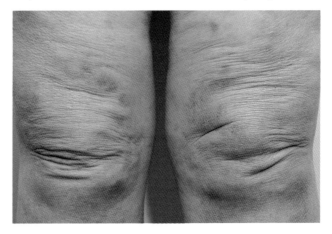

A. Systemic lupus erythematosus
B. Fungal infection (tinea corporis)
C. Pyoderma gangrenosum
D. Erythema nodosum
E. Pretibial myxoedema

Answers

BASIC SCIENCE

1. Answer A

Melanoma is a molecularly heterogenous malignancy. Systematic genome-wide screening has identified missense mutations in the B-raf gene, a component of the mitogen-activated protein kinase (MAPK) pathway in 66% of melanomas. An additional 15–20% of melanomas contain activating mutations in N-ras, a component of the MAPK pathway upstream of B-raf. These mutations are present in the majority of melanomas arising on skin intermittently exposed to the sun. B-raf and N-ras mutations in melanoma suggest that pharmacological inhibition of the MAPK pathway may provide therapeutic benefit. Inhibitors of the MAPK pathway are currently undergoing clinical investigation with some recent promising results (Sausville, 2012). Metastatic melanoma remains an aggressive malignancy conferring a very poor prognosis and standard chemotherapy has not demonstrated an overall survival benefit.

Sausville, E.A. (2012). Promises from trametinib in RAF active tumors. *N Engl J Med* 367, 171–172.
http://www.ncbi.nlm.nih.gov/pubmed/22663012

2. Answer A

Sunburn and direct damage to DNA is caused by ultraviolet B (UVB) radiation, but ultraviolet A (UVA) may be more damaging to the skin by free radical generation, photoageing, immunosuppression and photocarcinogenesis (Berwick, 2011). Terrestrial UV radiation consists of 5% UVB, which is mostly absorbed by the epidermis, and 95% UVA which can penetrate below the dermis.

Sunscreens may be organic or inorganic chemicals and should ideally block both wavebands, UVA and UVB. The sun protection factor (SPF) is mainly based on the effectiveness of the sunscreen in blocking UVB. It does not measure the effectiveness against UVA. It is determined by a highly controlled clinical test using lamps that simulate solar radiation on human volunteers. It measures the time taken for a minimal erythema to appear when sunscreen is applied compared to without sunscreen. Therefore, an SPF of 15 means that it takes 10 min for skin to start to burn without sunscreen compared to 150 min with that sunscreen. Sunscreens that have identical SPF ratings will have equal protection against UVB under the controlled conditions that are used to determine the SPF. One long-term study has found that regular use of sunscreen by adults can prevent the development of pre-cancerous actinic keratoses and skin cancers (squamous cell carcinoma and melanoma). While basal cell carcinomas (BCCs) did decrease, the results were not statistically significant, possibly because BCCs result from damage caused early in life.

Berwick, M. (2011). The good, the bad, and the ugly of sunscreens. *Clin Pharmacol Ther* 89, 31–33.
http://www.ncbi.nlm.nih.gov/pubmed/21170070

CLINICAL

3. Answer C

Stevens–Johnson syndrome (SJS) is an idiosyncratic, T-cell mediated, delayed (type IV) hypersensitivity reaction that results in widespread bright-red oedematous papules and plaques with blistering skin lesions (Stern, 2012). Trunk lesions predominate. Mucous membranes are nearly always involved with blisters and erosions. Eighty per cent of cases are drug-related. The onset is usually 4–21 days after the first dose of the drug. Epidermal necrosis is usually found on skin biopsy with full-thickness loss of epidermis. There is dense superficial dermal lymphocytic inflammation. Other features of SJS include temperature greater than 38.5°C, malaise, sore throat, dysphagia, dysuria or photophobia initially.

Stern, R.S. (2012). Exanthematous drug eruptions. *N Engl J Med* 366, 2492–2501.
http://www.ncbi.nlm.nih.gov/pubmed/22738099

4. Answer C

This patient has hyperkeratotic lesions typical of actinic keratosis in sun-exposed areas. Actinic keratosis is seen in areas of chronically sun-damaged skin and is considered a precursor lesion to the development of squamous cell carcinoma (SCC) (Madan et al., 2010).

Unlike basal cell carcinoma (BCC), SCC can have precursor lesions, such as actinic keratoses and SCC in situ (Bowen disease), which are considered premalignant. Although the rate of progression of individual actinic keratoses to invasive SCC has been estimated as 1–10% over 10 years, this risk could be much higher in patients with more than five actinic keratoses. Presence of actinic keratoses is an important marker of high UV exposure and increased risk of non-melanoma skin cancer generally. This marker can allow early identification and treatment of in-situ SCC to avoid metastasis and tissue destruction, since SCCs are more invasive than are BCCs. SCC usually develops on sun-exposed sites because of photodamage to the skin. Lesions of Bowen disease usually present as slowly enlarging erythematous scaly or crusted plaques and have a 3–5% risk of progression to SCC. Thus, it is important that the patient be followed regularly and evaluated by a dermatologist. The removal of these lesions through various techniques can prevent progression to cancer. Small SCCs arising from actinic keratosis lesions are less likely to metastasise than more atypical SCCs, such as those that are poorly differentiated or appear in non–sun-exposed areas or the oral or genital mucosa. Sunlight exposure is the most important risk factor for developing actinic keratosis and SCC, although radiation, chemical burns and chronic non-healing wounds may also predispose to SCC.

In white transplant recipients, risk of SCC increases 65–250-fold and risk of BCC 10–16-fold compared with the non-transplanted population. The ratio of SCC to BCC also reverses in iatrogenic immunosuppression, because SCC occurs more frequently in transplant recipients than does BCC, whereas in the general population BCC is three to six times more frequent than is SCC. Age, skin colour, male sex, UV dose and duration of immunosuppression are key components in pathogenesis of post-transplant non-melanoma skin cancer. However, complex genetic factors affecting the extent and consequences of immunosuppression can determine individual risk. Patients with HIV/AIDS or non-Hodgkin lymphoma, specifically chronic lymphocytic leukaemia, also have aggressive SCC.

Madan, V., Lear, J.T., and Szeimies, R.M. (2010). Non-melanoma skin cancer. *Lancet* 375, 673–685.
http://www.sciencedirect.com/science/article/pii/S014067360961196X

5. Answer E

Porphyria cutanea tarda (PCT) is due to an acquired deficiency of hepatic uroporphyrinogen decarboxylase (UROD) (Poh-Fitzpatrick, 2012). An inherited deficiency of UROD contributes in some cases. UROD is the fifth enzyme in the haem biosynthetic pathway. PCT results from a decrease in the activity of hepatic UROD to approximately 20% of normal. Markedly decreased activity of hepatic UROD leads to accumulation of large amounts of uroporphyrinogen and hepta-, hexa-, and penta-carboxyl porphyrinogen in the liver, which then appear in plasma and urine. Porphyrins that accumulate in the skin are photosensitising. PCT is usually associated with mild elevations in serum liver enzymes, especially serum alanine aminotransferase (ALT) and aspartate aminotransferase (AST). Advanced liver disease is uncommon at initial presentation, but may be seen in older patients with recurrent disease. PCT was initially described as a disease of males with alcohol abuse, and alcohol has been reported as an important and common susceptibility factor in many series.

Cutaneous manifestations of PCT include blisters, bullae, increased fragility, scarring and hyper- and hypo-pigmentation affecting sun-exposed areas of the body, such as the backs of the hands, forearms, face, ears, neck and feet. The chronic blistering skin manifestations are characteristic, but not specific. PCT is confirmed by demonstrating marked increase in porphyrins in plasma and/or urine, with a predominance of uroporphyrin and heptacarboxyl porphyrins. Erythrocyte porphyrins are usually normal. A total plasma porphyrin measurement may be most useful for initial screening. A skin biopsy reveals subepidermal bullae. Wood's lamp examination of the urine shows orange–red fluorescence.

Bullous pemphigoid is a subepidermal blistering disorder that most commonly occurs in older adults. The classic skin lesions are urticarial plaques and tense bullae on the trunk and extremities. Intense pruritus is common, and lesions typically do not scar. Cutaneous lichen planus is most commonly expressed as an eruption of shiny, flat, polygonal, violaceous papules. Dermatitis herpetiforms is an autoimmune blistering disease associated with coeliac disease and characterised by intensely itchy polymorphous vesicular lesions located over the extensor surfaces, back and scalp.

Poh-Fitzpatrick, M.B. (2012). Porphyria cutanea tarda: treatment options revisited. *Clin Gastroenterol Hepatol* 10, 1410–1411.
http://www.ncbi.nlm.nih.gov/pubmed/22982098

6. Answer A

The incidence of malignant melanoma is increasing. Significant advances have been made over the years in prevention, early detection and treatment of patients with melanoma. Patients with localised, early-stage disease have a favourable overall outcome with cure rates of up to 90%. The most important factor in the determination of the overall prognosis of a patient with malignant melanoma is the depth of invasion, as measured by the thickness of the lesion. Those less than 0.76 mm thick are less likely to metastasise, while those of greater thickness will do so with a frequency exceeding 30%. This measurement is part of the Breslow classification, which categorises the metastatic potential of a malignant melanoma according to its thickness. The other classification is that devised by Clark, in which the level of dermal or deeper invasion determines the likelihood of malignant spread. Ulceration of primary melanoma tumour carries a worse prognosis compared to non-ulcerated lesions.

Lymph node metastasis is one of the most important predictors of survival in melanoma patients. The techniques of sentinel lymph node (SLN) mapping and biopsy have permitted a more accurate assessment of the lymphatic drainage site from the primary site of the melanoma. It has been possible to identify more precisely a subset of patients with micrometastatic locoregional disease within the lymph nodes. Three factors are important in determining prognosis for advanced-stage melanoma: the site of metastasis, the number of metastatic sites and serum level of lactate dehydrogenase (LDH).

Australian Cancer Network Melanoma Guidelines Revision Working Party. Clinical Practice Guidelines for the Management of Melanoma in Australia and New Zealand. Cancer Council Australia and Australian Cancer Network, Sydney and New Zealand Guidelines Group, Wellington (2008).
http://www.nhmrc.gov.au/_files_nhmrc/publications/attachments/cp111.pdf

7. Answer B

Necrobiosis lipoidica diabeticorum is a chronic granulomatous dermatitis of unknown cause that is most often associated with diabetes mellitus (Marinella, 2002). However, in about 25% of patients with this condition, lesions develop before the onset of diabetes. The lesions appear as yellow–brown, telangiectatic plaques with central atrophy and raised violaceous borders. They occur most frequently on the shins or the dorsa of the feet. Ulcers, which exist in about 30% of lesions, are often induced by trauma. In rare cases, squamous cell carcinomas develop, typically in older, ulcerated lesions. Necrobiosis lipoidica is often associated with diabetic nephropathy and/or retinopathy.

Acanthosis nigricans has been reported in patients with insulin resistance syndrome; however, the lesions are velvety to the touch, black in colour and located predominantly in contact areas such as the axilla. Erythrasma is a fungal infection affecting the fifth intertriginous space. Contact dermatitis is very common and can be induced by allergic or irritant triggers. The distribution of the rash in contact dermatitis coincides with the specific areas of skin that were exposed to the irritant (e.g. in patients sensitive to nickel, rashes may appear on fingers on which rings containing nickel are worn; in patients sensitive to detergent, rashes may appear on areas covered by clothing containing detergent). Nearly 90% of psoriasis patients have plaque-type psoriasis, a form that is characterised by sharply demarcated, erythematous scaling plaques. The elbows, knees and scalp are the most commonly affected sites. The intergluteal cleft, palms, soles and genitals are also commonly affected, but psoriasis can involve any part of the body. Lesions frequently occur in a symmetrical pattern of distribution.

Marinella, M.A. (2002). Necrobiosis lipoidica diabeticorum. *Lancet* 360, 1143.
http://www.ncbi.nlm.nih.gov/pubmed/12387963

8. Answer B

Fixed drug reactions tend to recur at the same site and are typically followed by residual hyperpigmentation (Duarte de Sousa, 2011). Fixed drug eruptions are common, immune-mediated, cutaneous lesions that are typically of acute onset and appear as annular, oedematous, sometimes blistering, reddish–brown-to-violaceous macules or plaques. Their diagnostic hallmarks include residual hyperpigmentation after healing and recurrence at previously affected sites, with subsequent antigenic challenges. Treatment consists of topical glucocorticoids and avoidance of offending drug.

Discoid lupus lesions are characterised by discrete, erythematous, slightly infiltrated plaques covered by a well-formed adherent scale that extends into dilated hair follicles (follicular plugging). Lesions are most often present on the face, neck, and scalp, but also occur on the ears and, infrequently, on the upper torso. They tend to slowly expand with active inflammation at the periphery and then to heal, leaving depressed central scars, atrophy, telangiectasias and hyperpigmentation or hypopigmentation.

Pemphigus vulgaris is characterised by flaccid bullae that typically begin in the oropharynx and then may spread to involve the skin, with a predilection for the scalp, face, chest, axillae and groin.

Adult atopic dermatitis is characterised by thickened skin, increased skin markings (lichenification), and excoriated and fibrotic papules, especially over the flexural areas such as the neck, antecubital fossae and popliteal fossae.

Pityriasis rosea is an acute, self-limited, exanthematous skin disease characterised by the appearance of slightly inflammatory, oval, papulosquamous lesions on the trunk and proximal areas of the extremities.

Duarte de Sousa, I.C. (2011). Images in clinical medicine. Fixed drug eruption. *N Engl J Med* 365, e12.
http://www.ncbi.nlm.nih.gov/pubmed/21830962

9. Answer E

Hand eczema, also called hand dermatitis, is an inflammation of the skin of the hands characterised by redness, infiltration of the skin, scaling, oedema, vesicles, areas of hyperkeratosis, cracks (fissures) and erosions. It is common, with a point prevalence of 4% (Coenraads, 2012). Hydroxychloroquine is used for the suppression and treatment of acute attacks of malaria, systemic lupus erythematosus and rheumatoid arthritis. Potent topical glucocorticoids are first-line pharmacological treatment for hand eczema. Other treatments include topical tacrolimus and pimecrolimus, phototherapy and for resistant cases, systemic retinoids or immunosuppression may be appropriate.

Coenraads, P.J. (2012). Hand eczema. *N Engl J Med* 367, 1829–1837.
http://www.ncbi.nlm.nih.gov/pubmed/23134383

10. Answer D

The clinical presentation and biopsy is suggestive of erythema nodosum. The hallmark of erythema nodosum is tender, erythematous, subcutaneous nodules that typically are located symmetrically on the anterior surface of the lower extremities. Though usually considered idiopathic, the most common identifiable cause is streptococcal pharyngitis. It may be the first sign of a systemic disease such as tuberculosis, bacterial or deep fungal infection, sarcoidosis, inflammatory bowel disease or cancer. Certain drugs, including oral contraceptives and some antibiotics, also may be causative. Erythema nodosum is usually self-limiting or resolves with treatment of the underlying disorder.

9 Oncology

Questions

BASIC SCIENCE

Answers can be found in the Oncology Answers section at the end of this chapter.

1. Of the following, which one best describes the mechanism of chemoresistance associated with P-glycoprotein?
    A. Induction of mutations of the receptor that binds to cytotoxic agent
    B. Induction of angiogenesis
    C. Alterations in enzymes involved in DNA repair
    D. Recognition of the cytotoxic agent and pumping of the drug to the extracellular space
    E. Drug inactivation by glycosylation

2. Which one of the following statements regarding p53 protein is correct?
    A. p53 protein functions by directly repairing DNA molecules
    B. Activation of p53 results in DNA mutation
    C. p53 protein is an oncogene that is inactivated by cell hypoxia
    D. p53 mutations promote cellular apoptosis
    E. Activation of p53 leads to arrest in the G1 phase of the cell cycle

3. Which one of the following techniques in radiotherapy for lung cancers is used to counteract the effect of tumour motion due to breathing?
    A. Shunting
    B. Arc technique
    C. Gating
    D. Modulation
    E. Stereotactic

4. Which one of the following is a good prognostic factor for patients with breast cancer?
    A. Oestrogen receptor positivity
    B. Age greater than 70 years at the time of diagnosis
    C. Human epidermal growth factor receptor 2 (HER2) overexpression

Passing the FRACP Written Examination: Questions and Answers, First Edition. Jonathan Gleadle, Tuck Yong, Jordan Li, Surjit Tarafdar, and Danielle Wu.
© 2013 John Wiley & Sons, Ltd. Published 2013 by John Wiley & Sons, Ltd.

   D. Inflammatory breast cancer
   E. BRCA1 gene mutation

Theme: Gene mutation in cancers (for Questions 4 and 5)
   A. p53
   B. BRCA1
   C. BRCA2
   D. von Hippel–Lindau (VHL)
   E. APC
   F. KRAS
   G. MUTYH
   H. PTEN

For each of the following cancers, select the most likely gene mutation to be associated with it.

5. Which gene is frequently mutated in adult renal clear cell carcinoma?

6. Which gene mutation activates the mitogen-activated protein kinase (MAPK) signalling pathway and can lead to the development of colorectal cancers?

Theme: DNA damage response (for Questions 7 and 8)
   A. Direct DNA repair
   B. Base excision repair
   C. Nucleotide excision repair
   D. Mismatch repair
   E. Non-homologous end joining
   F. Homologous recombination repair
   G. Interstrand cross-link
   H. Single-strand break repair

Select the type of damage response that best fits the description provided below.

7. Which pathway corrects replication errors that cause the incorporation of the wrong nucleotide and nucleotide deletions and insertions?

8. Which pathway prevents unwanted mutations by removing ultraviolet-induced DNA damage?

CLINICAL

9. Which one of the following best describes bevacizumab in the treatment of metastatic colorectal carcinoma?
  - **A.** It is a monoclonal antibody that targets vascular endothelial growth factor (VEGF)
  - **B.** It is a monoclonal antibody that targets epidermal growth factor receptor (EGFR)
  - **C.** It is standard monotherapy for metastatic colorectal cancer
  - **D.** It has no proven survival benefit in patients with metastases
  - **E.** It is contraindicated in patients with hypertension

10. A 52-year-old man presents to hospital complaining of abdominal pain and watery diarrhoea over the past 2 months. He also has been increasingly breathless. He has stopped taking alcohol recently as he has noticed that on occasion his face and neck become red. On examination, there is pitting oedema of his ankles and tender hepatomegaly. He also has a pan-systolic murmur in the apex area and raised jugular venous pressure. Which one of the following investigations is likely to be the most useful diagnostically?
  - **A.** Plasma brain natriuretic peptide level
  - **B.** Plasma somatostatin levels
  - **C.** Plasma gastrin levels
  - **D.** 24-h urine for 5-hydroxyindoleacetic acid (5-HIAA)
  - **E.** 24-h urine for 4-hydroxymethoxymandelate (VMA)

11. A 50-year-old woman is receiving carboplatin-based combination chemo-therapy for ovarian cancer. Which one of the following is the most appropriate therapy to prevent acute emesis?
  - **A.** Intravenous NK1 receptor antagonist (aprepitant)
  - **B.** Metoclopramide and a 5-HT$_3$ serotonin antagonist
  - **C.** Dexamethasone, a 5-HT$_3$ serotonin antagonist and aprepitant
  - **D.** Metoclopramide and dexamethasone
  - **E.** Dexamethasone and aprepitant

12. Which one of the following describes the role of denosumab in the treatment of bone metastases of solid tumours?
  - **A.** Is superior to zoledronic acid for castration-resistant prostate cancer with bony metastasis
  - **B.** Is inferior to zoledronic acid for breast cancer with bony metastasis
  - **C.** Is renally cleared and contraindicated in patients with renal failure
  - **D.** Does not affect the serum calcium level
  - **E.** Is associated frequently with osteonecrosis of the jaw

13. Which one of the following statements is true of prostate cancer bony metastases and their complications?
   A. Most fractures occur as the result of trauma
   B. Pathological fractures of proximal long bones are more common than vertebral fractures
   C. Androgen deprivation therapy for prostate cancer may increase the risk of fracture
   D. Bisphosphonates may help to reduce bone pain but do not reduce the number of cancer-associated skeletal events
   E. Radiotherapy is the most effective way of preventing pathological fractures from bone metastases

14. A patient is referred for evaluation of a soft-tissue mass on his leg. The histopathology result is consistent with soft-tissue sarcoma. The patient wants to know how you would treat such a tumour. You will inform him that:
   A. Chemotherapy is contraindicated for soft-tissue sarcomas
   B. Local control of soft-tissue sarcomas consists of surgical resection, often with radiotherapy
   C. Localised soft-tissue sarcoma usually only requires radiotherapy
   D. Soft-tissue sarcomas are usually well encapsulated and are seen to have clear margins on resection
   E. The presence of necrosis on magnetic resonance imaging suggests a low-grade sarcoma

15. A 72-year-old man with unresectable lung cancer presents to the emergency department complaining of back pain. In addition, he reports having difficulty with ambulation for the past week (he is only able to stagger from bed to a nearby chair), but he denies having bladder or bowel problems. Physical examination reveals focal mid-thoracic vertebral body tenderness, 4 out of 5 strength in both legs and normal knee jerks bilaterally. Which one of the following management and imaging modalities of the spine is recommended for this presentation?
   A. Radionuclide bone scan and non-steroidal anti-inflammatory drugs
   B. Computed tomography of the spine and intravenous pamidronate
   C. Intravenous dexamethasone while awaiting plain films of the thoracic spine
   D. Intravenous pamidronate while awaiting radionuclide bone scan
   E. Intravenous dexamethasone while awaiting gadolinium-enhanced magnetic resonance imaging of the spine

16. A 63-year-old woman with no significant medical history presents to clinic with facial swelling. Physical examination confirms the patient's report of facial swelling and reveals distension of the jugular veins. She is alert and her vital signs are normal. A contrast-enhanced computed tomography of the chest reveals mediastinal lymphadenopathy and external compression of the superior vena cava

(SVC) by an enlarged node. What is the most appropriate step to take next in the management of this patient?
- A. Intravenous thrombolysis
- B. Fine-needle aspiration of an enlarged mediastinal lymph node
- C. Immediate initiation of mediastinal irradiation
- D. Thoracic magnetic resonance imaging
- E. Initiation of anti-coagulation with warfarin

17. Which one of the following factors increases the risk of venous thromboembolism in patients with cancer receiving chemotherapy?
- A. Use of erythropoiesis-stimulating agents
- B. Haemoglobin level of 120 g/L
- C. Low levels of circulating platelet microparticles
- D. Neutropenia
- E. Body mass index of 27 kg/m^2

18. A 30-year-old woman with non-Hodgkin lymphoma presents with fever after her second cycle of chemotherapy. She had her last chemotherapy session 10 days ago. She does not have cough, pleuritic chest pain, dysuria or abdominal pain. Her temperature is 39.0°C, pulse is 100 beats/min and respiration rate is 18 breaths/min. No rash is present, her chest is clear, no heart murmur is present and her abdomen is soft. Her urinary analysis is unremarkable. Chest X-ray is normal. The WBC is 0.7 x 10^9 cells/L (4.0–11.0 x 10^9 cells/L) and neutrophil count is 0.2 x 10^9 cells/L (1.8–7.5 x 10^9 cells/L). In addition to taking blood, sputum and urine cultures, what additional step is most appropriate for this patient?
- A. Granulocyte colony-stimulating factor
- B. Intravenous piperacillin–tazobactam
- C. Oral amoxicillin–clavulanate
- D. Intravenous ceftriaxone
- E. Intravenous vancomycin

19. A 55-year-old woman enquires about breast cancer mammographic screening. Which one of the following is the CORRECT information to give?
- A. Biennial mammography reduces the mortality from breast cancer by less than 10%
- B. The sensitivity of mammographic testing increases with age
- C. The number needed to screen to prevent one death from breast cancer is higher for older women (in their 60s) compared to those in their 50s
- D. Women between the age of 50 and 69 years without a family history of breast cancer should have screening mammography every 5 years
- E. The false-positive rate of screening mammography increases with age

20. A 65-year-old man presents with urinary hesitancy and incomplete bladder emptying. He reports no dysuria or haematuria. Rectal examination reveals a smoothly enlarged prostate. Other physical examination is normal. Urinalysis is

normal. The patient's prostate-specific antigen (PSA) level is 4.0 ng/mL (0–5 ng/mL). You should inform this patient that:
   A. Moderately elevated PSA (4–10 ng/mL) indicates that the prostate cancer is locally confined
   B. PSA is produced only by malignant prostatic epithelial cells
   C. With his level of PSA, the prostate biopsy will usually reveal prostate cancer
   D. A low PSA does not exclude prostate cancer
   E. A moderately elevated PSA (4–10 ng/mL) is rarely observed in benign prostate hypertrophy

21. Which one of the following is recommended for adjuvant treatment of early breast cancer?
   A. Aromatase inhibitors are replacing tamoxifen in pre-menopausal women due to better outcomes and greater tolerability
   B. Radiotherapy is indicated after breast conserving surgery only if more than four nodes are positive or the tumour is close to the resection margin
   C. Combination chemotherapy reduces recurrence and improves survival in selected patient groups
   D. Tamoxifen confers mortality benefit even in oestrogen receptor-negative tumours
   E. No survival benefit has been demonstrated with the use of trastuzumab in the adjuvant setting

22. A 71-year-old man has been treated with radiotherapy for prostate carcinoma. Which is the most common site of radiation injury with clinically apparent effects?
   A. Bladder
   B. Rectum
   C. Sigmoid colon
   D. Small intestine
   E. Ureter

23. A 24-year-old woman is concerned about her mother testing positive for the 'breast cancer genes'. She seeks general information regarding these tests and about the need for her and her family to be tested for these mutations. Which of the following is correct about BRCA1 and BRCA2 testing?
   A. If this patient tests negative for the BRCA1 and BRCA2 mutations, she will have no future need for routine breast cancer screening
   B. In individuals with BRCA mutations, ovarian cancer before breast cancer is more common
   C. Only 5–10% of cases of breast cancer are attributable to mutations in single genes, including BRCA1 and BRCA2
   D. If she is positive for BRCA1 or BRCA2 mutations, preventive mastectomy and chemoprevention is the most effective management

E. All women should have genetic testing for the BRCA1and BRCA2 mutations because measures to reduce cancer risk for individuals with these
   mutations are efficacious

Theme: Non-cytotoxic anti-neoplastics (for Questions 24–27)

A. Alemtuzumab
B. Bevacizumab
C. Cetuximab
D. Trastuzumab
E. Everolimus
F. Erlotinib
G. Imatinib
H. Sunitinib

Select the agent that best fits the description given below.

24. Which agent is a recombinant chimeric monoclonal antibody that binds to
the epidermal growth factor receptor (EGFR), thereby inhibiting proliferation and
inducing apoptosis of tumour cells that over-express EGFR?

25. Which agent is a recombinant humanised monoclonal antibody that binds
to human epidermal growth factor receptor 2 (HER2) and inhibits the proliferation
of tumour cells that over-express HER2?

26. Which agent is an inhibitor of tyrosine kinase targeting epidermal growth
factor receptor (EGFR)?

27. Which agent is an inhibitor of tyrosine kinase targeting vascular endothelial
growth factor (VEGF)?

Answers

BASIC SCIENCE

1. Answer D

Development of drug resistance is one of the major causes of cancer treatment failure. For a cytotoxic agent to reach a cancer cell, the drug must enter the bloodstream, be activated or escape inactivation by drug-metabolising enzymes, and arrive at the target in its active form. The drug–target interaction must then produce cell death. Resistance to cytotoxic therapy results from interference with one or more of these critical steps. Some of the factors affecting these steps are poor absorption or distribution of the drug; metabolism of the drug in the liver; decreased blood supply to the target organ; tumour microenvironment such as hypoxia; drug target modifications; and mechanisms that block the intracellular accumulation of the drug.

Multidrug resistance refers to the clinical and laboratory circumstances in which a tumour is no longer susceptible to several cytotoxic agents with different mechanisms or targets. P-glycoprotein is a member of the adenosine triphosphate (ATP)-binding receptor family. It spans the plasma membrane and recognises a broad spectrum of cytotoxic drugs. In the presence of ATP, P-glycoprotein pumps the drugs to the extracellular space so that an effective concentration at the intracellular target is never achieved.

2. Answer E

p53 is a tumour suppressor which plays a critical role in the maintenance of genomic integrity; hence its popular designation as 'guardian of the genome' (Meek, 2009). The p53 protein is normally expressed at low levels in all cells. However, genetic injuries, such as those that occur through ionising radiation, trigger the stabilisation and activation of p53 protein. p53 functions as a transcription factor, directing expression of p21, an inhibitor of the cyclin-dependent kinases that regulate the cell cycle. Activation of p53 leads to arrest in the G1 phase of the cell cycle, enabling cells to repair DNA damage before proceeding into S phase and DNA replication. In other cells, activation of p53 causes activation of multiple effectors, leading to apoptosis. Mutations of p53 are common in human cancers, being demonstrable in about 50% of cases, and increased levels of its negative regulators MDM2 and MDM4 (also known as MDMX) downregulate p53 function in many of the rest. Most mutations are amino acid substitutions within the DNA-binding domain of p53, resulting in its misfolding and binding to heat shock proteins. The rate of protein turnover is greatly slowed for these mutant p53 molecules. This explains the paradox that high levels of p53 protein in tumour specimens are commonly taken as evidence of a mutation in p53. A germline p53 mutation is associated with a familial syndrome of breast cancer, sarcomas and other neoplasms, known as Li–Fraumeni syndrome.

Meek, D.W. (2009). Tumour suppression by p53: a role for the DNA damage response? *Nat Rev Cancer* 9, 714–723.
http://www.ncbi.nlm.nih.gov/pubmed/19730431

3. Answer C

Accurately tracking tumour position is critically important when maximising radiation dose to the tumour and limiting normal tissue exposure. In certain locations in the body, such as the lungs, stomach and liver, tumours can move as the patient breathes. In the past, this movement has confounded the ability to precisely map the tumour location and to accurately deliver radiation therapy.

Gating is a system that tracks a patient's normal respiratory cycle with an infrared camera and chest/abdomen marker (Ahmad et al., 2012). The system is coordinated to only deliver radiation when the tumour is in the treatment field. This prevents unnecessary radiation exposure to normal structures. Lung cancers move with respiration and if this variation is great, four-dimensional CT can be used to obtain a series of CT scans at different phases of the respiratory cycle. The information can help define the motion of the tumour, which can then be targeted with respiratory gating. This involves tracking the patient's respiratory cycle, commonly using surface markers and delivering treatment at specific phases of the cycle.

Ahmad, S.S, Duke, S., Jena, R., Williams, M.V., and Burnet, N.G. (2012). Advances in radiotherapy. *BMJ* 345, e7765.
http://www.bmj.com/content/345/bmj.e7765?view=long&pmid=23212681

4. Answer A

Oestrogen receptor positivity is a good prognostic factor in breast cancer (Benson et al., 2009). Lymph node involvement is the most important adverse prognostic feature. Increasing grade of tumour and human epidermal growth factor receptor 2 (HER2) overexpression are also associated with poor prognosis. Inflammatory breast cancer has a poor prognosis. BRCA1 and 2 gene mutations as prognostic indicators have not been established

Two factors emerge as the principal determinants of local recurrence within the conserved breast: margin status and the presence or absence of an extensive in-situ component. Lymphatic invasion and young age (<35 years) are primary predictors for increased risk of ipsilateral breast tumour recurrence. Consistent associations have been recorded for larger tumour size (>2 cm) and higher histological grade, but not for tumour subtype or nodal status. Patterns of mRNA and microRNA expression in tumours are also predictive of outcome.

Benson, J.R., Jatoi, I., Keisch, M., Esteva, F.J., Makris, A., and Jordan, V.C. (2009). Early breast cancer. *Lancet* 373, 1463–1479.
http://www.ncbi.nlm.nih.gov/pubmed/19394537

5. Answer D

Renal cell carcinoma (RCC) arises from a complex series of mutation and selection events in cells located within the proximal tubules of nephrons, culminating in cancer cells that acquire characteristics allowing immortalisation, resistance to apoptosis, evasion of immunosurveillance, recruitment of angiogenic factors, and ultimately distant spread. A frequent event during the evolution of clear cell RCC is loss of function of the von Hippel–Lindau (VHL) gene, located on chromosome 3p (Gleadle, 2009). Inheritance of a defective copy of the VHL gene leads to VHL disease and is the most common cause for inherited clear-cell RCC in which a second hit or somatic mutation is presumed to occur in the cancerous cells. In addition, up to 75% of patients with sporadic clear-cell RCC have mutation or silencing by methylation of VHL. The VHL gene functions in several pathways linked to carcinogenesis, most notably the hypoxia-inducible pathway. In the absence of VHL, hypoxia-inducible factor α (HIF) accumulates, leading to production of several growth factors, including vascular endothelial growth factor and platelet-derived growth factor, and enhanced glycolysis. Many non-renal cancers are also characterised by hypoxia, enhanced HIF levels and increased expression of hypoxically-regulated genes that correlate both with tumour aggression and patient outcome.

Gleadle, J.M. (2009). Review article: How cells sense oxygen: lessons from and for the kidney. *Nephrology (Carlton)* 14, 86–93.
http://onlinelibrary.wiley.com/doi/10.1111/j.1440-1797.2008.01064.x/full

6. Answer F

The loss of genomic stability can drive the development of colorectal cancer by facilitating the acquisition of multiple tumour-associated mutations (Markowitz and Bertagnolli, 2009). Oncogenic mutations of RAS and BRAF, which activate the mitogen-activated protein kinase (MAPK) signalling pathway, occur in 37% and 13% of colorectal cancers, respectively. RAS mutations, principally in KRAS, activate the GTPase activity that signals directly to the RAF proto-oncogene serine/threonine-protein kinase. BRAF mutations signal BRAF serine–threonine kinase activity, which further drives the MAPK signalling cascade. BRAF mutations are detectable even in small polyps, and compared with RAS mutations, they are more common in hyperplastic polyps, serrated adenomas and proximal colon cancers. Patients with numerous and large hyperplastic lesions, a condition termed the hyperplastic polyposis syndrome, have an increased risk of colorectal cancer, with disease progression occurring through an intermediate lesion with a serrated luminal border on histological analysis.

Epidermal growth factor (EGF) is a soluble protein that has trophic effects on intestinal cells. Clinical studies have supported an important role of signalling through the EGF receptor (EGFR) in a subgroup of colorectal cancers. EGFR mediates signalling by activating the MAPK and PI3K signalling cascades. Recent clinical data have shown that advanced colorectal cancer with tumour-promoting mutations of these pathways, including activating mutations in KRAS, BRAF and the p110 subunit of PI3K, do not respond to anti-EGFR therapy.

Markowitz, S.D. and Bertagnolli, M.M. (2009). Molecular origins of cancer: Molecular basis of colorectal cancer. *N Engl J Med* 361, 2449–2460. http://www.ncbi.nlm.nih.gov/pmc/articles/PMC2843693/

7. Answer D

The DNA damage response (DDR) coordinates the repair of DNA and the activation of cell-cycle checkpoints to arrest the cell to allow time for repair. DNA is subject to a high level of endogenous damage and the DDR is essential for the maintenance of genomic stability and survival. Dysregulation of the DDR can lead to genomic instability that promotes cancer development, but this is exploitable with both conventional cytotoxic therapy and DDR inhibitors. Downregulated DDR pathways render the tumour sensitive to specific cytotoxic drugs and some DDR inhibitors. Upregulated DDR pathways confer therapeutic resistance. Inhibitors of the DDR have been developed to overcome resistance and to augment the activity of conventional therapy. Loss of a DDR pathway can lead to dependence on a compensatory pathway, and targeting this second pathway may render endogenous DNA damage cytotoxic by a process termed synthetic lethality, which is tumour-specific because the normal tissues have functional DNA repair.

Mismatch repair (MMR) corrects replication errors that cause the incorporation of the wrong nucleotide (a mismatch) and nucleotide deletions and insertions. Defective MMR increases mutation rates up to 1000-fold, results in microsatellite instability (MSI) and is associated with cancer development.

8. Answer C

Nucleotide excision repair (NER) removes helix-distorting adducts on DNA, e.g. those caused by ultraviolet (UV) radiation and tobacco smoke, and contributes to the repair of intrastrand and interstrand cross-links (ICLs); the xerodermapigmentosum (XP) proteins and DNA excision repair protein 1 (ERCC1) also have crucial roles in both the NER and ICL repair pathways. ERCC1 polymorphisms are associated with skin and lung cancer. Hereditary defects in NER cause UV sensitivity and skin cancer. Deficiency in NER confers sensitivity to platinum agent therapy, which reflects a reduced capacity to repair ICLs, and the measurement of levels of crucial NER enzymes could thus be used for patient stratification.

For Questions 7 and 8:

Curtin, N.J. (2012). DNA repair dysregulation from cancer driver to therapeutic target. *Nat Rev Cancer* 12, 801–817. http://www.ncbi.nlm.nih.gov/pubmed/23175119

CLINICAL

9. Answer A

Bevacizumab is a humanised monoclonal antibody that targets vascular endothelial growth factor (VEGF) (Kohne and Lenz, 2009). It has a high binding affinity to VEGF and interferes with binding of VEGF-A to the VEGF receptors VEGFR-1 and VEGFR-2, thus inhibiting VEGF-mediated intracellular signalling. Through inactivation of the VEGF–VEGFR pathway, this targeted agent can help prevent the formation of new blood vessels and tumour growth. It has been shown to improve survival in metastatic colorectal carcinoma when used in combination with chemotherapy. Bevacizumab is generally well tolerated when combined with other drugs, such as irinotecan. Hypertension, the only consistently observed bevacizumab-associated side effect that requires treatment, is manageable with standard oral anti-hypertensives (e.g. calcium-channel blockers, angiotensin converting enzyme inhibitors and diuretics).

Kohne, C.H. and Lenz, H.J. (2009). Chemotherapy with targeted agents for the treatment of metastatic colorectal cancer. *Oncologist* 14, 478–488.
http://theoncologist.alphamedpress.org/content/14/5/478.long

10. Answer D

The clinical picture is one of carcinoid syndrome secondary to a carcinoid tumour (Kulke and Mayer, 1999). The syndrome of facial flushing, watery diarrhoea, abdominal pain and cardiac abnormalities imply hepatic metastases of a carcinoid tumour. Common sites of carcinoid tumour in the bowel are the terminal ileum, rectum and appendix (25% of all tumours). Diagnosis is made from the clinical picture and 24-h collection of urine for levels of 5-HIAA, a metabolite of 5-HT (serotonin) that is postulated to be responsible for the cardiac manifestations of the disease and profuse watery diarrhoea.

The 24-h urine collection for the presence of VMA (metabolites of catecholamines) may be helpful in making the diagnosis of phaeochromocytoma, a rare catecholamine-producing tumour. In adults, 90% of tumours are in the adrenal medulla; 90% of these tumours are benign and 80% are unilateral.

Somatostatin is a peptide that inhibits hormone production by several tumours and its analogue octreotide is useful in the treatment of carcinoid syndrome.

Kulke, M.H. and Mayer, R.J. (1999). Carcinoid tumors. *N Engl J Med* 340, 858–868.
http://www.ncbi.nlm.nih.gov/pubmed/10080850

11. Answer C

The control of chemotherapy-induced nausea and vomiting (CINV) is an important issue for patients undergoing chemotherapy. The objective of anti-emetic therapy is the complete prevention of CINV, and this should be achievable in the majority of patients receiving chemotherapy. The type of chemotherapeutic agent is an important predictor of risk of acute emesis. Chemotherapy agents have been divided into four categories:

- Highly emetic: >90% risk of emesis
- Moderately emetic: 30–90% risk of emesis
- Low emetogenicity: 10–30% risk of emesis
- Minimally emetic: <10% risk of emesis.

The risk of acute emesis is high with carboplatin. In the high-risk group, the combination of dexamethasone and a $5-HT_3$ serotonin antagonist is superior to dexamethasone alone, $5-HT_3$ serotonin antagonist alone and various combinations containing metoclopramide. Recently, the introduction of the NK1 (neurokinin) receptor antagonist aprepitant has significantly improved the ability to prevent both acute and delayed CINV in patients receiving highly and moderately emetic chemotherapy. The benefit of combining aprepitant with $5-HT_3$ receptor antagonists and glucocorticoids for the prevention of CINV was shown in phase III trials that included 1099 patients receiving cisplatin-containing chemotherapy. Although aprepitant improved control of CINV when combined with a $5-HT_3$ receptor antagonist and dexamethasone, aprepitant plus dexamethasone alone was not as effective as the three-drug combination regimen. A $5-HT_3$ receptor antagonist remains necessary in patients receiving cisplatin-based chemotherapy.

Roila, F., Herrstedt, J., Aapro, M., et al. (2010). Guideline update for MASCC and ESMO in the prevention of chemotherapy- and radiotherapy-induced nausea and vomiting: results of the Perugia consensus conference. *Ann Oncol* 21 Suppl 5, v232–243.
http://annonc.oxfordjournals.org/content/21/suppl_5/v232.long

12. Answer A

Skeletal morbidity is a substantial burden in many patients with advanced solid tumours. Pathological fractures, pain, spinal cord compression and hypercalcaemia are among the potential complication of bone metastases. Zoledronic acid is the most potent bisphosphonate available. It has been the standard bone-targeted treatment for the prevention of skeletal-related events (SREs) in patients with solid tumours that have metastasised to bone.

Denosumab represents a new class of osteoclast-targeted therapy as it inhibits the receptor activator of nuclear factor κB (RANK) signalling pathway (Saylor, 2011). Denosumab is superior to zoledronic acid in reducing SREs in men with castration-resistant prostate cancer that has metastasised to bone. Denosumab is non-inferior to zoledronic acid in patients with metastases due to non-prostate and non-breast cancer in reducing SREs and may be superior in women with metastatic breast cancer. In patients with renal dysfunction, denosumab offers a potential advantage. Denosumab clearance is not dependent on kidney function. Hypocalcaemia can occur with any potent osteoclast inhibitor, although it seems to be more common with denosumab. Osteonecrosis of the jaw is a rare but important potential toxic effect of both drugs.

Saylor, P.J. (2011). Targeted therapies: denosumab – a new option for solid tumors metastatic to bone. *Nat Rev Clin Oncol* 8, 322–324.
http://www.ncbi.nlm.nih.gov/pubmed/21556026

13. Answer C

The most common symptom of bone metastases from prostate cancer is pain (Lee et al., 2011). Metastases to vertebral bones can cause spinal cord compression, compression fractures, nerve root compression and cauda equina syndrome. Pathological fractures of proximal long bones occur but are less common than vertebral fractures. Excessive osteoblastic bone deposition can cause hypocalcaemia and secondary hyperparathyroidism. Anaemia due to ineffective erythropoiesis can be caused by both bone metastases and cancer therapies.

Androgen deprivation therapy (ADT) with a gonadotropin-releasing hormone (GnRH) agonist is the standard initial hormonal treatment for metastatic prostate cancer. ADT causes severe hypogonadism and significantly increases the risk of fracture. Pathological fractures may occur without trauma. Prophylactic orthopaedic intervention may be required for bone lesions at high risk of fracture. Bisphosphonates may help to reduce bone pain and reduce the number of cancer-associated skeletal events. A minority of cases with spinal cord compression may be suitable for surgical intervention.

Lee, R.J., Saylor, P.J., and Smith, M.R. (2011). Treatment and prevention of bone complications from prostate cancer. *Bone* 48, 88–95.
http://www.ncbi.nlm.nih.gov/pmc/articles/PMC3010497

14. Answer B

The goals of the treatment of sarcomas are local and systemic control of the sarcoma; preservation of the limb or organ function; and quality of life (Clark et al., 2005). Surgery, supplemented when necessary by adjuvant radiotherapy, is often curative for localised soft-tissue sarcomas. Although local treatment of primary soft-tissue sarcoma of the limbs influences the likelihood of local recurrence, limb salvage and functional outcome, the metastatic potential is mainly determined by the grade and size of the primary tumour. Low-grade tumours push aside contiguous structures, whereas high-grade tumours invade adjacent organs and have large areas of necrosis. Soft-tissue sarcomas grow along histological planes and are usually pseudo-encapsulated (i.e. microscopic projections of tumour extend beyond the apparent tumour capsule). Any excision that merely 'shells out' the apparently encapsulated tumour generally leaves behind microscopic residual tumour, resulting in regrowth of the tumour in 80% of cases.

Radiotherapy alone is considered when surgery is inappropriate or declined and achieves rates of local control of 30–60%. Whereas the goal of surgery and radiotherapy is local control of the tumour, the aim of chemotherapy is systemic control, which may be therapeutic, adjuvant or palliative. Multimodality therapy, including chemotherapy, is routine therapy for rhabdomyosarcomas and Ewing sarcoma. The use of adjuvant chemotherapy generally does little to influence the natural history of other sarcomas. Encouraging progress is occurring with the use of therapies directed against specific molecular targets associated with soft-tissue sarcoma.

Post-treatment surveillance [by means of clinical examination and chest radiography or computed tomography (CT)] is recommended to detect treatable recurrence and metastasis. Recurrence rates of 5–10% might be expected after optimal treatment of soft-tissue sarcomas of the limbs. The utility of CT and magnetic resonance imaging for detecting subclinical local recurrence has not been established, but these approaches may be more useful for detecting deep lesions. Since two-thirds of recurrences occur within 2 years, follow-up should be most intense during this period.

Clark, M.A., Fisher, C., Judson, I., and Thomas, J.M. (2005). Soft-tissue sarcomas in adults. *N Engl J Med* 353, 701–711.
http://www.ncbi.nlm.nih.gov/pubmed/16107623

15. Answer E

This patient is likely to have spinal cord compression due to metastatic lung cancer (Abrahm et al., 2008). Gadolinium-enhanced magnetic resonance imaging (MRI) of the spine is the most sensitive and specific method of evaluation. Myelography is invasive and may be uncomfortable for the patient with severe bone pain; in addition, radiologists experienced in its interpretation may not be available. CT of the spine should not be performed, because its ability to scan the entire spinal axis efficiently and its sensitivity in identifying epidural disease are inferior to those of gadolinium-enhanced MRI. The current recommendation for the radiographic evaluation of patients with suspected epidural compression is gadolinium-enhanced MRI of the entire spinal axis.

Before diagnosis, 83–95% of patients experience back pain, which often is referred, obscuring the site(s) of the compression(s). Prediction of subsequent walking ability depends on a patient's ambulatory status before therapy and time between developing motor defects and starting therapy. Ambulatory patients with no visceral metastases and less than 15 days between developing motor symptoms and receiving therapy have the best rate of survival. To preserve ambulation and optimise survival, MRI should be performed for cancer patients with new back pain despite normal neurological findings. At diagnosis, counselling, pain management and corticosteroids are begun. Most patients are offered radiation therapy. Surgery followed by radiation is considered for selected patients with a single high-grade epidural lesion caused by a radio-resistant tumour and who have an estimated survival of more than 3 months.

Abrahm, J.L., Banffy, M.B., and Harris, M.B. (2008). Spinal cord compression in patients with advanced metastatic cancer: 'all I care about is walking and living my life'. *JAMA* 299, 937–946.
http://jama.jamanetwork.com/article.aspx?articleid=181514

16. Answer B

Recent reviews have suggested that superior vena cava (SVC) syndrome is not a true emergency and that histological diagnosis should be quickly established first and then treatment promptly initiated (Wilson et al., 2007). SVC syndrome is most commonly caused by extrinsic compression of the thin-walled, low pressure SVC by a malignant mediastinal mass such as bronchogenic carcinoma (especially small-cell lung cancer) and non-Hodgkin lymphoma. Before a histological diagnosis is established, emergency treatment with mediastinal irradiation is only warranted in children and, occasionally, in adults who have mental status alteration, other life-threatening manifestations of increased intracranial pressure, cardiovascular collapse or evidence of upper airway obstruction. In the absence of such conditions, as with this patient, the next step in the management of SVC syndrome should focus on efforts to obtain a histological diagnosis of the underlying condition so that appropriate therapy may be initiated. Obtaining further radiological studies will not assist in making a histological diagnosis and these are therefore not the priority in the management of this patient.

Wilson, L.D., Detterbeck, F.C., and Yahalom, J. (2007). Superior vena cava syndrome with malignant causes. *N Engl J Med* 356, 1862–1869.
http://www.ncbi.nlm.nih.gov/pubmed/17476012

17. Answer A

Patients with cancer-associated thrombosis are more likely to have experienced a medical inpatient stay, but are less likely to have a history of venous thromboembolism (VTE), thrombophilia, intravenous drug abuse or smoking than cancer-free patients (Young et al., 2012). High white blood cell counts and anaemia at presentation are also reported to be associated with increased risk of VTE, as are increased platelets. High levels of circulating platelet microparticles in patients with cancer may also be a useful surrogate marker for VTE risk. Very high levels of D-dimer in patients with cancer and VTE are also associated with poor outcomes and may reflect either the biology of the tumour or the extent of venous thrombosis.

The relative risk for thromboembolic events is increased by 67% in patients treated with erythropoietin-stimulating agents (ESAs) compared with placebo. The use of ESAs should be carefully reconsidered in patients with a high risk of thromboembolic events, such as a previous history of thrombosis, surgery, prolonged immobilisation or limited activity, and in patients with multiple myeloma and treated with thalidomide or lenalidomide in combination with doxorubicin and corticosteroids. There are no data on the preventive use of anti-coagulants or aspirin.

Young, A., Chapman, O., Connor, C., Poole, C., Rose, P., and Kakkar, A.K. (2012). Thrombosis and cancer. *Nat Rev Clin Oncol* 9, 437–449.
http://www.ncbi.nlm.nih.gov/pubmed/22777060

18. Answer B

This patient with chemotherapy-induced neutropenia has a fever, but her examination does not suggest a clear cause. Initial evaluation should address the presence of systemic compromise, and whether the patient is at high or low risk for medical complications to determine the choice of antibiotic therapy. She should receive antibiotics that provide coverage of Gram-negative rods, including *Pseudomonas aeruginosa*, as well as Gram-positive coverage. There is no one optimal treatment regimen. Piperacillin–tazobactam is an appropriate agent for the treatment of neutropenic fever (Tam et al., 2011). It performed better than cefepime and similar to carbapenems in systematic reviews comparing regimens. Pharmacokinetic/pharmacodynamic studies support the use of 6-hourly piperacillin–tazobactam for *Pseudomonas* infection. In this patient, amoxicillin–clavulanate would not provide broad enough coverage against Gram-negative rods. Several studies have suggested that oral quinolone therapy may be an option in selected patients. Ceftriaxone would not offer *Pseudomonas* coverage.

As the median time to defervescence in patients successfully treated with frontline antibiotics is 3–5 days, escalation of antibiotic coverage should not occur prior to this in the absence of clinical instability, isolation of a resistant organism or emergence of new infective foci. Any modifications to the initial choice of antibiotic should be guided by repeat clinical assessment (e.g. emergence of focal sites of infection) and microbiological culture results.

Tam, C.S., O'Reilly, M., Andresen, D., et al (2011). Use of empiric anti-microbial therapy in neutropenic fever. *Intern Med J* 41, 90–101.
http://www.ncbi.nlm.nih.gov/pubmed/21272173

19. Answer B

The most important benefits of breast cancer screening are a reduction in the risk of death and the number of life-years gained. Screening mammography for women aged between 50 and 69 years is universally recommended. In this age group, data have consistently shown a 14–32% reduction in mortality from breast cancer with annual or biennial mammography, provided their life expectancy is 5 years or more. There is a greater reduction among the older women in this age group, which reflects the increasing sensitivity of mammographic testing with age and is associated with a decrease in breast density and slower tumour growth. There is also a higher incidence of breast cancer in the older age group. False-positive results are inversely related to age with a rate of about 98 per 1000 women screened in the 39–49-year age group and about 69 per 1000 women in the 70–79-year age group.

Warner, E. (2011). Breast-cancer screening. *N Engl J Med* 365, 1025–1032.
http://www.ncbi.nlm.nih.gov/pubmed/21916640

20. Answer D

Prostate-specific antigen (PSA), a glycoprotein with serine protease activity in the kallikrein family, is abundant in semen, where it dissolves seminal coagulum. Both normal and malignant prostatic epithelial cells produce PSA; production may actually be higher in normal cells than in malignant cells. A problem with PSA-based screening is that an elevated PSA level lacks specificity. Most abnormal PSA values are false-positive results that can be caused by benign prostatic hyperplasia (BPH), prostatitis or cystitis, ejaculation, perineal trauma, or the recent use of instruments for testing or surgery in the urinary tract. Moreover, a normal PSA value does not rule out prostate cancer (Hoffman, 2011).

Despite the increased likelihood of prostate cancer in men with a moderately elevated serum PSA level (i.e. a level 4–10 ng/mL), biopsy usually reveals BPH rather than prostate cancer. Determination of the free PSA level (i.e. the percentage of PSA that is unbound to serum proteins) is also a potential means of distinguishing malignancy from benign hyperplasia. PSA derived from malignant epithelial cells tends to bind more avidly to serum proteins. Thus, in men with an elevated serum PSA level, cancer is more likely when the percentage of free PSA is low. However, the clinical usefulness of these strategies remains unproved.

Hoffman, R.M. (2011). Screening for prostate cancer. *N Engl J Med* 365, 2013–2019.
http://www.nejm.org/doi/full/10.1056/NEJMcp1103642

21. Answer C

The indication for adjuvant systemic therapy after definitive surgery is based on established prognostic factors, including age, co-morbidities, axillary lymph node involvement, tumour size and tumour grade.

Combination chemotherapy reduces recurrence and improves survival in selected patient groups when given as adjuvant treatment for breast cancer. Guidelines recommend adjuvant chemotherapy for healthy patients with axillary node involvement and for node-negative disease when tumours are larger than 1 cm or in the presence of other adverse prognosticators (e.g. age <35 years, negative oestrogen receptor or progesterone receptor status, high-grade tumour). All patients within a subgroup are assumed to derive similar benefit from chemotherapy, but many are overtreated and do not have micrometastatic disease at presentation. Identification of patients with distant microscopic spread is particularly relevant in patients with node-negative, oestrogen receptor- or progesterone receptor-positive breast cancer (Benson et al., 2009).

Radiotherapy is indicated for all patients after breast-conserving surgery. Long-term follow-up of breast-conservation trials confirm significantly increased rates of local relapse when radiotherapy is omitted. Omission of radiotherapy should be cautioned at present since it can lead to rates of ipsilateral breast tumour recurrence approaching 30% for small tumours of favourable grade, and local control does affect overall survival. Older women benefit in terms of breast cancer-specific survival from radiotherapy after breast-conservation surgery, and tamoxifen alone cannot substitute for radiotherapy.

Aromatase inhibitors are replacing tamoxifen in post-menopausal women due to the lower rate of recurrence and their greater tolerability. Head-to-head comparison of tamoxifen and anastrazole shows no difference in overall survival. Significant survival benefit has been demonstrated with the use of trastuzumab (Herceptin) in the adjuvant setting. In patients with human epidermal growth factor receptor 2 (HER2)-positive early-stage breast cancer, trastuzumab improves rates of disease-free and overall survival independent of age, axillary node metastases, and oestrogen receptor or progesterone receptor status.

Benson, J.R., Jatoi, I., Keisch, M., Esteva, F.J., Makris, A., and Jordan, V.C. (2009). Early breast cancer. *Lancet* 373, 1463–1479.
http://www.ncbi.nlm.nih.gov/pubmed/19394537

22. Answer B
Radiation injury to surrounding tissues is relatively common after radiotherapy for prostate carcinoma. The gastrointestinal tract is particularly radiosensitive and small and large bowel damage may occur. The small bowel is partially protected by the peristaltic movement in and out of the field of radiation and has a lower risk of injury than the colon. The rectum, a fixed structure lying in close proximity to the prostate, is most vulnerable to injury. The sigmoid colon is more remote from the treatment field and radiation proctitis is the most common complication of pelvic irradiation. Implants deliver smaller amounts of focused radiation and cause less damage to the gastrointestinal tract than external beam radiation. Tumours that require higher doses of radiation, such as pelvic tumours, are associated with a greater risk of damage.

Yeoh, E.K., Holloway, R.H., Fraser, R.J., et al. (2012). Pathophysiology and natural history of anorectal sequelae following radiation therapy for carcinoma of the prostate. *Int J Radiat Oncol Biol Phys* 84, e593–599.
http://www.ncbi.nlm.nih.gov/pubmed/22836050

23. Answer C
The efficacy of measures to reduce cancer risk for individuals with BRCA1 and BRCA2 cancer-predisposing mutations is unknown (Robson and Offit, 2007). Breast cancer, like other common disorders such as coronary artery disease, diabetes mellitus and Alzheimer disease, is regarded as a complex disorder. Complex disorders have multiple aetiologies, including heritable single genes, multiple genes with an additive effect through interaction with often undefined environmental influences, and acquired environmental or genetic changes. Single heritable genes may represent a relatively small contribution to the overall incidence and morbidity from common diseases, including breast cancer, which affects one in nine women. Only 5–10% of cases of breast cancer are attributed to mutations in single genes, including BRCA1 and BRCA2. For a woman whose relatives have

a known BRCA1 and BRCA2 mutation but who herself has tested negative for the mutation known to be in the family, the chance of the development of breast cancer is still one in nine. This patient therefore has the same need for close surveillance as women in the general population.

In women with a BRCA mutation, screening should begin by the age of 25–30 years. Although no studies have shown a mortality benefit, magnetic resonance imaging (MRI) screening is recommended in addition to mammography for women with a BRCA mutation or for women who have a lifetime breast-cancer risk of at least 20–25% on the basis of family history. Ultrasonography and breast examination may increase detection rates slightly, but at a cost of more false-positive results and additional evaluations. Preventive mastectomy and salpingo-oophorectomy for BRCA mutation carriers are options that should be discussed with women who are at increased risk. Oophorectomy is performed after child-bearing, since the greatest increase in the risk of ovarian cancer occurs later than that of breast cancer in BRCA mutation carriers. Risks and benefits of chemopre-vention (e.g. with tamoxifen or raloxifene) should also be discussed. The patient should be made aware of the inherited nature of breast cancer risks and should be encouraged to refer family members for consideration of genetic testing and of strategies for prevention and early detection.

 Robson, M. and Offit, K. (2007). Clinical practice. Management of an inherited predisposition to breast cancer. *N Engl J Med* 357, 154–162.
http://www.ncbi.nlm.nih.gov/pubmed/17625127

24. Answer C

Cetuximab is a recombinant chimeric monoclonal antibody that binds to the epidermal growth factor receptor (EGFR), thereby inhibiting proliferation and inducing apoptosis of tumour cells that over-express EGFR. It is used for the treat-ment of head and neck squamous cell cancer or EGFR-positive, KRAS wild-type metastatic colorectal cancer. Cetuximab is unlikely to be effective for tumours with a KRAS mutation. It is indicated only for colorectal cancer without this mutation.

25. Answer D

Trastuzumab (Herceptin) is a recombinant humanised monoclonal antibody that binds to human epidermal growth factor receptor 2 (HER2) and inhibits the pro-liferation of tumour cells that over-express HER2. It can be used in the treatment of HER2-positive cancers, e.g. breast cancer, gastric cancer and, gastro-oesophageal junction cancer. The use of trastuzumab results in a small-to-modest risk for cardiotoxicity. Trastuzumab-related cardiotoxicity is most often manifested by an asymptomatic decrease in left ventricular ejection fraction (LVEF) and less often by clinical overt heart failure. In contrast to cardiotoxicity from anthracyclines, trastuzumab-related cardiotoxicity does not appear to be related to cumulative dose. It is often reversible with treatment discontinuation, and rechallenge is often tolerated after recovery. In addition, cardiac biopsy specimens after trastuzumab exposure do not show the significant myocyte destruction characteristic of anthracycline-induced dysfunction. Patients' cardiac status must be assessed before starting trastuzumab, including history and physical examination, electrocardiogram, echocardiogram and measurement of LVEF. Thereafter, cardiac function is monitored at least every 3 months.

26. Answer F

Erlotinib is a reversible tyrosine kinase inhibitor that acts on the epidermal growth factor receptor (EGFR) and it is used in the treatment of non–small-cell lung cancer (NSCLC) and pancreatic cancer. NSCLC with activating EGFR mutations may be more responsive to erlotinib (the rate of these mutations is higher in Asians, never-smokers, women and those with adenocarcinoma); erlotinib is unlikely to be effective if there is a KRAS mutation. Erlotinib has shown a survival benefit in the treatment of NSCLC in phase III trials. Rash occurs in the majority of patients treated with erlotinib. This resembles acne and primarily involves the face and neck. It is self-limited and resolves in the majority of cases, even with continued use. Interestingly, some clinical studies have indicated a correlation between the severity of the skin reactions and increased survival, though this has not been quantitatively assessed. In other words, rash seems to be a surrogate marker of clinical benefit, but this finding needs to be confirmed in future studies.

27. Answer H

Sunitinib is an inhibitor of tyrosine kinase and targets multiple receptors, including vascular endothelial growth factor (VEGF) receptors 2 and 3, platelet-derived growth factor receptor B (PDGFR B), FLT-3 and c-KIT. These receptors play a role in both tumour angiogenesis and tumour cell proliferation. The simultaneous inhibition of these targets therefore leads to both reduced tumour vascularisation and cancer cell apoptosis, and ultimately tumour shrinkage.

Sunitinib is used in the treatment of renal cell carcinoma (RCC), gastrointestinal stromal tumour and pancreatic neuroendocrine tumour. First-line treatment options for patients with metastatic RCC with good or intermediate prognosis are sunitinib, bevacizumab plus interferon-alpha, or pazopanib. Temsirolimus (a derivative of sirolimus, mTOR inhibitor) and sunitinib can be used for those in the poor-risk prognostic group.

10 Infectious diseases

Questions

BASIC SCIENCE

Answers can be found in the Infectious diseases Answers section at the end of this chapter.

1. Which cells does the Epstein–Barr virus establish a latent infection in?
   A. Erythrocytes
   B. Neutrophils
   C. B lymphocytes
   D. Basophils
   E. T lymphocytes

2. Which one of the following is a Gram-positive organism that exists intracellularly?
   A. *Listeria monocytogenes*
   B. *Clostridium difficile*
   C. *Staphylococcus aureus*
   D. *Clostridium perfringens*
   E. *Streptococcus pyrogenes*

3. What cell type is preferentially infected by JC virus in progressive multifocal leucoencephalopathy?
   A. Astrocyte
   B. Ependyma
   C. Microglia
   D. Oligodendrocyte
   E. Schwann cell

4. Human immunodeficiency virus-1 (HIV-1) infection has been associated with which one of the following changes?
   A. Depletion of mucosal CD4 cells
   B. Increased numbers of CD4 naïve cells
   C. Increased production of CD34 progenitor cells in the bone marrow

Passing the FRACP Written Examination: Questions and Answers, First Edition. Jonathan Gleadle, Tuck Yong, Jordan Li, Surjit Tarafdar, and Danielle Wu.
© 2013 John Wiley & Sons, Ltd. Published 2013 by John Wiley & Sons, Ltd.

D. Increased proliferation of thymocytes
E. Complement-mediated B-lymphocyte death

Theme: Toxins produced by microorganisms
(for Questions 5–9)
A. *Bacillus anthracis* toxin
B. Botulinum toxin
C. *Clostridium difficile* toxin
D. *Clostridium tetani* toxin
E. Cyanobacteria toxin
F. Staphylococcal toxins
G. *Vibrio cholera* toxin
H. Aspergillus aflatoxin

For each of the following questions select the most likely responsible toxin.

5. Which toxin causes paralysis by blocking release of acetylcholine in the peripheral nerve synapses?

6. Which toxin activates large numbers of T lymphocytes?

7. Which toxin acts by preventing the release of the inhibitory neurotransmitter gamma-aminobutyric acid (GABA) and glycine, leading to sustained excitatory discharge by motor neurones?

8. Which toxin acts by causing persistent activation of adenylate cyclase?

9. Which toxin is carcinogenic?

CLINICAL

10. A 45-year-old resident of Northern Queensland presents with a 3-day history of fever (39.5° C), myalgia, headache, protracted vomiting and a macular rash. A blood test shows thrombocytopaenia and there is prolonged bleeding at the venipuncture site. A provisional diagnosis of dengue is made and confirmed by a positive RT-PCR test for dengue non-structural protein 1 (NS1). What treatments should be administered?
  A. A broad-spectrum cephalosporin and an aminoglycoside
  B. Supportive care, including monitoring for the development of shock and a systemic vascular leak syndrome
  C. Supportive care, including monitoring for the development of shock and a systemic vascular leak syndrome, and high-dose corticosteroids
  D. Intravenous valganciclovir
  E. Intramuscular artesunate

11. A 38-year-old man with previously treated early syphilis and hepatitis C infection presents to a hospital complaining of tender right inguinal lymphadenopathy for the past 3 months. An excisional biopsy showed the formation of necrotising granuloma indicative of lymphogranuloma venereum. What should he be treated with?
  A. Benzylpenicillin
  B. Clindamycin
  C. Ciprofloxacin
  D. Doxycycline
  E. Sulphamethoxazole–trimethoprim (Bactrim)

12. A 78-year-old woman is diagnosed to have herpes zoster ophthalmicus. Her other medical history included myelodysplastic syndrome and type 2 diabetes. Which one of the following statements about her treatment is correct?
  A. Aciclovir is effective in treating post-herpetic neuralgia
  B. Aciclovir is beneficial when therapy is initiated within 72 h of onset of the skin lesions
  C. Famciclovir has been shown to more effective than aciclovir, leading to a shorter duration of symptoms
  D. Aciclovir is contraindicated in patients with myelodysplastic syndrome
  E. Topical steroid eye drops should be administered

13. A 42-year-old man with human immunodeficiency virus (HIV) infection on combination highly active anti-retroviral treatment (HARRT) including zidovudine complains of leg weakness and incontinence. Physical examination reveals reduced strength in the legs with accompanying mild spasticity. There is also diminished sensation in the feet and legs bilaterally. Despite treatment, his most recent CD4 count is 45 cells/μL. Lumbar puncture shows:

Opening pressure	10 cmH$_2$0
Lymphocyte count	4 × 10^6/L (<5 × 10^6/L)
Glucose	3.8 mmol/L (serum glucose 5.6 mmol/L)
Total protein	0.33 g/L (0.10–0.65 g/L)
Gram stain	No organisms seen

Additional laboratory investigations show normal haematological parameters, normal vitamin B$_{12}$ levels and negative serology for syphilis. Magnetic resonance imaging of the head is normal. Which one of the following is the most likely diagnosis?

    A. HIV-associated dementia
    B. HIV-associated myelopathy
    C. Cryptococcal meningoencephalitis
    D. Cytomegalovirus polyradiculopathy
    E. Zidovudine-related toxicity

14. A 64-year-old woman presents with fever and speech disturbance over the past week. Her temperature is 37.9°C. The patient is alert and oriented with respect to time but unable to name objects properly. Dysarthria and occasional word substitution are noted. The patient is able to follow simple but not three-step commands. Part of her magnetic resonance imaging of the brain is shown below. What is the most likely diagnosis?

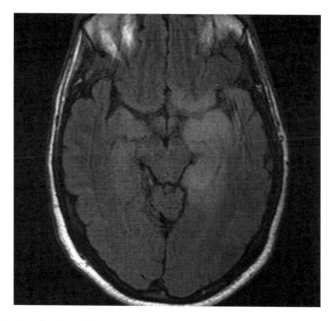

    A. Cerebral toxoplasmosis
    B. Herpes simplex encephalitis

C. Meningococcal meningitis
D. Multiple sclerosis
E. Progressive multifocal leucoencephalopathy

15. A patient with human immunodeficiency virus (HIV) is concerned about changing facial appearance after receiving highly active anti-retroviral therapy (HAART). Which one of the following anti-retroviral drugs is most likely to cause lipoatrophy?
   A. Delavirdine
   B. Zidovudine
   C. Nevirapine
   D. Didanosine
   E. Abacavir

16. Regarding *Clostridium difficile* infection, which one of the following is INCORRECT?
   A. Judicious use of antibiotics, minimisation of cross-infection by observing careful hand hygiene and barrier precautions can prevent acquisition of *C. difficile* infection in hospitalised patients
   B. There is significant antibiotic resistance in patients previously treated with oral metronidazole or oral vancomycin
   C. Oral metronidazole is recommended as a first-line therapy for mild *C. difficile* infection because of its lower cost and concerns about the proliferation of vancomycin-resistant bacteria
   D. Oral vancomycin is the recommended first-line agent for treating severe *C. difficile* infection due to the more prompt symptom resolution and a lower risk of treatment failure
   E. Faecal transplantation remains unpopular for practical and aesthetic reasons despite proven efficacy in case series

17. In patients with human immunodeficiency virus (HIV) infection the definite indications for offering anti-retroviral therapy (ART) are:
   A. CD4 cell count of 550 cells/μL in patients with previous history of *Pneumocystis jiroveci* pneumonia
   B. CD8 cell counts of <400 cells/μL
   C. Thrombocytopenia (platelet count <150 × 10^9 cells/L)
   D. Age younger than 50 years
   E. Diabetes in HIV-infected patient

18. Overwhelming post-splenectomy infection defines fulminating sepsis, meningitis or pneumonia in splenectomised and hyposplenic individuals. The most common causative organism is:
   A. *Neisseria meningitides*
   B. *Escherichia coli*
   C. *Pseudomonas aeruginosa*
   D. *Enterococcus* spp
   E. *Streptococcus pneumoniae*

19. An 18-year-old girl was studying for examinations together with a friend who was hospitalised 2 days ago with meningitis. The blood cultures in her friend grew meningococcus group A. Which one of the following actions should be taken for the girl who was in contact with the patient with meningitis?
  A. No treatment is required
  B. Immunisation with meningococcus vaccine
  C. Single-dose intramuscular ceftriaxone 250 mg
  D. Single dose intramuscular ceftriaxone 250 mg and immunisation with meningococcus vaccine
  E. Single-dose oral rifampicin and immunisation with meningococcus vaccine

20. A 29-year-old indigenous man was admitted with a 6-day history of abdominal pain, vomiting and diarrhoea. His medical history included chronic alcohol-related liver disease, co-infection with hepatitis B and human T-cell lymphotropic virus type 1 (HTLV-1). Blood cultures grew *Escherichia coli*. Rhabditiform larvae were seen on stool microscopy. He was given intravenous ceftriaxone. Forty-eight hours after admission, he became hypotensive and transferred to the intensive care unit. He was treated for septic shock. Apart from fluid resuscitation, intravenous ceftriaxone and inotropic support, which one of the following treatments is most appropriate?
  A. Intravenous ganciclovir
  B. Intravenous hydrocortisone
  C. Intravenous metronidazole
  D. Oral albendazole
  E. Oral ivermectin

21. Which one of the following statements best describes the evaluation or management of patients with syphilis in Australia and New Zealand?
  A. Screening for syphilis in Australia utilises enzyme immune assay (EIA) treponemal tests
  B. Cerebrospinal fluid (CSF) analysis is not essential to confirm neurosyphilis
  C. Azithromycin is the first-line treatment for all stages of syphilis in Australia
  D. Different antibiotic regimens are indicated in HIV-positive patients with syphilis co-infection
  E. Contacts presenting within 3 months of exposure to syphilis do not require treatment unless serologically positive

22. A 70-year-old man was admitted to the intensive care unit because of septic shock caused by *Pseudomonas aeruginosa* urinary tract infection. He received intravenous ceftazidime and amikacin via a central venous line. After 7 days of antibiotics he developed fever and blood culture was positive for Gram-positive cocci in chains, which were catalase negative. Vancomycin was started but the blood cultures remained positive for the same organism even after 3 days of therapy. The most likely organism causing this infection is:

A. *Staphylococcus aureus*
B. *Pseudomonas aeruginosa*
C. *Enterococcus faecalis*
D. Coagulase-negative staphylococcus
E. *Streptococcus pyogenes*

Theme: Opportunistic infections (for Questions 23–26)

A. *Pneumocystis jirovecii*
B. *Candida albicans*
C. Toxoplasmosis
D. Cryptosporidium
E. Cryptococcus
F. Varicella zoster
G. Cytomegalovirus
H. *Mycobacterium avium intracellulare*

For each of these patients, select the most likely organism.

23. A 43-year-old woman who is known to be human immunodeficiency virus (HIV) positive presents with nausea, dizziness, confusion and a stiff neck of 1 week's duration. Her temperature is 38.5°C and mild neck stiffness is present; all other examination is normal. Complete blood count and routine chemistries are normal, except for mild leukopenia. Computed tomography of the head is unremarkable. Lumbar puncture is performed, with the following results: an opening pressure of 32 cmH$_2$O; a low glucose level; an elevated protein level; and an elevated white cell count, with neutrophil predominance. What is the most likely infective organism responsible for this presentation?

24. A 46-year-old man who is HIV positive (CD4+ T-cell count of 42 cells/μL) presents after having a seizure. He reports that for the past 3 weeks he has been experiencing worsening tremor, visual disturbances and headaches. Computed tomography of the head with contrast showed a single thin-walled cavitating lesion with ring enhancement and oedema of the surrounding white matter. Which one of the infective organism can cause his clinical presentation?

25. A 45-year-old woman has been HIV positive for the past 10 years. Despite receiving highly active anti-retroviral therapy (HAART), her most recent CD4+ T-cell count was 180 cells/μL. Which opportunistic infection is this patient most at risk of developing?

26. A 39-year-old man who is HIV positive (CD4+ T-cell count 100 cells/μL) presents with a complaint of profuse, watery diarrhoea. He has had these symptoms for 2 weeks. Conservative treatment measures have been unsuccessful. Evaluation of the stool reveals oocysts. What is the most likely organism that can explain his presentation?

Answers

BASIC SCIENCE

1. Answer C

The Epstein–Barr virus (EBV) is a γ-herpes virus that establishes a latent infection in B lymphocytes and epithelial cells. Under certain conditions such as immuno-suppression, the virus may reactivate its full latent repertoire in the infected B cell to induce lymphoproliferative diseases which, under normal conditions, would lead to destruction of the cell by virtue of the expression of various latent proteins that unmask the infected cell to the immune system. Depending on the cell type and the immunological environment, EBV establishes different types of latent infection.

About 95% of all adults worldwide show serological markers of EBV infection. In most people, EBV infection is symptomless, but the virus occasionally induces infectious mononucleosis, a self-limiting lymphoproliferation with elevated lymphocytes and atypical monocytes. EBV is found in virtually all cases of undifferentiated nasopharyngeal carcinoma and nasal NK/T-cell lymphoma, in about 95% of cases of endemic Burkitt lymphoma (BL), in some subsets of Hodgkin lymphoma, in approximately 15% of diffuse large B-cell lymphoma and in about 10% of gastric carcinoma. In contrast to the endemic form, EBV is found only in 15–30% of sporadic BL. EBV is present in up to 90% of post-transplant lymphoma (PTLD) under immunosuppression (Lim et al., 2006).

 Lim, W.H., Russ, G.R., and Coates, P.T. (2006). Review of Epstein–Barr virus and post-transplant lymphoproliferative disorder post-solid organ transplantation. *Nephrology (Carlton)* 11, 355–366.
http://onlinelibrary.wiley.com/doi/10.1111/j.1440-1797.2006.00596.x/full

2. Answer A

Listeria monocytogenes is a small Gram-positive facultative intracellular bacillus. Listeria has the ability to spread from cell to cell without entering the extracellular environment. It does this by using an actin polymerisation propulsion system. Other pathogenic bacteria that can exist intracellularly include mycobacterium, brucella, rickettsia and chlamydia.

Endotoxins are part of the outer membrane of the cell wall of Gram-negative bacteria and are invariably associated with Gram-negative bacteria whether the organisms are pathogenic or not. *Listeria monocytogenes* is the only Gram-positive bacteria that produce endotoxins.

Listeria can cause meningoencephalitis, sepsis and gastroenteritis. Infection in pregnancy can lead to premature birth or fetal death. Immunosuppressed and elderly patients, pregnant women and newborns of infected mothers are typically affected by *L. monocytogenes*. Listeria is most commonly transmitted via unpasteurised dairy products, meat and vegetables. Also, it can spread transplacentally during delivery. Ampicillin is the treatment of choice. Listeria is always resistant to cephalosporins.

3. Answer D
Progressive multifocal leucoencephalopathy (PML) is a potentially fatal demyelinating disease of the central nervous system that predominantly affects immunocompromised patients. The aetiological agent, JC virus (JCV), is a widespread polyomavirus with a very particular target, the myelin-producing oligodendroglia of the brain. During periods of immune suppression, the virus can be reactivated from lymphoid tissues and kidney, causing targeted myelin destruction and corresponding neurological deficits. The incidence of PML has increased in recent years, due to HIV infection and the growing number of patients receiving immunosuppressant treatment, including natalizumab treatment of multiple sclerosis. Serological studies have shown that more than 80% of the human population has antibodies to JCV.

4. Answer A
Depletion of CD4 cells in human immunodeficiency virus (HIV) infection may occur as a result of direct infection and death of CD4 cells or by indirect mechanisms. HIV-1 infection has been associated with:
- Impaired production of CD34 progenitor cells in the bone marrow
- Reduced proliferation of thymocytes and direct infection of CD4 thymocytes leading to reduced numbers of recent thymic emigrants and CD4 naïve cells
- Direct infection of circulating CD4 memory cells but at low frequency
- Depletion of mucosal CD4 cells by direct infection of both $CCR5^+$ and $CCR5^-$ CD4 cells, dendritic cells and macrophages
- High levels of immune activation that increase the proliferation and death of both CD4 and CD8 cells, which are linked to lymph node fibrosis and retention of T cells in the lymph nodes (Cohen et al., 2011; Moir et al., 2011).

 Cohen, M.S., Shaw, G.M., McMichael, A.J., and Haynes, B.F. (2011). Acute HIV-1 Infection. *N Engl J Med* 364, 1943–1954.
http://www.ncbi.nlm.nih.gov/pubmed/21591946

 Moir, S., Chun, T.W., and Fauci, A.S. (2011). Pathogenic mechanisms of HIV disease. *Annu Rev Pathol* 6, 223–248.
http://www.ncbi.nlm.nih.gov/pubmed/21034222

5. Answer B
Botulinum toxin is absorbed from the gut and carried via the blood to peripheral nerve synapses where it blocks release of acetylcholine. The toxin is a polypeptide encoded by a lysogenic phage. There are eight immunological types of toxin; A, B and E are the most common in human illness. Very small amounts of this toxin are effective in the treatment of certain spasmodic muscle disorders, such as torticollis and diffuse oesophageal spasm.

6. Answer F

S. aureus exotoxins cause disease because they are superantigens. Superantigens are molecules that are able to activate large numbers of T cells, often up to 20% of all T cells at one time, resulting in massive cytokine production. In typical T-cell recognition, an antigen is taken up by an antigen-presenting cell, processed, expressed on the cell surface in complex with class II major histocompatibility complex (MHC) in a groove formed by the alpha and beta chains of class II MHC, and recognised by an antigen-specific T-cell receptor. By contrast, superantigens do not require processing by antigen-presenting cells, but instead interact directly with the invariant region of the class II MHC molecule. The superantigen–MHC complex then interacts with the T-cell receptor at the variable (V) part of the beta chain. Thus, all T cells with a recognised V beta region are stimulated. Activated T cells then release interleukin (IL)-1, IL-2, tumour necrosis factor (TNF)-alpha and TNF-beta, and interferon (IFN)-gamma in large amounts, resulting in the signs and symptoms of toxic shock syndrome.

7. Answer D

The tetanus toxin is transported from the peripheral to the central nervous system by retrograde axonal transport. It interferes with the exocytosis of inhibitory neurotransmitters so that alpha motor neurones are therefore under no inhibitory control and undergo sustained excitatory discharge, causing the characteristic muscle spasms of tetanus. The toxin exerts its effects on the spinal cord, the brain stem, peripheral nerves, at neuromuscular junctions and directly on muscles. Tetanus toxin is highly homologous to the family of botulinum neurotoxins, which like tetanus toxin, inhibit neurotransmitter release by cleavage of proteins involved in vesicle fusion. The difference in clinical symptoms between botulism and tetanus is due to the location of toxin action. Botulinum toxin is not transported to the central nervous system and remains at the periphery where it inhibits the release of acetylcholine. This results in an acute flaccid paralysis.

8. Answer G

Following ganglioside-mediated binding to enterocytes, components of the cholera toxin catalyses the ADP-ribosylation of a GTP-binding protein, leading to persistent activation of adenylate cyclase. The increase of cAMP in the intestinal mucosa leads to increased chloride secretion and decreased sodium absorption, producing the massive fluid and electrolyte loss characteristic of cholera.

9. Answer H

Aflatoxins are mycotoxins produced by aspergillus fungi and can occur in foods (including wheat, soybeans and peanuts). They have been associated with the development of hepatocellular carcinoma and may be associated with high rates of p53 mutation.

CLINICAL

10. Answer B

Dengue is caused by an RNA virus transmitted by the mosquito *Aedes aegypti*. Anti-bacterial antibiotics are therefore of no benefit unless there is secondary infection, there is no place for anti-malarials, and no evidence of benefit from existing anti-viral therapies or corticosteroids. Treatment is supportive, with particular emphasis on careful fluid management (Simmons et al., 2012).

Patients who are significantly unwell or who are unable to tolerate oral fluids should be hospitalised and observed closely. Patients with severe dengue infection should be treated in high-dependency or intensive care units where frequent clinical observations by experienced staff and repeated haematocrit measurements can ensure that fluid therapy is carefully titrated. The most concerning complication is the development of the dengue shock syndrome with systemic vascular leakage. If shock develops, prompt fluid resuscitation to restore plasma volume is vital, followed by cautious ongoing fluid therapy with isotonic crystalloid; and isotonic colloid solutions should be reserved for profound shock or lack of a response to initial therapy. Blood transfusion can be required for patients with severe haemorrhage, but it should be undertaken with care because of the risk of fluid overload. Platelet concentrates, fresh-frozen plasma and cryoprecipitate may also be needed depending on the coagulation tests.

Simmons, C.P., Farrar, J.J., Nguyen, V., and Wills, B. (2012). Dengue. *N Engl J Med* 366, 1423–1432.
http://www.ncbi.nlm.nih.gov/pubmed/22494122

11. Answer D

Lymphogranuloma venereum (LGV) is a sexually transmitted disease caused by *Chlamydia trachomatis* (White, 2009). It causes a papule or ulcer that may occur on the penis, urethra or cervix. Proctocolitis may also be present, mimicking inflammatory bowel disease. Regional lymphadenopathy develops in the secondary stage of disease when there may be systemic symptoms. Confirmation of a diagnosis of LGV requires serological tests or PCR on genitourinary specimens. Prolonged treatment with doxycycline or roxithromycin for 3 weeks is required for affected patients.

White, J.A. (2009). Manifestations and management of lymphogranuloma venereum. *Curr Opin Infect Dis* 22, 57–66.
http://www.ncbi.nlm.nih.gov/pubmed/19532081

12. Answer B

Oral aciclovir has been shown to shorten the duration of signs and symptoms, as well as to reduce the incidence and severity of herpes zoster ophthalmicus complications (Steiner et al., 2007). While aciclovir can reduce the pain during the acute phase, it has no demonstrated effect on reducing the incidence or severity of post-herpetic neuralgia. Aciclovir appears to benefit patients the most when therapy is initiated within 72 h of onset of the lesions. Both famciclovir and valaciclovir have been shown to be as effective as aciclovir in the treatment of herpes zoster and to reduce complications. Famciclovir is a prodrug that is metabolised to an active metabolite, penciclovir. Aciclovir is not haematotoxic and can be used in patients with myelodysplastic syndrome.

Topical steroids alone do not reactivate the virus, but may exacerbate spontaneous recurrences. In addition, while steroid eye drops may be beneficial for herpes zoster ophthalmicus, they are helpful only in certain ocular diseases and can exacerbate others such as epithelial keratitis. Therefore, ophthalmologic consultation is mandatory prior to initiating ocular steroid therapy.

Steiner, I., Kennedy, P.G., and Pachner, A.R. (2007). The neurotropic herpes viruses: herpes simplex and varicella-zoster. *Lancet Neurol* 6, 1015–1028.
http://www.ncbi.nlm.nih.gov/pubmed/17945155

13. Answer B

Human immunodeficiency virus (HIV)-associated myelopathy is one of the most common neurological complications of acquired immunodeficiency syndrome (AIDS) (McArthur et al., 2005). There is degeneration of the spinal tracts in the posterior and lateral columns, which have a vacuolated microscopic appearance. Although the morphological changes and clinical manifestations are similar to those associated with vitamin B_{12} deficiency, the pathogenetic mechanism is probably not related to dietary deficiencies. Since there is no specific clinical or laboratory test available for the diagnosis of this syndrome, HIV-associated myelopathy remains a diagnosis of exclusion.

HIV-associated dementia manifests with progressive memory loss, alterations in fine motor control, urinary incontinence and altered mental status.

Cytomegalovirus (CMV) polyradiculopathy may simulate HIV myelopathy and is a relatively frequent complication of AIDS. It can be excluded by the results of cerebrospinal fluid (CSF) analysis. CMV infection commonly leads to a neutrophilic pleocytosis in the CSF.

Cryptococcal meningoencephalitis would lead to signs and symptoms of meningitis. The CSF would show the fungal organism, which can be detected by India ink stains and culture studies.

Zidovudine-related toxicity would lead to proximal muscle weakness and tenderness, due mainly to a myopathic process.

McArthur, J.C., Brew, B.J., and Nath, A. (2005). Neurological complications of HIV infection. *Lancet Neurol* 4, 543–555.
http://www.ncbi.nlm.nih.gov/pubmed/16109361

14. Answer B

Herpes simplex viruses (HSV-1 and HSV-2) produce a variety of infections involving mucocutaneous surfaces, the central nervous system (CNS) and, occasionally, the visceral organs. HSV encephalitis is the most common identified cause of acute, sporadic viral encephalitis that is usually localised to the temporal and frontal lobes in adults. Typically, it causes a flu-like illness with headache and fever followed by seizures, cognitive impairment, behavioural changes and focal neurological signs, as in this case. However, its presentation is variable (Sabah et al., 2012).

If herpes simplex encephalitis is suspected, brain imaging (magnetic resonance imaging if possible, otherwise computed tomography) and cerebrospinal fluid (CSF) analysis (if lumbar puncture is not contraindicated, such as by mass effect or coagulopathy) should be performed urgently. Definitive diagnosis of herpes simplex encephalitis is made by the detection of viral nucleic acid in the CSF by polymerase chain reaction (PCR). This test has a sensitivity of 96–98% and specificity of 95–99% and has removed the need for brain biopsy. It remains positive for at least 5–7 days after starting anti-viral therapy. Viral DNA may be undetectable in early disease, but, if so, a repeat examination by PCR on CSF 3–7 days later can confirm the diagnosis.

Pending the confirmation of the diagnosis of herpes simplex encephalitis, all adults with suspected encephalitis should be given aciclovir empirically, at a dose of 10 mg/kg, administered as intravenous infusions over 1 h and repeated every 8 h for 14–21 days if renal function is normal.

Sabah, M., Mulcahy, J., and Zeman, A. (2012). Herpes simplex encephalitis. *BMJ* 344, e3166.
http://www.bmj.com/content/344/bmj.e3166?view=long&pmid=22674925

15. Answer B

Lipodystrophy, including subcutaneous adipose tissue wasting (subcutaneous lipoatrophy), central adipose tissue accumulation (central lipohypertrophy), severe dyslipidaemia and abnormalities in glucose metabolism are common among HIV-infected patients receiving highly active anti-retroviral therapy (HAART) (Brown and Glesby, 2012). Facial lipoatrophy, which begins in the malar region and extends to the buccal and temporal regions with increasing severity, can reduce quality of life and compromise adherence to HAART.

Exposure to the thymidine analogue nucleoside reverse transcriptase inhibitors (NRTIs) zidovudine and stavudine is the most important risk factor for the development of lipoatrophy. These medications cause mitochondrial dysfunction in adipocytes, leading to adipocyte apoptosis. Other patient factors, such as male sex, older age and more advanced HIV disease have also been associated with the development of lipoatrophy, and certain mitochondrial haplotypes and nuclear genetic polymorphisms may increase susceptibility. The low incidence of lipoatrophy in HIV-infected individuals not receiving thymidine analogue NRTIs supports the primary role of these medications in its pathogenesis.

The most effective treatment for lipoatrophy is avoidance of or switching from treatment with thymidine analogue NRTIs. Fortunately, with the availability of other NRTIs without adverse effects on body composition (e.g. abacavir and teno-fovir), use of thymidine analogue NRTIs has decreased considerably in the developed world.

Didanosine causes pancreatitis. Nevirapine and delavirdine are non-nucleoside reverse transcriptase inhibitors (NNRTI) with Stevens–Johnson syndrome/rash as their main side effect.

Brown, T.T. and Glesby, M.J. (2012). Management of the metabolic effects of HIV and HIV drugs. *Nat Rev Endocrinol* 8, 11–21.
http://www.ncbi.nlm.nih.gov/pmc/articles/PMC3371609/

16. Answer B

Anti-microbial resistance to vancomycin has never been reported in *C. difficile* and resistance to metronidazole is rare. The same antibiotic agent used to treat the initial episode of *C. difficile* infection can be used for a first recurrence of infection. However, there is no standard or proven therapy for multiple recurrences. Regimens that incorporate tapering or pulsed administration of vancomycin have significantly fewer recurrences (Kelly and LaMont, 2008).

C. difficile infection causes significant morbidity and mortality in elderly and frail hospital and nursing home patients. The careful selection of antibiotics and the avoidance of antibiotic use when possible remain the mainstays of prevention. Probiotics can reduce the incidence of simple antibiotic-associated diarrhoea, but their efficacy in preventing *C. difficile* infection is inconsistent.

Markers of severe *C. difficile* infection include pseudomembranous colitis on endoscopy, marked peripheral leucocytosis, acute renal failure and hypotension.

There is no significant difference in response rate between vancomycin (98%) and metronidazole (90%) in patients with mild infection ($P = 0.36$). However, in patients with severe infection, vancomycin has a significantly better response rate (97%) compared to metronidazole (76%) ($P = 0.02$).

Kelly, C.P. and Lamont, J.T. (2008). *Clostridium difficile* – more difficult than ever. *N Engl J Med* 359, 1932–1940.
http://www.ncbi.nlm.nih.gov/pubmed/18971494

17. Answer A

According to the Australasian Society of HIV Medicine (ASHM), Australia follows the USA Department of Health and Human services (DHHS) guidelines for the treatment of AIDS. As per the DHHS guidelines, anti-retroviral therapy (ART) is recommended for all HIV-infected individuals. The strength of this recommendation depends on the pre-treatment CD4 cell count:

- CD4 count <350 cells/μL (AI)
- CD4 count 350–500 cells/mm³ (AII)
- CD4 count >500 cells/mm³ (BIII)

where the rating of recommendations is A = strong, B = moderate and C = optional, and rating of evidence is I = data from randomised controlled trials, II = data from well-designed non-randomised trials or observational cohort studies with long-term clinical outcomes, and III = expert opinion.

Regardless of the CD4 count, initiation of ART is strongly recommended for individuals with the following conditions:

- Pregnancy
- History of an AIDS-defining illness
- HIV-associated nephropathy
- Age older than 60 years
- HIV/hepatitis B virus (HBV) co-infection
- Effective ART also has been shown to prevent transmission of HIV from an infected individual to a sexual partner; therefore, ART should be offered to patients who are at risk of transmitting HIV to sexual partners.

The use of Antiretroviral Agents in HIV-1-Infected Adults and Adolescents. Available from:
http://arv.ashm.org.au/

18. Answer E

Overwhelming post-splenectomy infection (OPSI) is a medical emergency requiring prompt diagnosis, and immediate treatment can reduce mortality (Sabatino et al., 2011). The mortality rate is 50–70% and most deaths occur within the first 24 h.

Bacteraemia commonly has an unknown origin; after a brief prodrome characterised by fever, rigor, myalgia, vomiting, diarrhoea and headache, septic shock develops within a few hours with anuria, hypotension, hypoglycaemia, disseminated intravascular coagulation and massive adrenal haemorrhage, and progresses to multiorgan failure and death.

Streptococcus pneumoniae is the most common causal organism (50–90% of cases) followed by *Haemophilus influenzae* type b and *Neisseria meningitides*. *Salmonella* spp. can infect patients with sickle-cell disease, which mostly causes osteomyelitis. Less frequent causative organisms include *Escherichia coli*, *Pseudomonas aeruginosa*, *Capnocytophaga canimorsus* and, rarely, *Enterococcus* spp., *Bacteroides* spp. and *Bartonella* spp.

In patients at risk and with indicative symptoms of OPSI, treatment with empirical antibiotics is essential; third-generation cephalosporins combined with gentamicin or ciprofloxacin if possible urinary or intestinal focus is suspected, or vancomycin in case of resistance to benzylpenicillin.

Up to 84% of splenectomised individuals are thought to be unaware of their increased susceptibility to severe infection.

Sabatino, A.D., Carsetti, R., and Corazza, G.R. (2011).
Post-splenectomy and hyposplenic states. *Lancet* 378, 86–97.
http://www.ncbi.nlm.nih.gov/pubmed/21474172

19. Answer D

A single dose of intramuscular ceftriaxone is very effective (97%) in eradicating pharyngeal meningococci from carriers and more effective than oral rifampicin 600 mg twice a day for 2 days (75–81%). For eradication the recommended dose of antibiotic for adults is 250 mg intramuscularly, as a single dose. Other treatment options include a single oral dose of 500 mg of ciprofloxacin. Ceftriaxone is the preferred agent for pregnant women. Because compliance is likely to be good and because it is readily available, it should also be considered as the preferred agent in rural and remote communities, especially in indigenous communities.

Due to the prolonged risk of secondary cases in household settings or close contact, vaccination is indicated for unimmunised household and sexual/close contacts of cases of confirmed vaccine-preventable invasive meningococcal disease. Vaccination should be offered to these contacts as soon as the serogroup is confirmed, and within 4 weeks of onset of disease in the case. There are two different types of meningococcal vaccine: the meningococcal C conjugate vaccines (MenCCVs) and the tetravalent meningococcal polysaccharide vaccines (4vMenPVs). They differ in the way they stimulate an immune response. MenCCVs confer protection only against serogroup C disease, but 4vMenPVs provide protection against serogroups A, C, W_{135} and Y. Household contacts (or equivalent) of cases of vaccine-preventable strains should be provided with a letter advising that they should receive vaccination, and that they should visit their usual health-care provider at the earliest opportunity to receive this.

Communicable Diseases Network Australia. Guidelines for the early clinical and public health management of meningococcal disease in Australia.
Commonwealth Department of Health and Ageing, 2007.
http://www.health.gov.au/internet/main/publishing.nsf/content/cda-pubs-other-mening-2007.htm

20. Answer E

This patient has disseminated strongyloidiasis. *Strongyloides stercoralis* is a nematode human parasite that can maintain long-term infection by means of an autoinfective life cycle. *S. stercoralis* is particularly prevalent in indigenous Australians (Einsiedel and Fernandes, 2008). The autoinfective life cycle permits prolonged infection and has the potential to produce a hyperinfective syndrome in immunocompromised patients. Mortality rates of 87% have been reported in immunocompromised patients. Death frequently results from bloodstream infection with enteric pathogens due to carriage of bacteria by the nematode or ulceration of the bowel wall. Complicated strongyloidiasis is usually a complication of malignancy, malnutrition in the setting of excessive alcohol consumption, immunosuppression and co-infection with HTLV-1. Before commencement of immunosuppression, indigenous patients and patients at risk for strongyloidiasis should be screened for strongyloidiasis and their HTLV-1 serostatus determined. The diagnosis of complicated strongyloidiasis should be considered for all indigenous patients who present with sepsis due to infection with enteric bacterial pathogens or where pulmonary and gastrointestinal systems are involved and no causative organism can be found.

Previous studies from areas not endemic for HTLV-1 have clearly shown the inferiority of albendazole compared with ivermectin for the treatment of uncomplicated disease. The optimal treatment of disseminated disease and hyperinfection is uncertain. In immunocompromised patients with disseminated disease, reduction of immunosuppressive therapy is an important adjunct to any anthelminthic therapy. In such cases, it is also usually necessary to prolong or repeat ivermectin therapy. Some experts give ivermectin for 5–7 days in disseminated disease, or combine ivermectin with albendazole until the patient responds. Others suggest daily ivermectin until symptoms resolve and stool tests have been negative for at least 2 weeks (one autoinfection cycle), or longer if the patient remains immunosuppressed. If the patient is unable to receive oral therapy due to ileus or obtundation, alternative regimens, including subcutaneous ivermectin (200 µg/kg), per rectal ivermectin administration and a parenteral veterinary formulation of ivermectin, have been used with variable success.

Einsiedel, L. and Fernandes, L. (2008). Strongyloides stercoralis: a cause of morbidity and mortality for indigenous people in Central Australia. *Intern Med J* 38, 697–703.
http://www.ncbi.nlm.nih.gov/pubmed/19143887

21. Answer A
Syphilis has been resurgent in Australian and New Zealand cities for the last decade (Read and Donovan, 2012). Screening for syphilis in Australia utilises sensitive and specific treponemal tests, such as enzyme immune assay (EIA) that may contain both immunoglobulin G and immunoglobulin M components. These are then confirmed by supplementary specific tests, such as *Treponema pallidum* particle agglutination assay (TPPA) or fluorescent treponemal antibody absorption test (FTA-Abs). However, these tests do not give any indication of disease activity and will normally remain positive for life regardless of treatment. A non-specific test, such as the rapid plasma regain (RPR) or Venereal Disease Research Laboratory (VDRL) test, is used to provide a titre to stage the infection, assess treatment response and detect re-infection.

Neurosyphilis is the most serious complication of syphilis. Cerebrospinal fluid (CSF) analysis is required to confirm the diagnosis. The CSF white cell count (usually lymphocytes) is typically raised at more than 5 cells/mm^3, protein levels are increased and glucose is normal. CSF VDRL confirms the diagnosis if positive.

Penicillin has remained the first-line treatment for all stages of syphilis. Azithromycin has been shown to be at least as effective in producing serological cure as penicillin. However, in Sydney, the prevalence of the azithromycin resistance gene A2058G on the 23S ribosome of *T. pallidum* is present in over 85% of samples. Treatment response is monitored using the RPR or VDRL titres, and a four-fold reduction within 6–12 months is considered a cure.

Syphilis is more common in HIV-positive than in HIV-negative individuals in Australia. Contact tracing is the responsibility of the diagnosing clinician. Contacts presenting within 3 months of exposure to syphilis should be treated empirically as primary syphilis because serology may be falsely negative during this period.

Read, P.J. and Donovan, B. (2012). Clinical aspects of adult syphilis. *Intern Med J* 42, 614–620.
http://www.ncbi.nlm.nih.gov/pubmed/22697151

22. Answer C

Catalase-negative Gram-positive cocci are characteristic of either *Streptococcus* or *Enterococcus*. Enterococci are common causes of hospital-acquired infections and are resistant to third-generation cephalosporins and sometimes to vancomycin (Courvalin, 2006).

Vancomycin interferes with the synthesis of peptidoglycan in the production of the bacterial cell wall. Vancomycin does not penetrate into the cytoplasm; therefore, interaction with its target can take place only after translocation of precursors to the outer surface of the membrane. Because vancomycin does not interact with cell wall biosynthetic enzymes, but forms complexes with peptidoglycan precursors, its activity is not determined by the affinity for a target enzyme but by the substrate specificity of the enzymes that determine the structure of peptidoglycan precursors. Resistance to vancomycin is due to the presence of operons that encode enzymes for synthesis of low-affinity precursors, in which the C-terminal D-Ala residue is replaced by D-lactate (D-Lac) or D-serine (D-Ser), thus modifying the vancomyin-binding target or for elimination of the high-affinity precursors that are normally produced by the host, thus removing the vancomycin-binding target.

Six types of vancomycin resistance have been characterised in enterococci. Five of these types (VanA, B, D, E and G) correspond to acquired resistance; one type (VanC) is an intrinsic property of *Enterococcus gallinarum* and *E. casseliflavus–E. flavescens*. The vanA gene cluster has been found mainly in *E. faecium* and *E. faecalis*. VanA-type resistance is characterised by inducible high levels of resistance to vancomycin and teicoplanin, is the most frequently encountered type of glycopeptide resistance in enterococci and, to date, is the only one to be detected in *Staphylococcus aureus*.

Courvalin, P. (2006). Vancomycin resistance in gram-positive cocci. *Clin Infect Dis* 42 Suppl 1, S25–34.
http://cid.oxfordjournals.org/content/42/Supplement_1/S25.long

23. Answer E

Cryptococcus is a yeast widely disseminated in nature. In immunocompetent patients, the organism is inhaled and asymptomatic pulmonary infection develops. In patients with compromised cell-mediated immunity, pulmonary infection may progress to central nervous system infection because cerebrospinal fluid (CSF) lacks several soluble anti-cryptococcal factors that are present in serum, such as complement components. Patients with cryptococcal meningitis often present with non-specific complaints, such as headache, nausea, dizziness and irritability. They may or may not have the usual signs of neck stiffness and fever. Diagnosis is made on the basis of CSF evaluation: an elevated opening pressure, an elevated white cell count with neutrophil predominance, an elevated protein level and a decrease in the glucose level. Latex agglutination alone detects antigen in 90% of patients with cryptococcal meningitis and can provide a definitive diagnosis when confirmed by culture. India ink smear detects cryptococci in only 25–60% of patients, and antigen titres are only used to follow the course of disease. CT or MRI may be normal or result in findings that are non-specific for meningitis.

24. Answer C

Most cases of toxoplasmosis in patients with HIV result from reactivation of latent toxoplasma cysts acquired before infection with HIV; reactivation is particularly likely when the CD4+ T-cell count falls below 100 cells/μL. Infection with the protozoan *Toxoplasma gondii* can cause encephalitis and cerebral abscesses, which can be misdiagnosed as primary cerebral tumour, lymphoma or stroke (Tan et al., 2012). The symptoms are of a space-occupying lesion, may cause seizure, focal neurological deficit, confusion and personality change. MRI is the investigation of choice in suspected toxoplasma infection and is superior to CT scanning. Serum antibody tests cannot be relied on in the diagnosis of primary toxoplasmosis in patients with HIV; antibody titres do not reach the high levels typical of immunocompetent patients with toxoplasmosis, nor are IgM antibodies present in patients with HIV. However, antibodies against *Toxoplasma* are present in the cerebrospinal fluid in nearly two-thirds of HIV patients with cerebral toxoplasmosis, and their detection may assist in the diagnosis.

Treatment with pyrimethamine in combination with sulphadiazine and folinic acid for at least 6 weeks can produce remarkable improvements in clinical condition. With appropriate therapy, clinical and radiological improvement is often observed within 1–2 weeks.

If patients respond poorly to treatment and are seronegative or belong to population groups at high risk for tuberculosis, biopsy should be strongly considered. Patients with HIV who have been treated for toxoplasmosis require prolonged suppressive therapy. If the CD4+ T-cell count rises above 200 cells/μL for 3 months, secondary prophylaxis for toxoplasmosis can be stopped.

Tan, I.L., Smith, B.R., von Geldern, G., Mateen, F.J., and McArthur, J.C. (2012). HIV-associated opportunistic infections of the CNS. *Lancet Neurol* 11, 605–617. http://www.ncbi.nlm.nih.gov/pubmed/22710754

25. Answer A

The risk of various opportunistic infections can be categorised on the basis of the patient's CD4+ T-cell count. A CD4+ T-cell count of less than 350 cells/μL places the patient at risk for *Mycobacterium tuberculosis* infection. When the CD4+ T-cell count is less than 200 cells/μL, there is a dramatic increase in risk of *Pneumocystis jiroveci* pneumonia (PJP) [formally called *Pneumocystis carinii* pneumonia (PCP) (Thomas and Limper, 2007)]; Kaposi sarcoma is also seen in patients with this level of immunosuppression. *Pneumocystis jiroveci* pneumonia is one of the most common life-threatening infections in HIV. It is a marker of severity of immunosuppression as it is rarely seen with CD4+ T-cell counts higher than 200 cells/μL. Prophylaxis when CD4+ T-cell counts drop below 200 cells/μL is given and co-trimoxazole (trimethoprim–sulphamethoxazole) is the agent of choice. For patients whose CD4+ T-cell counts are less than 100 cells/μl, the risk of central nervous system (CNS) toxoplasmosis and cryptococcal meningitis is increased. With very severe immunosuppression (i.e. CD4+ T-cell counts of <50 cells/μL), other infections and malignancies should be considered; these include disseminated *Mycobacterium avium* infection, cytomegalovirus retinitis, CNS lymphoma and progressive multifocal leucoencephalopathy.

Thomas, C.F., Jr. and Limper, A.H. (2007). Current insights into the biology and pathogenesis of Pneumocystis pneumonia. *Nat Rev Microbiol* 5, 298–308.
http://www.ncbi.nlm.nih.gov/pubmed/17363968

26. Answer D

In immunocompromised patients, cryptosporidiosis can be persistent and severe (O'Connor R et al., 2011). In HIV-infected patients with CD4+ T-cell levels greater than 180 cells/μl, cryptosporidiosis can be self-limiting. With more profound immunocompromise, however, the secretory diarrhoea, which is chronic and profuse, is usually unremitting. In these patients, Cryptosporidium organisms may cause hepatobiliary disease, including cholecystitis, cholangitis and papillary stenosis. An effective regimen for treatment of cryptosporidiosis has not been established. For some HIV-infected patients, paromomycin may be at least partially beneficial in treating cryptosporidiosis, though in small controlled trials, no benefit was seen with this approach, as compared with placebo.

O'Connor R, M., Shaffie, R., Kang, G., and Ward, H.D. (2011). Cryptosporidiosis in patients with HIV/AIDS. *AIDS* 25, 549–560.
http://www.ncbi.nlm.nih.gov/pubmed/21160413

11 Haematology

Questions

BASIC SCIENCE

Answers can be found in the Haematology Answers section at the end of this chapter.

1. Which one of the following is a correct description of erythropoiesis and thalassaemia?
   A. Patients with thalassaemia are more susceptible to malarial infection
   B. Mutation of one beta-globin gene leads to beta-thalassaemia with severe anaemia
   C. Beta-globin synthesis is normally controlled by four beta genes
   D. Production of alpha-like and beta-like globins is normally balanced at each stage of development
   E. In beta-thalassaemia, beta chains precipitate in erythroid precursor cells, causing dyserthropoiesis

2. Granulocyte colony-stimulating factor (G-CSF) causes an increase in the production of which one of the following cells in the bone marrow?
   A. Dendritic cells
   B. Eosinophils
   C. Monocytes
   D. Neutrophils
   E. T lymphocytes

3. Thrombopoietin (TPO):
   A. Is synthesised by platelets
   B. Activates the erythropoietin receptor
   C. Promotes survival and differentiation of megakaryocytes
   D. Promotes the formation of thrombin
   E. Levels are inappropriately high in immune thrombocytopenia

Passing the FRACP Written Examination: Questions and Answers, First Edition. Jonathan Gleadle, Tuck Yong, Jordan Li, Surjit Tarafdar, and Danielle Wu.
© 2013 John Wiley & Sons, Ltd. Published 2013 by John Wiley & Sons, Ltd.

4. Prothrombin complex concentrate and fresh frozen plasma are used in warfarin reversal. Which one of the following coagulation factors is present in fresh frozen plasma, but only at low levels in prothrombin complex concentrate?
   A. Factor II
   B. Factor V
   C. Factor VII
   D. Factor IX
   E. Factor X

5. Protein C acts by:
   A. Inactivating thrombin
   B. Inactivating factor V
   C. Activating endogenous heparin
   D. Activating anti-thrombin III
   E. Activating protein S

6. How does hepcidin regulate iron absorption through duodenal enterocytes?
   A. Helps duodenal crypt cells to sense the body iron stores
   B. Decreases iron transfer to the circulation by degrading ferroportin
   C. Inhibits the haemochromatosis protein HFE
   D. Inhibits beta 2-microglobulin
   E. Inhibits hepatic production of aminotranferases

7. Which one of the following best describes the mechanism of action of imatinib mesylate?
   A. Blocks the action of P-glycoprotein
   B. Inhibits BCR–ABL translocation
   C. Inhibits c-kit kinase
   D. Inhibits the kinase activity of BCR–ABL
   E. Stimulates platelet-derived growth factor receptor (PDGFR)

8. Which one of the following best describes the role of von Willebrand factor (vWF) in blood coagulation?
   A. Activates thrombin by reducing its degradation
   B. Activates factor VIII
   C. Binds to factor VIII and reduces its degradation
   D. Inactivates endogenous heparin
   E. Activates factor V

Theme: Haemostasis (for Questions 9–12)
   A. Factor XII
   B. Factor VIII
   C. Factor IX
   D. Factor X
   E. Fibrin

F. Plasmin

G. Prostacyclin

H. Thrombin

For each of the following questions, select the factor most likely to be responsible.

9. Which one of the above activates prothrombin?

10. Which one of the above inhibits platelet aggregation?

11. The deficiency of which factor is responsible for haemophilia A?

12. The deficiency of which factor is responsible for haemophilia B?

CLINICAL

13. A previously healthy 68-year-old woman presents with a spontaneous bleed into her psoas muscle. The results of coagulation tests are shown below. Which of the following best accounts for these results?

	Value	Reference range
Activated partial thromboplastin time (APTT) (s)	79	26–38
APTT correction (immediate mix) (s)	38	26–38
APTT correction (2-h incubation) (s)	79	26–38
International normalised ratio (INR)	1.1	0.9–1.2
Fibrinogen (g/L)	3.2	2.0–4.0

    A. Von Willebrand disease
    B. Disseminated intravascular coagulation (DIC)
    C. Acquired factor VIII inhibitor
    D. Chronic liver disease
    E. Haemophilia B

14. A 78-year-old woman is found incidentally to have a lymphocyte count of 20.0×10^9/L (0.5–3.5×10^9 cells/L) on full blood count examination before her elective right knee replacement. On examination, there is no lymphadenopathy, splenomegaly or hepatomegaly. Her haemoglobin is 114 g/L (115–155 g/L) and platelet count is 220×10^9/L (120–400×10^9 cells/L). Lymphocyte surface markers reveal expression of CD5, CD19, CD20 and CD28. What management should she receive?
    A. Chlorambucil after bone marrow biopsy
    B. Alemtuzumab after computed tomography scan for staging
    C. Observation without bone marrow biopsy
    D. Fludarabine without bone marrow biopsy
    E. Lenalidomide after molecular study

15. A 32-year-old woman presents to the emergency department with an 8-h history of severe right upper quadrant pain. An abdominal ultrasound reveals several mobile gallstones and gallbladder wall thickening, which is consistent with acute cholecystitis. The liver is unremarkable but the spleen measures 14 cm. The cholecystitis improves with conservative management. On further questioning, she tells you that her father had his spleen removed. The results of investigations and the blood film are shown below. Which one of the following tests is the most appropriate next investigation?

	Value	Reference range
Haemoglobin (g/L)	111	115–155
Mean corpuscular volume (fL)	101	80–98
White blood cells (/L)	8.1×10^9	$4.0–11.0 \times 10^9$
Platelet count (/L)	190×10^9	$150–400 \times 10^9$
Reticulocyte count (%)	7	1–3
Bilirubin (µmol/L)	27	2–24

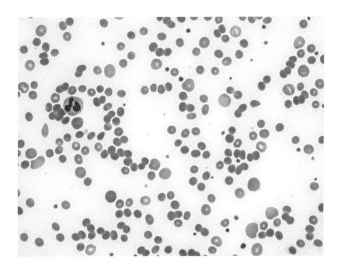

A. Autoimmune profile
B. Bone marrow biopsy
C. Coombs test
D. Osmotic fragility test
E. Haemoglobin electrophoresis

16. Which one of the following is correct in a patient with severe aplastic anaemia?

A. Patients with severe aplastic anaemia usually present with severe infection at initial presentation

B. Megakaryocytes are not helpful in distinguishing myelodysplastic syndrome from severe aplastic anaemia

C. Aplastic anaemia and paroxysmal nocturnal haemoglobinuria rarely overlap (<1% of cases)

D. The appearance of bone marrow in inherited and acquired aplastic anaemia is identical

E. Change in leucocytes telomere length is not associated with severe aplastic anaemia

17. A 60-year-old man has recently been diagnosed with B-cell non-Hodgkin lymphoma. He is waiting for chemotherapy to commence in 2 days. He suddenly develops headache, confusion, visual deterioration and epistaxis. Fundoscopy reveals retinal haemorrhages. Which one of the following investigations should be included in the evaluation?

    A. Complement levels
    B. C-reactive protein
    C. Plasma electrophoresis
    D. Serum free light chains
    E. Serum viscosity

18. Which one of the following factors should be taken into account when determining the dose of an iron-chelating agent in a patient who is red blood cell transfusion dependent because of myelodysplastic syndrome?

    A. Presence of cardiac iron overload
    B. Presence of splenomegaly
    C. Haemoglobin level
    D. Mean corpuscular volume
    E. Pain at the site of subcutaneous infusion

19. Which one of the following statements best describes the role of ^{18}F-fluorodeoxyglucose (^{18}F-FDG) positron emission tomography (PET) in the evaluation of adults with Hodgkin lymphoma?

    A. Detects metabolically inactive tumour tissue
    B. Determines the most appropriate combination chemotherapy
    C. Diagnosis of the condition
    D. Disease staging
    E. Identifies patients who need chemotherapy only

20. A 34-year-old primigravida is found to have a low platelet count (see below) on a full blood examination performed at 34 weeks of gestation. Her platelet count was 180×10^9/L at 12 weeks of gestation. She has no significant past medical history and is not taking any medications. Her blood pressure is 105/70 mmHg. Her other investigation results are shown below. Her liver function tests are normal. Which of one of the following is the most likely cause of her thrombocytopenia?

	Value	Reference range
Haemoglobin (g/L)	108	115–160
White blood cell count (cells/L)	4.3×10^9	$3.2–11.0 \times 10^9$
Platelet count (cells/L)	80×10^9	$150–450 \times 10^9$
Mean corpuscular volume (fL)	80	82–98
Reticulocyte count (%)	1.8	0.8–2.0
Urinary analysis (mg/L)	Protein 30	Negative
Serum creatinine (μmol/L)	61	70–110
Lactate dehydrogenase (IU/L)	173	70–250

A. Haemolysis, elevated liver enzymes and low platelet (HELLP) syndrome
B. Pre-eclampsia
C. Evan syndrome
D. Thrombotic thrombocytopenic purpura
E. Gestational thrombocytopenia

21. A 52-year-old woman who had an ischemic stroke 12 months ago but no residual neurological deficits was referred for evaluation of recurrent episodes of proximal deep venous thrombosis (DVT) of the lower limbs in the last 10 months. The results of investigations are shown below. A bone marrow biopsy showed a mild hyperplasia of erythrocytic bone marrow. Urine dipstick for blood was +++. What is the most likely diagnosis?

	Value	Reference range
Haemoglobin (g/L)	82	115–155
Mean corpuscular volume (fL)	98	80–98
Mean corpuscular haemoglobin (pg)	31	27–33
White blood cells (cells/L)	4.0×10^9	$4.0–11.0 \times 10^9$
Platelet count (cells/L)	93×10^9	$150–400 \times 10^9$
Reticulocytes (%)	5.4	0.5–1.5
Total bilirubin (µmol/L)	50	2–24
Lactate dehydrogenase (U/L)	944	110–230
Coombs test	Negative	

A. Anti-thrombin III deficiency
B. Haemolytic uraemic syndrome
C. Paroxysmal nocturnal haemoglobinuria
D. Homocysteinaemia
E. Protein C deficiency

22. Which one of the following factors is the most important risk factor for acute graft-versus-host disease after allogeneic haemopoietic cell transplantation?
A. Age of the recipient
B. CD4+ cell count in the recipient at time of transplantation
C. Cytomegalovirus status of recipient
D. Mismatch between donor and recipient in human leucocyte antigens (HLAs)
E. Total CD34+ cells transplanted

23. Which one of the following best describes rituximab use in the treatment of B-cell lymphomas?
A. Rituximab is only used as a single agent
B. Rituximab is a chimeric monoclonal antibody that recognises human CD38 antigen

C. Patients should be screened for Epstein–Barr virus before rituximab treatment

D. Rituximab when combined with chemotherapy improves progression-free survival of aggressive non-Hodgkin lymphoma

E. Rituximab-induced lymphopenia usually lasts more than 18 months

24. A 65-year-old woman with headache, flushing and unexplained (anaphylactoid) shock was found to have a high serum tryptase level. Collateral history from her husband revealed previous allergic reactions to multiple medications, including penicillin, cephalosporins and aspirin. Which one of the following tests is the cornerstone of diagnosis this patient's condition?

A. Lymphocyte surface markers

B. Radioallergosorbent test (RAST)

C. Cytogenetic study

D. Bone marrow biopsy

E. Rechallenge the patient with the medications that she was allergic to

25. A 54-year-old obese woman presents with extensive deep venous thrombosis of her left leg. She has a family history of venous thromboembolism. She was started on low-molecular-weight heparin and warfarin 10 mg daily for 2 days. Within 72 h, she developed necrotic-looking skin lesions on her thighs without trauma. What underlying condition is she most likely to have?

A. Anti-thrombin III deficiency

B. Protein S deficiency

C. Anti-phospholipid syndrome

D. Protein C deficiency

E. Homozygous factor V Leiden mutation

26. A 58-year-old man presents with a 3-month history of worsening breathlessness, confusion, headache and bleeding gums. His investigation results are shown below. Bone marrow biopsy reveals marrow infiltration by small lymphocytes showing plasma cell differentiation. What is the next appropriate treatment for this patient?

	Value	Reference range
Haemoglobin (g/L)	95	135–175
White cell count (cells/L)	3.0×10^9	$4.0–11.0 \times 10^9$
Platelet count (cells/L)	135×10^9	$150–450 \times 10^9$
IgA (g/L)	3.0	0.9–3.4
IgG (g/L)	6.0	5.0–16.0
IgM (g/L)	31.0	0.5–3.0
Serum viscosity (cP)	4.2	1.3–1.8

A. Chlorambucil

B. Cyclophosphamide

C. Plasma exchange
D. Rituximab
E. Thalidomide

27. Epstein–Barr virus is associated with which of the following subtypes of non-Hodgkin lymphoma?
A. Gastric mucosa-associated lymphoid tissue lymphoma
B. Follicular lymphoma
C. Nasal natural killer cell lymphoma
D. Chronic lymphocytic leukaemia
E. Splenic marginal-zone lymphoma

28. Which one of the following is used to treat mild haemophilia A without the risk of transmitting infectious diseases?
A. Factor VIII concentrate
B. Factor IX concentrate
C. Prothrombin complex concentrate
D. Tranexamic acid
E. Desmopressin

29. Which one of the following is correct concerning atypical haemolytic uraemic syndrome (aHUS)?
A. It is only an acute disease
B. It is predominantly (>80%) a condition affecting children
C. It is associated with mutations in genes encoding complement regulatory proteins
D. It is due to mutations in the gene encoding ADAMTS13
E. Plasma exchange is the only effective treatment

30. The results of a patient's biochemistry profile after chemotherapy for Burkitt lymphoma are shown below. He was transferred to the intensive care unit for cardiac monitoring and treatment. Which one of the following treatment options should be used to lower uric acid level?

	Value	Reference range
Potassium (mmol/L)	6.8	3.4–4.5
Phosphate (mmol/L)	2.4	0.70–0.95
Corrected calcium (mmol/L)	1.60	2.10–2.55
Urate (mmol/L)	0.87	0.45–0.60
Creatinine (μmol/L)	348	60–120

A. Aggressive intravenous diuretics
B. Allopurinol
C. Rasburicase
D. Urinary alkalinisation
E. Prednisolone

31. A 68-year-old woman is recovering from an elective knee replacement surgery for osteoarthritis. She has been receiving unfractionated heparin 5000 units twice a day. On day 10 she is breathless and computed tomographic pulmonary angiography shows bilateral pulmonary embolism. Laboratory investigation reveals a haemoglobin of 95 g/L (115–155 g/L) and platelet count of 45×10^9 cells/L (150–450×10^9 cells/L). What additional diagnostic investigation should be undertaken?
- **A.** Extractable nuclear antibodies
- **B.** Activated partial thromboplastin time
- **C.** Anti-phospholipid antibodies
- **D.** Anti-platelet factor-4/heparin antibodies
- **E.** Anti-thrombin III levels

Theme: Anaemia (for Questions 32–35)
- **A.** Haemolytic anaemia
- **B.** Pure red cell aplasia
- **C.** Iron-deficiency anaemia
- **D.** Pernicious anaemia
- **E.** Beta-thalassaemia minor
- **F.** Sideroblastic anaemia
- **G.** Anaemia of chronic disease
- **H.** Sickle cell disease

32. Which disorder is predisposed to salmonella osteomyelitis?

33. A 30-year-old woman with known hypoparathyroidism and Addison disease has been found to have a mutation in the autoimmune regulator (AIRE) gene and has become progressively anaemic. What cause of anaemia should be considered?

34. A 70-year-old woman with a 10-year history of myasthenia gravis adequately controlled with pyridostigmine, presents with general fatigue secondary to severe anaemia [haemoglobin of 62 g/L (115–155 g/L)]. A computed tomography (CT) scan of the thorax revealed the presence of an anterior mediastinal mass. Bone marrow aspirate showed severe erythroid hypoplasia associated with normal myeloid and megakaryocytic cell lines. What is the most likely diagnosis?

35. A 29-year-old man presents with an 8-day history of fever and productive cough. The patient was previously healthy and was not using any drugs. On physical examination, the patient appears ill and his temperature is 39.8°C. Chest examination showed bilateral basal crackles. The results of initial investigations are shown below. His chest X-ray shows bilateral basal opacities. Anti-mycoplasma antibody titre by complement fixation was high at 1:10240. What is the most likely cause of his anaemia?

	Value	Reference range
Haemoglobin (g/L)	93	115–155
Mean corpuscular volume (fL)	94	80–98
Mean corpuscular haemoglobin (pg)	31	27–33
White blood cells (cells/L)	18.1×10^9	$4.0–11.0 \times 10^9$
Platelet count (cells/L)	203×10^9	$150–400 \times 10^9$
Reticulocytes (%)	3.4	0.5–1.5
Lactate dehydrogenase (U/L)	758	110–230

Answers

BASIC SCIENCE

1. Answer D

For an adult to maintain a normal red blood cell count, about 2–3 million new red blood cells are produced every second. For severe forms of thalassaemia, many erythroblasts and mature red blood cells are damaged, increasing erythropoiesis by 20–30 times.

At a molecular level, haemoglobin synthesis is controlled by two multigene clusters on chromosome 16 (encoding alpha-like globins) and on chromosome 11 (encoding beta-like globins) (Higgs et al., 2012). At each stage of development, the production of alpha-like and beta-like globins is balanced. Beta-globin synthesis is normally controlled by the two beta genes (one on each copy of chromosome 11). In thalassaemia, there are defects in the production of either the alpha-like (alpha-thalassaemia) or the beta-like (beta-thalassaemia) globin chains. The main pathophysiology in beta-thalassaemia results from the synthesis of insufficient beta chains to partner the alpha-globin chains to generate adult haemoglobin ($\alpha_2\beta_2$). Excess alpha chains precipitate in erythroid precursor cells causing dyserthropoiesis, and in mature red blood cells causing membrane damage and haemolysis. If only one of the beta-globin genes bear a mutation, patients suffer from minor microcytic anaemia. If both genes have mutations, this leads to severe microcytic, hypochromic anaemia, which if untreated causes anaemia, splenomegaly, severe bone deformities and death before age 20. Treatment consists of periodic blood transfusion; splenectomy if splenomegaly is present, and treatment of iron overload caused by transfusion. Cure is possible by bone marrow transplantation.

Worldwide about 1.5% of the population are carriers of beta-thalassaemia and these individuals mostly originate from the Mediterranean, Middle East, central Asia, India and southern China, which suggests a selective advantage to carrying such a mutation in these areas. Individuals with either alpha- or beta-thalassaemia trait are somewhat protected in areas where falciparum malaria is or has been endemic, thus explaining the high carrier frequency via natural selection.

Higgs, D.R., Engel, J.D., and Stamatoyannopoulos, G. (2012). Thalassaemia. *Lancet* 379, 373–383.
http://www.ncbi.nlm.nih.gov/pubmed/21908035

2. Answer D

Granulocyte colony-stimulating factor (G-CSF) is a colony-stimulating factor hormone. G-CSF is produced by endothelium, macrophages and a number of other immune cells. The G-CSF receptor is present on precursor cells in the bone marrow, and, in response to stimulation by G-CSF, initiates proliferation and differentiation into mature granulocytes (Kaushansky, 2006).

G-CSF promotes the survival and stimulates the proliferation of neutrophil progenitors and their differentiation into mature neutrophils. In addition, the cytokine causes premature release of neutrophils from bone marrow and enhances their phagocytic capacity, generation of superoxide anions and bacterial killing. The administration of G-CSF causes toxic granulation of neutrophils in the peripheral blood, which is a morphological correlate of their heightened functional state, and a leftward shift (immaturity) in the leucocyte differential count. Activation of neutrophils in the bone marrow by G-CSF causes them to release matrix metalloproteases. This helps to explain the mobilisation of haematopoietic stem cells from the bone marrow in response to the administration of G-CSF, a finding that facilitates the collection of haematopoietic stem cells for transplantation.

3. Answer C
Thrombopoietin (TPO) is the major physiological regulator of megakaryocyte growth and differentiation, and therefore of platelet production (Kaushansky, 2006). It is synthesised and secreted mainly by the liver, and its production is constant, with no translational or post-translational regulation and levels can fall in liver failure. When TPO is released into the circulation, most of the protein binds to TPO receptors (c-Mpl or CD110) on platelets and is destroyed with the platelets. The remaining TPO binds to receptors on bone marrow precursors. Therefore, the rising and dropping platelet concentrations regulate the TPO levels. Low platelets lead a higher degree of TPO exposure to the undifferentiated bone marrow cells and thus their differentiation into megakaryocytes and further maturation of these cells. TPO levels are inappropriately low for the degree of thrombocytopenia in the majority of patients with immune thrombocytopenia (ITP), providing the rationale for treatment with TPO-receptor agonists. Trials of a modified recombinant form, megakaryocyte growth and differentiation factor (MGDF), were stopped when healthy volunteers developed autoantibodies to endogenous thrombopoietin and then developed thrombocytopenia themselves. Romiplostim and eltrombopag, structurally unrelated peptide mimetics which stimulate the same pathway, are being increasingly used in the treatment of thrombocytopenia.

Genetic causes of thrombocytosis and thrombocytopenia have been associated with activating and disruptive mutations of thrombopoietin and c-Mpl.

For Questions 2 and 3

Kaushansky, K. (2006). Lineage-specific hematopoietic growth factors. *N Engl J Med* 354, 2034–2045.
http://www.ncbi.nlm.nih.gov/pubmed/16687716

4. Answer B
Fresh frozen plasma (FFP) contains all the coagulation factors. Prothrombin complex concentrate (PCC) contains factors II, VIII, IX and X, but low levels of factor V (Baker et al., 2004).

Warfarin inhibits the vitamin K-dependent synthesis of the four factors contained in PCC as well as protein C and protein S. To reverse the effects of warfarin, vitamin K can be given but immediate reversal is achieved with PCC and/or FFP. Vitamin K is essential for sustaining the reversal achieved by PCC and FFP.

Baker, R.I., Coughlin, P.B., Gallus, A.S., Harper, P.L., Salem, H.H., and Wood, E.M. (2004). Warfarin reversal: consensus guidelines, on behalf of the Australasian Society of Thrombosis and Haemostasis. *Med J Aust 181*, 492–497.
http://www.ncbi.nlm.nih.gov/pubmed/15516194

5. Answer B

All endothelial cells except those in the cerebral microcirculation produce thrombomodulin. Thrombin, which is normally a procoagulant, becomes an anticoagulant after binding to thrombomodulin. The thrombin–thrombomodulin complex activates protein C, which in the presence of its cofactor protein S inactivates factors V and VIII.

Unfractionated heparin binds to anti-thrombin III and converts it into a rapid inactivator of several clotting proteins, chiefly factor Xa. In order to inactivate thrombin (factor II), heparin must bind simultaneously to both anti-thrombin III and thrombin, an effect which occurs with the long unfractionated heparin but not the shorter low-molecular-weight heparin (LMWH). Therefore, LMWH exerts its anti-coagulant effect primarily via factor Xa.

6. Answer B

Systemic regulation of iron absorption is mediated by hepcidin. It binds to and internalises the iron channel ferroportin, leading to its destruction in the intestinal epithelial cells (Fleming and Ponka, 2012).

The body iron status is sensed by the intestinal crypt cells via an interaction between circulating transferrin-bound iron and the transferrin receptor. This interaction is facilitated by a complex between the HFE protein and beta 2-microglobulin. When the body iron stores are sensed to be low, there is upregulation of mRNA expression for the divalent metal transporter 1 (DMT1). The crypt cells eventually migrate up the villous and mature into adult enterocytes, and the elevated DMT1 in these cells causes increased iron absorption from the intestinal lumen. Absorbed iron is exported into the circulation at the basolateral surface by ferroportin. Hepcidin is produced in the liver and is an acute-phase reactant that binds to and internalises the ferroportin into the enterocytes. This degradation of ferroportin inhibits further absorption of iron. Hepatocellular hepcidin production is regulated by signals affecting inflammation, iron status, erythropoietic activity and oxygen tension.

Impairment of the hepcidin–ferroportin axis characterises hereditary haemochromatosis, resulting in inadequate or ineffective hepcidin-mediated down-regulation of ferroportin.

Fleming, R.E., and Ponka, P. (2012). Iron overload in human disease. *N Engl J Med* 366, 348–359.
http://www.ncbi.nlm.nih.gov/pubmed/22276824

7. Answer D

Imatinib mesylate (Gleevec, Novartis) is an inhibitor of multiple tyrosine kinases, including ABL, BCR–ABL, platelet-derived growth factor receptor (PDGFR) and c-kit. By preventing the phosphorylation by BCR–ABL, imatinib selectively inhibits downstream signalling and the growth of BCR–ABL-positive cells, inducing apoptosis of these cells (Schiffer, 2007).

Chronic myeloid leukaemia (CML) is a myeloproliferative disorder that is a consequence of an acquired mutation affecting haematopoietic stem cells. This mutation results in a balanced translocation between chromosomes 9 and 22 [t(9;22)(q34;q11)], termed the Philadelphia (Ph) chromosome. This translocation results in the juxtaposition of a portion of the human homologue of the Abelson murine leukaemia (ABL) gene from chromosome 9 and the breakpoint cluster region (BCR) gene of chromosome 22, resulting in the formation of a BCR–ABL fusion protein. The BCR–ABL protein contains the active tyrosine kinase region of ABL, producing a cytokine-independent, constitutive proliferative signal, and affects a variety of downstream pathways. This signal results in continuous cell growth and replication.

Imatinib is a substrate for the CYP3A4 metabolic pathway and can inhibit other cytochrome P-450 pathways. Careful monitoring of the international normalised ratio in patients receiving warfarin is advisable. Single-nucleotide mutations in the BCR–ABL gene producing conformation changes in the BCR–ABL protein, which can affect the binding of imatinib to specific activation or kinase sites, can be detected in approximately half the patients who are resistant to imatinib. As a result, newer inhibitors of BCR–ABL have been developed; dasatinib and nilotinib.

 Schiffer, C.A. (2007). BCR-ABL tyrosine kinase inhibitors for chronic myelogenous leukemia. *N Engl J Med 357*, 258–265.
http://www.ncbi.nlm.nih.gov/pubmed/17634461

8. Answer C

Von Willebrand factor (vWF) acts as a carrier for factor VIII in the circulation. It helps to maintain the level of factor VIII by increasing its half-life by five-fold.

vWF also performs the important task of helping normal platelets to bind to exposed collagen in the blood vessels. On disruption of normal endothelium, platelets bind to the exposed collagen both directly by glycoprotein 1a (GP1a) membrane receptor and indirectly by binding to vWF by GP1b receptor, which in turn binds to the collagen. Following adhesion, platelets undergo shape change from a disc to a sphere and release the contents of their cytoplasmic granules: dense bodies [containing adenosine diphosphate (ADP) and serotonin] and alpha-granules (containing platelet-derived growth factor, platelet factor 4, fibrinogen and other factors). The release of ADP leads to a conformational change in the glycoprotein IIb–IIIa receptor on the surface of the adherent platelet, allowing it to bind fibrinogen and eventually leading to the formation of a clot.

Hereditary or acquired defects of vWF lead to von Willebrand disease (vWD), a bleeding diathesis of the skin and mucous membranes, causing epistaxis, menor-rhagia and gastrointestinal bleeding. The point at which the mutation occurs determines the severity of the bleeding diathesis. There are three types (I, II and III), and type II is further divided in several subtypes. Treatment depends on the nature of the abnormality and the severity of the symptoms. Most cases of vWD are hereditary, but abnormalities of vWF may be acquired; aortic valve stenosis, for instance, has been linked to vWD type IIA, causing gastrointestinal bleeding, an association known as Heyde syndrome.

9. Answer D

Factor X is synthesised in the liver and requires vitamin K for its synthesis. The half-life of factor X is 40–45 h. Factor X is activated into factor Xa by both factor IX (with its cofactor, factor VIII, in a complex known as intrinsic Xase) and factor VII (with its cofactor, tissue factor, a complex known as extrinsic Xase). It is there-fore the first member of the final common pathway or thrombin pathway (Furie and Furie, 2008).

Factor Xa acts by cleaving prothrombin in two places, which yields active thrombin. This process is optimised when factor Xa is complexed with activated co-factor V in the prothrombinase complex. Factor Xa is inactivated by protein Z-dependent protease inhibitor (ZPI), a serine protease inhibitor (serpin). The affin-ity of this protein for factor Xa is increased 1000-fold by the presence of protein Z. Defects in protein Z lead to increased factor Xa activity and a propensity for thrombosis.

Inborn deficiency of factor X is very rare (1 in 500000), and may present with epistaxis, haemarthrosis and gastrointestinal blood loss. Apart from congenital deficiency, low factor X levels may occur occasionally in a number of disorders such as amyloidosis, where factor X is absorbed to the amyloid fibrils in the vasculature.

Deficiency of vitamin K or antagonism by warfarin leads to the production of an inactive factor X. In warfarin therapy, this is desirable to prevent thrombosis. Inhibiting factor Xa would offer an alternate method for anti-coagulation and direct Xa inhibitors, such as apixaban and rivaroxaban, are another way of inter-fering with the thrombotic process.

10. Answer G

Prostacyclin is produced in endothelial cells from prostaglandin H_2 (PGH_2) by the action of the enzyme prostacyclin synthase. Although prostacyclin is considered an independent mediator, it is called PGI_2 (prostaglandin I_2) in eicosanoid nomen-clature, and is a member of the prostanoids (together with the prostaglandins and thromboxane). Prostacyclin chiefly prevents formation of the platelet plug involved in primary haemostasis (a part of blood clot formation). It does this by inhibiting platelet activation. It is also an effective vasodilator.

11. Answer B

12. Answer C
Commentary for Questions 11 and 12

Haemophilia A is an X-linked recessive bleeding disorder caused by a deficiency in the activity of coagulation factor VIII (Berntorp and Shapiro, 2012). The disorder has a variable severity, depending on the plasma levels of coagulation factor VIII: mild, with levels 6–30% of normal; moderate, with levels 2–5% of normal; and severe, with levels less than 1% of normal. Patients with mild haemophilia usually bleed excessively only after trauma or surgery, whereas those with severe haemophilia may have 20–30 episodes of spontaneous or excessive bleeding a year after minor trauma, particularly into joints and muscles. These symptoms differ from those of bleeding disorders due to platelet defects or von Willebrand disease, in which mucosal bleeding predominates.

Haemophilia B is due to factor IX deficiency and is clinically indistinguishable from haemophilia A. In both haemophilia A and B there is prolongation of activated partial thromboplastin time (APTT).

Berntorp, E. and Shapiro, A.D. (2012). Modern haemophilia care. *Lancet* 379, 1447–1456.
http://www.ncbi.nlm.nih.gov/pubmed/22456059

Furie, B., and Furie, B.C. (2008). Mechanisms of thrombus formation. *N Engl J Med 359*, 938–949.
http://www.ncbi.nlm.nih.gov/pubmed/18753650

CLINICAL

13. Answer C

The sudden appearance of a large haemorrhage into the muscle in an elderly person with an elevated activated partial thromboplastin time (APTT) should always raise the suspicion of an acquired factor VIII inhibitor (Franchini and Lippi, 2008).

Patients often present with large haematomas, extensive ecchymoses or severe mucosal bleeding, including epistaxis, gastrointestinal bleeding and gross haematuria. Spontaneous haemarthroses, which are common in haemophilia A (hereditary factor VIII deficiency) or B (hereditary factor IX deficiency), are unusual. The cause is usually circulating autoantibodies directed against functional epitopes of factor VIII, causing neutralisation and/or its accelerated clearance from the plasma. There are associations with post-parturition, rheumatoid arthritis, systemic lupus erythematosus and underlying malignancies.

The APTT assay is a reliable screening test for factor VIII inhibitor detection as it is typically prolonged when factor VIII activity decreases to 45% of the mean normal level or less. Furthermore, mixing studies with patient plasma and normal plasma do not normalise the APTT. Weak autoantibodies, however, may not prolong the APTT unless the mixture is incubated for at least 1 or 2 h at 37°C. As a result, while mixing studies may show initial normalisation of APTT, repeat studies after 1–2 h of incubation typically shows that the APTT is prolonged again.

Although von Willebrand disease may be diagnosed at an older age and is associated with prolonged APTT with normal PT and INR, there is usually personal and family history of bleeding. In coagulopathy due to chronic liver disease there will usually be an elevated INR and APTT. Haemophilia B, which usually presents at an early age with characteristic spontaneous haemarthroses, is associated with prolonged APTT with normal PT and INR. In acute disseminated intravascular coagulopathy (DIC) both APTT and INR are prolonged, while the fibrinogen levels are low due to rapid consumption.

Franchini, M. and Lippi, G. (2008). Acquired factor VIII inhibitors. *Blood* 112, 250–255.
http://bloodjournal.hematologylibrary.org/content/112/2/250.full

14. Answer C

This patient most likely has chronic lymphocytic leukaemia (CLL) (Gribben, 2010). CLL is characterised by the progressive accumulation of functionally incompetent lymphocytes which are of monoclonal origin. Peripheral blood film shows lymphocytosis with typically small, mature-appearing lymphocytes, but they are fragile when smeared onto a glass slide, giving an appearance of broken cells, called smudge cells. Flow cytometry characteristically shows that the atypical lymphocytes express CD19, dim CD20, dim CD5, CD23, CD43 and CD79a, and weakly express surface immunoglobulin IgM and IgD.

A bone marrow biopsy is not usually required at diagnosis of CLL. Bone marrow biopsy is commonly performed at the time of requirement for treatment or when patients present with cytopenias. Bone marrow examination is useful in evaluating whether cytopenias are immune mediated or caused by marrow replacement. Staging of CLL is performed by clinical examination and results of blood counts only, and for this reason the guidelines do not recommend computed tomography (CT) scan at diagnosis. The molecular profile of CLL provides insight into the underlying pathogenesis of the disease and provides predictors of time to progression, time to need for therapy and overall survival. It is not used in selecting treatment regimens currently, but it is an area of active research.

As this patient is asymptomatic with near-normal haemoglobin and platelet counts, she does not merit any pharmacological intervention. She should not be treated based purely upon a high lymphocyte count alone. Indications for therapy in CLL are symptomatic disease, bulky progressive adenopathy, marrow failure or B-type symptoms (fever, night sweats and weight loss).

Gribben, J.G. (2010). How I treat CLL up front. *Blood* 115, 187–197.
http://bloodjournal.hematologylibrary.org/content/115/2/187.full

15. Answer D

This patient's history is strongly suggestive of hereditary spherocytosis, which is associated with increased haemolysis and subsequent raised risk of gallstones, as seen here. Spherocytosis is caused by inherited defects in the membrane of red blood cells that reduce cell deformability. This leads to cells being removed by the spleen, which causes progressive splenic enlargement.

Disease is mild in 20–30% of patients. As in this case, hereditary spherocytosis can present later in life. However, 60–70% of patients have more severe anaemia and splenomegaly, which leads to presentation in childhood.

Hereditary spherocytosis is most commonly associated with dominant inheritance (75%). Mutations of genes encoding ankyrin, spectrin or Band 3 red cell proteins account for most cases.

The diagnosis of hereditary spherocytosis is usually made on clinical grounds, based upon the presence of spherocytes on blood film. A number of tests are available for identifying individuals with hereditary spherocytosis:
- Osmotic fragility testing
- Ektacytometry
- Acidified glycerol lysis test (AGLT)
- Cryohaemolysis test
- Eosin-5-maleimide binding test (EMA binding test).

Elective splenectomy is often required in severe cases, but patients with mild hereditary spherocytosis may require no intervention at all.

16. Answer D

Patients with severe aplastic anaemia (AA) usually present with symptomatic anaemia or haemorrhage (Scheinberg and Young, 2012). Infection at presentation is infrequent. Megakaryocytes are the most reliable lineage to use in distinguishing myelodysplastic syndrome (MDS) from severe AA: small mononuclear or aberrant megakaryocytes are typical of MDS, whereas megakaryocytes are markedly reduced or absent in severe AA. Aplastic anaemia and paroxysmal nocturnal haemoglobinuria (PNH) overlap in approximately 40–50% of cases (AA/PNH syndrome). The appearance of the marrow in inherited and acquired aplastic anaemia syndromes is identical. Blood leucocyte telomere length may be reduced and is particularly associated with genetic abnormalities such as DKC1, TERT and TERC mutations.

Scheinberg, P. and Young, N.S. (2012). How I treat acquired aplastic anemia. *Blood* 120, 1185–1196.
http://www.ncbi.nlm.nih.gov/pubmed/22517900

17. Answer E

This patient's presentation is suspicious for hyperviscosity syndrome in the setting of a lymphoproliferative disorder and cryoglobulinaemia is a possible cause (Ramos-Casals et al., 2012).

B-cell lymphoproliferative diseases are the major cause of cryoglobulinaemia associated with malignancy. Type I cryoglobulinaemia is reported predominantly in patients with Waldenström macroglobulinaemia, multiple myeloma or chronic lymphocytic leukaemia. Mixed cryoglobulinaemias occur mainly in B-cell lymphomas.

Two major mechanisms are involved to a varying extent in the different types of cryoglobulinaemia: cryoglobulin precipitation in the microcirculation, and vascular immune complex-mediated inflammation. Vascular occlusion is more frequent in type I cryoglobulinaemia, which is usually accompanied by high cryoglobulin concentrations, and can be associated with hyperviscosity syndrome and cold-induced acral necrosis. Immune complex-mediated vasculitis is more frequent in mixed cryoglobulinaemias, particularly type II, in which the monoclonal IgM component generates large immune complexes with IgG and complement fractions.

Hyperviscosity syndrome develops mainly in patients with type I cryoglobulinaemia associated with haematological malignancies, and is uncommon in patients with mixed cryoglobulinaemia (<3%). The key symptoms are neurological (headache, confusion), ocular (blurred vision, visual loss) and ear and nose (epistaxis, hearing loss). The physical examination should include fundoscopy to exclude hyperviscosity-related retinal changes, including haemorrhages. In patients in whom hyperviscosity syndrome is suspected, serum viscosity should be measured. Patients usually become symptomatic at viscosity measurements greater than 4.0 centipoise (cP), but some patients are symptomatic with lower viscosities. Symptomatic hyperviscosity requires urgent treatment with plasma exchange.

Low complement levels (particularly C4) and raised titres of serum rheumatoid factor are commonly observed in mixed cryoglobulinaemias and can correlate with clinical symptoms. Cryoglobulin detection can be difficult given the requirement to maintain blood at 37°C prior to analysis. Hepatitis C (HCV) testing is important (antibodies and serum HCV-RNA detection) in patients with mixed cryoglobulinaemia. Testing for other viruses (hepatitis B virus, HIV) and autoimmune diseases (anti-nuclear, anti-DNA, anti-Ro/La, anti-citrullinated antibodies) is recommended, even in patients known to have HCV.

Ramos-Casals, M., Stone, J.H., Cid, M.C., and Bosch, X. (2012). The cryoglobulinaemias. *Lancet* 379, 348–360.
http://www.ncbi.nlm.nih.gov/pubmed/21868085

18. Answer A

Long-term treatment with red blood cell transfusion can sustain patients with chronic congenital and acquired refractory anaemia. Since humans lack an effective means to eliminate excess iron, long-term transfusion alone will lead to the clinical problem of iron overload (Bird et al., 2012; Brittenham, 2011).

Iron-chelating therapy should be considered in all patients who require long-term red cell transfusion. Ideally, iron-chelating therapy should be initiated prophylactically before clinically significant iron accumulation has occurred. Treatment should begin when patients have received between 10 and 20 units of red cell transfusion. The dose of an iron-chelating agent is determined by three principal factors: the presence or absence of cardiac iron overload, the rate of transfusional iron loading and the body iron burden.

The effectiveness of iron-chelating therapy is best monitored by periodic measurements of cardiac iron concentrations by magnetic resonance imaging (MRI), and by the actual rate of iron loading. Serum ferritin concentrations are usually measured at least quarterly. Hepatic, cardiac and endocrine function should be assessed periodically along with nutritional status.

Bird, R.J., Kenealy, M., Forsyth, C., et al. (2012). When should iron chelation therapy be considered in patients with myelodysplasia and other bone marrow failure syndromes with iron overload? *Intern Med J* 42, 450–455.
http://www.ncbi.nlm.nih.gov/pubmed/22498118

Brittenham, G.M. (2011). Iron-chelating therapy for transfusional iron overload. *N Engl J Med* 364, 146–156.
http://www.ncbi.nlm.nih.gov/pubmed/21226580

19. Answer D

Functional imaging with ^{18}F-fluorodeoxyglucose (^{18}F-FDG) positron emission tomography (PET) is increasingly used to stage Hodgkin lymphoma, delineate margins of radiotherapy, provide a baseline for subsequent assessment (interim and end-of-treatment assessments) and follow-up surveillance, but its precise role has not been fully defined (Townsend and Linch, 2012). Most tumours are metabolically active and preferentially take up and utilise glucose for anaerobic metabolism (the Warburg effect).

End-of-treatment ^{18}F-FDG PET can be used to distinguish between fibrotic and residual active disease. There is much interest in the potential use of ^{18}F-FDG PET for interim assessment to identify those who have responded completely or need escalation of treatment.

Bone marrow involvement is found in 5–8% of patients with Hodgkin lymphoma but the frequency is lower (<1%) in early disease and is usually felt too low to justify performing a bone marrow biopsy. ^{18}F-FDG PET is sensitive for focal bone marrow infiltration and its increasing use may reduce the number of staging trephine biopsies done. Currently, combined modality therapy (chemotherapy and radiotherapy) has replaced radiotherapy alone in localised Hodgkin lymphoma because it substantially reduces relapse rate through the chemotherapeutic eradication of occult disease outside the radiation field and allows for smaller radiation fields.

Townsend, W. and Linch, D. (2012). Hodgkin's lymphoma in adults. *Lancet* 380, 836–847.
http://www.ncbi.nlm.nih.gov/pubmed/22835602

20. Answer E

Asymptomatic mild gestational thrombocytopenia is typically seen late in pregnancy (Myers, 2012). Gestational thrombocytopenia is seen in about 5% of pregnancies near term and is typically mild with full resolution post partum and no neonatal thrombocytopenia.

Haemolysis, elevated liver enzymes and low platelet (HELLP) syndrome, which is seen after 20 weeks of gestation, is associated with microangiopathic haemolytic anaemia, abnormal liver function tests and thrombocytopenia.

Pre-eclampsia, which is seen after 20 weeks of gestation, is associated with hypertension and proteinuria.

Evan syndrome is an autoimmune haemolytic anaemia with idiopathic thrombocytopenia.

Thrombotic thrombocytopenic purpura is characterised by thrombocytopenic purpura, fever, fluctuating cerebral dysfunction, haemolytic anaemia with red cell fragmentation and often renal failure.

Myers, B. (2012). Diagnosis and management of maternal thrombocytopenia in pregnancy. *Br J Haematol* 158, 3–15.
http://www.ncbi.nlm.nih.gov/pubmed/22551110

21. Answer C

Paroxysmal nocturnal haemoglobinuria (PNH) is a rare haematopoietic stem cell disorder caused by a somatic mutation in a gene known as phosphatidylinositol glycan class A (PIGA) (Brodsky, 2009). It may arise de novo or in the setting of acquired aplastic anaemia. The product of the PIGA gene is required for the biosynthesis of a glycolipid anchor that attaches a class of membrane proteins known as glycosylphosphatidyl inositol (GPI)-anchored proteins to the cell surface. The absence of GPI-anchored proteins leads to complement-mediated intravascular haemolysis, because two important complement regulatory proteins (CD55 and CD59) are missing from PNH cells.

Clinical presentations include acute intravascular haemolytic crisis, especially nocturnal, chronic haemolytic anaemia, haemoglobinuria, bone marrow failure and thrombosis. Haemolysis in PNH occurs intravascularly, leading to release of free haemoglobin, a potent nitric oxide scavenger. Depletion of nitric oxide contributes to fatigue, oesophageal spasm, thrombosis and male erectile dysfunction.

In the past, PNH was diagnosed indirectly based upon the sensitivity of PNH red cells to lysis by complement (e.g. Ham test). However, the recognition of a deficiency of GPI-linked proteins in PNH has resulted in the development of flow cytometric methods for diagnosis. Thrombosis, the leading cause of death from PNH, most commonly occurs in abdominal and cerebral veins, but arterial thrombotic episodes can occur. Therapeutic options include bone marrow transplantation and monoclonal antibody therapy with the terminal complement inhibitor, eculizumab. Eculizumab decreases haemolysis in PNH by binding to C5 and blocking the terminal portion of the complement cascade.

Brodsky, R.A. (2009). How I treat paroxysmal nocturnal hemoglobinuria. *Blood* 113, 6522–6527.
http://www.ncbi.nlm.nih.gov/pmc/articles/PMC2710914/

22. Answer D

Graft-versus-host disease (GvHD) is one of the main complications of haemopoietic cell transplantation (HCT) (Ferrara et al., 2009). It is an immunological disorder, which affects many organ systems, including the gastrointestinal tract, liver, skin and lung. GvHD can be classified as acute or chronic. At the onset of GvHD, affected regions include the skin (~80%), gastrointestinal tract (~50%) and liver (~50%). GvHD can develop in various clinical settings when tissues containing T cells (blood products, bone marrow and solid organs) are transferred from one person to another who is unable to eliminate those cells. GvHD arises when donor T cells respond to genetically-defined proteins on host cells, the most important of which are human leucocyte antigens (HLAs). These antigens are highly polymorphic and are encoded by the major histocompatibility complex (MHC). The frequency of acute GvHD is directly related to the degree of mismatch between HLA proteins and thus ideally, donors and recipients are matched at HLA A, B, C and DRB1 loci (referred to as 8/8 matches), but mismatches can be tolerated for umbilical cord blood grafts. The prevalence of GvHD ranges from 35–45% in recipients of full-matched sibling donor grafts to 60–80% in people receiving one-antigen HLA-mismatched unrelated-donor grafts.

About 40% of recipients of HLA-identical grafts develop systemic acute GvHD that needs treatment with high-dose steroids. This is a result of genetic differences that lie outside the HLA loci and that encode proteins referred to as minor histocompatibility antigens.

Ferrara, J.L., Levine, J.E., Reddy, P., and Holler, E. (2009). Graft-versus-host disease. *Lancet* 373, 1550–1561.
http://www.ncbi.nlm.nih.gov/pmc/articles/PMC2735047/

23. Answer D

Rituximab is a chimeric monoclonal antibody that recognises the human CD20 antigen. CD20 is a B-cell-specific differentiation antigen that is expressed on mature B cells and in most B-cell non-Hodgkin lymphomas (Maloney, 2012). CD38 is a marker of plasma cells. Rituximab causes the death of tumour cells through several mechanisms.

Rituximab has been investigated in both aggressive and indolent non-Hodgkin lymphoma (NHL), as either a single agent or in combination with standard chemotherapy regimens for lymphoma, such as cyclophosphamide, doxorubicin, vincristine and prednisolone (CHOP regimen). In aggressive NHL, the 3-year rate of progression-free survival was 85% with the addition of rituximab compared to 68% with chemotherapy alone.

The initial dose is associated with infusion-related symptoms such as flu-like symptoms and urticaria in more than half of patients. Although these symptoms are usually modest, more serious reactions, including hypotension, bronchospasm and angio-oedema can occur in 10% of patients. Rituximab-induced lymphopenia occurs in most patients, typically lasting about 6 months; a full recovery of B lymphocytes in the peripheral blood is usually seen 9–12 months after therapy has ceased.

Maloney, D.G. (2012). Anti-CD20 antibody therapy for B-cell lymphomas. *N Engl J Med* 366, 2008–2016.
http://www.nejm.org/doi/full/10.1056/NEJMct1114348

24. Answer D

The clinical features are suggestive of systemic mastocytosis with symptoms associated with release of mast cell mediators. Systemic mastocytosis is more commonly seen in adults and cutaneous mastocytosis is more common in the paediatric population. Patients with systemic mastocytosis invariably have bone marrow involvement. Beyond bone marrow, abnormal growth and accumulation of neoplastic mast cells in various extracutaneous organs can cause pathology in the liver, spleen and bone. Careful histological with immunohistochemical study of the bone marrow is the cornerstone of establishing the diagnosis of systemic mastocytosis. Other tests such as mast cell immunophenotyping, cytogenetic/ molecular studies and serum tryptase levels are useful in confirming the diagnosis. Mast cells express CD25 and/or CD2 and these surface markers are used as part of the World Health Organization (WHO) minor diagnostic criteria for systemic mastocytosis.

In normal bone marrow, the mast cell burden is very low (<0.1%). A mast cell burden of more than 10% suggests a high disease burden and may be associated with aggressive or advanced mast cell disorders. Patients with cutaneous and low mast cell burden can be managed symptomatically. Recent advances in cytogenetics/molecular studies have identified the cohort of patients with high mast cell burden who are more likely to benefit from cytoreductive therapy.

Patnaik, M., Rindos, M., Kouides, P., Tefferi, A., and Pardanani, A. (2007). Systemic mastocytosis: A concise clinical and laboratory review. *Arch Pathol Lab Med* 131, 784–791.
http://www.ncbi.nlm.nih.gov/pubmed/17488167

25. Answer D

Protein C deficiency is associated with recurrent familial thrombosis (Seligsohn and Lubetsky, 2001). It is inherited as an autosomal dominant trait and heterozygotes present with venous thrombotic manifestations. A family history is essential in assessing the association of a patient's deficiency with their risk of thrombosis.

Patients with protein C deficiency are at high risk for warfarin-induced skin necrosis during initiation of therapy. Warfarin-induced skin necrosis occurs in the feet, buttocks, thighs, breasts, upper extremities and genitalia. The lesions usually begin as maculopapular lesions several days after initiation of warfarin and progress into bullous, haemorrhagic and necrotic lesions. The mechanism is thought to be that, following the initiation of warfarin, both protein C antigen and activity levels drop rapidly, compared with levels of other vitamin K-dependent factors, such as factors IX and X and prothrombin. Therefore, administration of warfarin to protein C-deficient individuals causes a temporary exaggeration of the balance between pro-coagulant and anti-coagulant pathways; that is the early suppressive action of warfarin on protein C may not be counterbalanced by the anti-coagulant effect created by the decline in other vitamin K-dependent factors, thereby leading to a relative hypercoagulable state at the start of treatment. This leads to thrombotic occlusions of the microvasculature with resulting necrosis. Protein S deficiency and anti-thrombin III are rarely associated with warfarin-induced skin necrosis.

Seligsohn, U. and Lubetsky, A. (2001). Genetic susceptibility to venous thrombosis. *N Engl J Med* 344, 1222–1231.
http://www.ncbi.nlm.nih.gov/pubmed/11309638

26. Answer C

Waldenström macroglobulinaemia (WM) is a malignant lymphoplasmo-proliferative disorder with monoclonal pentameric IgM production. Patients with WM have symptoms attributable to:

- Tumour infiltration leading to cytopenias and progressive anaemia
- Circulating IgM leading to an increase in vascular resistance and viscosity
- Tissue deposition of IgM
- Autoantibody activity of IgM.

Symptoms of hyperviscosity usually appear when serum viscosity is greater than 4.08 cP (corresponding to a serum IgM level of at least 30 g/L) and include constitutional symptoms, bleeding and ocular, neurological and cardiovascular manifestations.

Plasma exchange is indicated for the acute management of patients with symptoms of hyperviscosity because 80% of the IgM protein is intravascular. The main choices for primary treatment of WM are alkylating agents (chlorambucil, cyclophosphamide, melphalan), purine analogues (cladribine, fludarabine) and monoclonal antibody [rituximab (anti-CD20)]. Alkylating agents deplete stem cells and hence should not be used among patients who may be eligible for autologous transplantation. The roles of allogeneic or non-myeloablative allogeneic transplantation and thalidomide in the treatment of WM are being explored.

 Vijay, A. and Gertz, M.A. (2007). Waldenström macroglobulinaemia. *Blood* 109, 5096–5103.
http://bloodjournal.hematologylibrary.org/content/109/12/5096.long

27. Answer C

Epstein–Barr virus (EBV) has been recognised in association with nasal natural killer (NK) cell, Burkitt and T-cell lymphomas. Hepatitis C is associated with splenic marginal-zone lymphoma. *Helicobacter pylori* is implicated in the pathogenesis of gastric mucosa-associated lymphoid tissue (MALT) lymphoma. Nasal NK-cell and T-cell lymphoma associated with EBV are more frequent in East Asia than in other regions, as is adult T-cell lymphoma associated with infection by human T-cell lymphotropic virus type 1.

 Shankland, K.R., Armitage, J.O., and Hancock, B.W. (2012). Non-Hodgkin lymphoma. *Lancet* 380, 848–857.
http://www.ncbi.nlm.nih.gov/pubmed/22835603

28. Answer E

In mild factor VIII deficiency, administration of the synthetic vasopressin analogue desmopressin acetate increases plasma concentrations of coagulation factor VIII and von Willebrand factor two–six times through endogenous release. Desmopressin can be administered intravenously, as an intranasal spray or subcutaneously. It is an attractive therapeutic option because it does not carry a risk of transmission of infectious diseases. Desmopressin is a widely used haemostatic agent; it has been used for prevention of bleeding with invasive procedures and for treatment of bleeding. Not all patients with haemophilia A achieve a haemostatic activity level with this drug. The clinical use depends on the post-treatment plasma factor VIII concentration, which generally depends on the patient's baseline factor VIII activity. Anti-fibrinolytic drugs are useful to control bleeding after dental extractions and other mucocutaneous bleeds; simultaneous use of tranexamic acid and factor VIII increases clot resistance to fibrinolysis. Fibrin sealants promote haemostasis during surgery in patients with haemophilia and reduce the need for replacement therapy.

Berntorp, E. and Shapiro, A.D. (2012). Modern haemophilia care. *Lancet* 379, 1447–1456.
http://www.ncbi.nlm.nih.gov/pubmed/22456059

29. Answer C
Atypical haemolytic uraemic syndrome (aHUS) is a genetic, chronic, systemic and potentially life-threatening disease affecting both adults and children. It is associated with mutations in genes encoding both complement regulators (factor H, factor I, membrane cofactor protein and thrombomodulin) and activators (factors B and C3), and autoantibodies against factor H. Diagnosis of aHUS does not require identification of a genetic mutation, as genetic mutations are not identified in 40% of patients with aHUS. Due to permanent genetic mutations, aHUS is an ongoing, lifelong disease of systemic complement-mediated thrombotic microangiopathy (TMA). Approximately half of the patients with aHUS are adults. Renal injury occurs in aHUS but other vital organ systems, including the cardiac and neurological system, are also affected. The related condition thrombotic thrombocytopenic purpura (TTP) results from a deficiency of ADAMTS13, a plasma metalloprotease that cleaves von Willebrand factor.

Kavanagh, D. and Goodship, T.H. (2011). Atypical hemolytic uremic syndrome, genetic basis, and clinical manifestations. *Hematology* 2011, 15–20.
http://asheducationbook.hematologylibrary.org/content/2011/1/15.long

30. Answer C
The patient's clinical tumour lysis syndrome is a result of chemotherapy for a highly aggressive mature B-cell lymphoma. As such, the patient developed acute kidney injury, hyperkalaemia, hyperphosphataemia, secondary hypocalcaemia (caused by hyperphosphataemia) and hyperuricaemia. Tumour lysis syndrome (Howard et al., 2011) is seen in patients treated for bulky tumours and extensive metastasis, or with a high rate of proliferation of cancer cells, cancer cell sensitivity to therapy and an intensive cancer treatment regimen.

A persistently high uric acid level increases the risk of crystal formation and acute renal injury. Supportive treatment, including intravenous fluids (not diuretics!) and cautious monitoring of the electrolyte imbalance to prevent cardiac dysrhythmias and neuromuscular irritability, should be supplemented with treatment to lower the level of uric acid.

Rasburicase removes uric acid by enzymatically degrading it into allantoin, a highly soluble product that has no known adverse effects. The use of rasburicase can preserve or improve renal function and lower phosphorus levels as a secondary beneficial effect.

Allopurinol is a xanthine oxidase inhibitor. It prevents the conversion of hypoxanthine and xanthine into uric acid but does not remove existing uric acid. Allopurinol has also shown to worsen serum creatinine level (by 12%) compared to rasburicase, which improved creatinine level (by 31%).

Where rasburicase is available, it is the recommended solution over the use of allopurinol in patients with high risk of or clinically established tumour lysis syndrome.

Howard, S.C., Jones, D.P., and Pui, C.H. (2011). The tumor lysis syndrome. *N Engl J Med* 364, 1844–1854.
http://www.ncbi.nlm.nih.gov/pmc/articles/PMC3437249/

31. Answer D

Heparin-induced thrombocytopenia (HIT) is caused by antibodies against complexes of platelet factor 4 (PF4) and heparin (Arepally and Ortel, 2006). Patients classically present with a low platelet count or a relative decrease of 50% or more from baseline. Thrombotic complications develop in approximately 20–50% of patients. Risk of thrombosis remains high for days to weeks after discontinuation of heparin, even after normalisation of platelet count. The incidence of HIT is 10 times higher in patients treated with unfractionated heparin compared to those receiving low-molecular-weight heparin. The incidence of HIT appears particularly high after orthopaedic surgery. Venous thromboses predominate in medical and orthopaedic patients, whereas arterial and venous thromboses occur at similar frequency in patients who have undergone cardiac or vascular surgery.

Laboratory tests play an important role in the diagnosis of HIT because of the challenges of clinical diagnosis. When HIT is suspected, testing for heparin-dependent antibodies is indicated with immunological assays, which identify circulating anti-PF4/heparin antibodies irrespective of their capacity to active platelets or functional assays, which detect patient antibodies that induce heparin-dependent platelet activation or both. Immunological assays detect circulating IgG, IgM and IgA antibodies and are the first-line screening test. The major shortcoming of the immunological assays is limited specificity. False-positive results are common and may result from detection of non-pathogenic anti-PF4/heparin antibodies or anti-phospholipid antibodies against either PF4 or PF4-bound beta-2 glycoprotein I. Functional assays measure platelet activation and detect heparin-dependent antibodies capable of binding to and activating Fc receptors on platelets. The most extensively studied functional tests for HIT diagnosis are the ^{14}C-serotonin release assay (SRA) and heparin-induced platelet activation assay

(HIPA). Both tests are significantly more specific than existing immunoassays and are useful for confirming a positive immunological assay. Unfortunately, technical requirements restrict their use to a small number of reference laboratories. As such, they commonly do not provide results in the real time necessary to guide initial management.

Arepally, G.M. and Ortel, T.L. (2006). Clinical practice. Heparin-induced thrombocytopenia. *N Engl J Med* 355, 809–817.
http://www.ncbi.nlm.nih.gov/pubmed/16928996

32. Answer H
Sickle cell disease patients are prone to bone infarcts and osteomyelitis, especially from salmonella (Almeida and Roberts, 2005). The increased susceptibility of sickle cell disease patients to infections, including osteomyelitis, has long been recognised, with several mechanisms postulated, including hyposplenism, impaired complement activity and the presence of infarcted or necrotic bone. The most common cause of osteomyelitis in sickle cell disease is salmonella (especially the non-typical serotypes *Salmonella typhimurium*, *S. enteritidis*, *S. choleraesuis* and *S. paratyphi B*), followed by *Staphylococcus aureus* and Gram-negative enteric bacilli.

Diagnosis of osteomyelitis can be difficult in sickle cell disease: failure to identify it may result in severe bone damage and life-threatening infection, while an erroneous diagnosis subjects the patient to lengthy and unnecessary intravenous and oral antibiotics. Osteomyelitis usually presents with pain, swelling and tenderness over the affected area. The most common sites are the diaphysis of long bones, such as the femur, tibia or humerus. Most patients also have fever and elevated inflammatory markers, but the fever may be modest. These signs and symptoms are similar to those found in vaso-occlusive crises, making the distinction between a painful crisis and osteomyelitis extremely difficult; indeed osteomyelitis may not be suspected until the signs and symptoms of a typical painful crisis have failed to resolve after 1–2 weeks of standard therapy. Blood cultures are often sterile when taken at this stage, as it is common practice to treat patients upon admission with vaso-occlusive crises with broad-spectrum antibiotics, especially if they are febrile. Thus, confident diagnosis of osteomyelitis in such patients tends to rely on various imaging techniques. However, in some cases, osteomyelitis presents late as a more indolent process often with abscess formation.

Almeida, A. and Roberts, I. (2005). Bone involvement in sickle cell disease. *Br J Haematol* 129, 482–490.
http://www.ncbi.nlm.nih.gov/pubmed/15877730

33. Answer D
Mutations in an autoimmune-suppressor gene (AIRE, for autoimmune regulator), which encodes a transcription factor, is responsible for autoimmune polyendocrine

syndrome type I (Michels and Gottlieb, 2010). Individuals with any two of the following conditions – mucocutaneous candidiasis, hypoparathyroidism and Addison disease – are likely to have AIRE mutations. Mutations to this gene cause many autoimmune diseases and affected patients are at risk for the development of multiple autoimmune diseases over time, including type 1 diabetes, hypothyroidism, pernicious anaemia, alopecia, vitiligo, hepatitis, ovarian atrophy and keratitis.

Michels, A.W. and Gottlieb, P.A. (2010). Autoimmune polyglandular syndromes. *Nat Rev Endocrinol* 6, 270–277.
http://www.ncbi.nlm.nih.gov/pubmed/20309000

34. Answer B

Myasthenia gravis (MG) and pure red cell aplasia (PRCA) can be associated with thymoma (Sawada et al., 2008). MG appears in about 20–40% of patients with thymoma and PRCA develops in about 2–5% of those patients. On the other hand, thymoma is detected in 10–17% of patients with MG and in 5–13% of patients with PRCA. However, the simultaneous occurrence of MG, PRCA and thymoma is rare.

PRCA in adults can be diagnosed when isolated anaemia is found in the presence of normal white cell and platelet counts. The bone marrow biopsy shows almost complete absence of erythroblasts but normal myeloid cells and megakaryocytes. Evaluations for the possible causes of PRCA should include a previous history of drug use and toxins or infections, liver and kidney functions, immunological examination including autoantibodies, bone marrow examination including morphology, chromosome and rearrangement of T-cell receptor (TCR) analysis, peripheral blood flow cytometry, virological examination including parvovirus B19 DNA, and computed tomography and/or magnetic resonance imaging examinations to rule out the presence of thymoma and neoplasms.

Sawada, K., Fujishima, N., and Hirokawa, M. (2008). Acquired pure red cell aplasia: updated review of treatment. *Br J Haematol* 142, 505–514.
http://www.ncbi.nlm.nih.gov/pmc/articles/PMC2592349/

35. Answer A

Cold antibody haemolytic anaemia (CAHA) may occur as a secondary disorder in association with a number of different underlying disorders, such as certain infectious diseases (e.g. mycoplasma infection and infectious mononucleosis) and lymphoproliferative diseases (e.g. non-Hodgkin lymphoma and chronic lymphocytic leukaemia) (Gertz, 2006). An increase in cold agglutinin titres is frequently observed with *Mycoplasma pneumoniae* infection; it has been reported that 50–60% of these patients have cold agglutinins, which appear 1 week after the onset of the illness and decline toward undetectable levels after 2–6 weeks. Cold agglutinins appear to be more specific for Iantigen of the red blood cell surface and often result in mild, subclinical haemolysis and mild reticulocytosis.

Severe haemolytic anaemia is rare and is usually associated with marked pulmonary involvement. Post-*M. pneumoniae* pneumonia CAHA is usually self-limiting and most patients recover with supportive care. Antibiotics are likely to be of limited value in mycoplasma-associated haemolytic anaemia; however, treatment of the underlying mycoplasma infection has been associated with more rapid resolution of the haemolytic process. Furthermore, in the setting of an autoimmune haemolytic anaemia, packed red blood cell transfusions can potentiate haemolysis and their use should be limited.

Gertz, M.A. (2006). Cold hemolytic syndrome. *Hematol Am Soc Hematol Educ Program*, 19–23.
http://asheducationbook.hematologylibrary.org/content/2006/1/19.long

12 Clinical immunology

Questions

BASIC SCIENCE

Answers can be found in the Clinical immunology Answers section at the end of this chapter.

1. Major histocompatibility complex (MHC) class II antigens are expressed by:
  A. Renal tubular cells
  B. Erythrocytes
  C. Antigen-presenting cells
  D. Hepatocytes
  E. Osteoclasts

2. Which one of the following options correctly describes these three primary immunodeficiency diseases: DiGeorge syndrome, chronic granulomatous disease and severe combined immunodeficiency?

	DiGeorge syndrome	Chronic granulomatous disease	Severe combined immunodeficiency
A	Defects in neutrophils	Defects in lymphocytes	Absent thymus
B	Absent thymus	Defects in lymphocytes	Defects in neutrophils
C	Defects in neutrophils	Absent thymus	Defects in lymphocytes
D	Defects in lymphocytes	Absent thymus	Defects in neutrophils
E	Absent thymus	Defects in neutrophils	Defects in lymphocytes

3. Toll-like receptors function in which one of the following?
  A. Regulation of B-cell activation by antigen binding
  B. Activation of the complement pathway
  C. Recognition of microorganisms by the innate immune system
  D. Activation of immunoglobulin chain switching
  E. Inhibition of eosinophils

Passing the FRACP Written Examination: Questions and Answers, First Edition. Jonathan Gleadle, Tuck Yong, Jordan Li, Surjit Tarafdar, and Danielle Wu.
© 2013 John Wiley & Sons, Ltd. Published 2013 by John Wiley & Sons, Ltd.

4. Which one of the following is an advantage of killed viral vaccines compared with live viral vaccines?
   A. Killed viral vaccines produce a CD8 cytotoxic T-cell response
   B. Killed viral vaccines can be given by the natural route of infection and induce an immunoglobulin G and A response
   C. Killed viral vaccines often confer life-long protection
   D. Killed viral vaccines do not revert to virulence
   E. Killed viral vaccines can be given pre-exposure to disease-causing agents

5. Which one of the following is the main difference between cytotoxic (type II) and immune complex (type III) hypersensitivity?
   A. Distribution of antigen–antibody complexes
   B. Involvement of T cells
   C. Involvement of complement
   D. Antibody isotype
   E. Difference in triggers

6. Which one of the following correctly describes immunoglobulin A (IgA) in humans?
   A. It is the rarest immunoglobulin isotype
   B. The two subclasses of IgA, IgA1 and IgA2, differ in their light chains
   C. IgA2 is present more abundantly than IgA1 in the airways
   D. Secretory IgA can reduce the motility of *Salmonella* species, thus affecting the bacterial virulence
   E. IgA2 is the predominant subclass in the serum

7. Which one of the following describes the involvement of human natural killer (NK) cells in innate immunity?
   A. NK cells are activated directly by macrophages
   B. NK cells express antigen-specific receptors
   C. NK cells contribute to the delayed T-cell response following infection
   D. NK cells do not mediate antibody-dependent cellular cytotoxicity
   E. NK cells are found only in the lymph nodes

8. A 24-year-old man is stung by a bee and experiences respiratory distress within minutes and lapses into unconsciousness. This reaction is probably mediated by:
   A. IgG antibody
   B. IgE antibody
   C. IgM antibody
   D. Complement
   E. Sensitised T cells

9. Which one of the following is a mechanism in the development of immune tolerance?
   A. Clonal amplification of B cells in the thymus
   B. Failure of B cells bearing low-affinity receptors to recognise self-antigens in the thymus

   C. T cells in the thymus with high affinity for self-antigen undergo positive selection
   D. Regulatory T cells actively activate an immune response to an antigen
   E. Acquisition of anergy after T-cell receptor ligation without co-stimulation

10. A 56-year-old bee-farmer was admitted after an anaphylactic reaction to bee stings. He underwent immunotherapy/desensitisation to prevent future adverse reactions associated with bee stings. Which one of the following mechanisms explains the principle of immunotherapy?
   A. Reduces allergen-specific IgE
   B. Acts by induction of 'blocking' IgG antibodies
   C. Works by altering T-cell reactivity to specific antigen, which in turn causes a reduction in release of pro-allergic/inflammatory cytokines
   D. Works by inactivating B cells, which then alters T-cell reactivity to the specific antigen
   E. Acts by blocking the antigen-presenting cells directly, so the foreign antigen is not detected by the immune system of the patient

11. Interferon-gamma is produced by:
   A. Type 1 helper T cells
   B. Type 2 helper T cells
   C. B lymphocytes
   D. Plasma cells
   E. Eosinophils

Theme: Cytokines and immune cells (for Questions 12 and 13)
   A. Neutrophils
   B. Eosinophils
   C. B lymphocytes
   D. T lymphocytes
   E. Macrophages
   F. Dendritic cells
   G. Natural killer cells
   H. Plasma cells

12. Which cell is the main source of interleukin-1?

13. Which cell is the main source of interleukin-2?

CLINICAL

14. A 24-year-old man with a history of hereditary angio-oedema (HAE) presents with acute breathlessness and on examination is found to have laryngeal, pharyngeal and tongue oedema. In addition to securing his airway, which drug should be administered urgently?

- **A.** Intravenous methylprednisolone
- **B.** Intravenous frusemide
- **C.** Anti-histamine
- **D.** Fresh frozen plasma (FFP)
- **E.** Nebulised salbutamol

15. A 20-year-old woman presents with dyspnoea, angio-oedema, urticaria and hypotension after eating shellfish. She is successfully treated with epinephrine (adrenaline), anti-histamines, corticosteroid and intravenous fluids. She has a history of asthma. She takes inhaled beclomethasone. Radioallergosorbent (RAST) testing reveals the presence of shellfish-specific IgE. Which one of the following statements regarding this patient's condition is the most accurate?

- **A.** This allergy is likely to disappear in a few years
- **B.** She should avoid other highly allergenic foods, such as peanuts and tree nuts
- **C.** She is at high risk for developing a more severe anaphylactic reaction in the future if she ingests shellfish
- **D.** She had a type II hypersensitivity reaction
- **E.** She had a type IV hypersensitivity reaction

16. A 30-year-old Aboriginal woman received a tetanus vaccination today. She had her diphtheria/pertussis/tetanus injection following the birth of her first child. She asks whether she should have any other immunisations. Which one of the following is the immunisation recommendation for Aboriginal and Torres Strait Islanders?

- **A.** Immunisation with pneumococcal and annual influenza vaccine for all Aboriginal and Torrens Strait Islanders who are 15 years of age and older
- **B.** Immunisation with pneumococcal and annual influenza vaccine for all Aboriginal and Torrens Strait Islanders who are 50 years of age and older
- **C.** Immunisation with pneumococcal and annual influenza vaccine for all Aboriginal and Torrens Strait Islanders who are 65 years of age and older
- **D.** Immunisation with pneumococcal vaccine for all Aboriginal and Torrens Strait Islanders who are 50 years of age and older and influenza vaccine for those who are 65 years of age and older
- **E.** Immunisation with annual influenza vaccine for all Aboriginal and Torrens Strait Islanders who are 50 years of age and older and pneumococcal vaccine for those who are 65 years of age and older

17. A 21-year-old man presents with recurrent bacterial infections. Investigations show low immunoglobulin (IgG, IgA and IgM) levels and comparison with previous results shows decreasing levels with age. His full blood count is normal. Which one of the following is the most likely diagnosis?

    A. Myeloperoxidase deficiency

    B. Common variable immunodeficiency

    C. Chronic granulomatous disease

    D. Hyper-IgM syndrome

    E. C1 inhibitor deficiency

18. An 80-year-old man presents with a urinary tract infection. After receiving a dose of intravenous cephazolin, his systolic blood pressure falls from 170 mmHg to 90 mmHg. This patient has a known allergy to penicillin. Hypotension caused by anaphylaxis is suspected. Serum tryptase level is checked. Which one of the following is correct in the interpretation of tryptase results?

    A. Peak tryptase levels occur at 4 h after an anaphylactic event

    B. Tryptase is more useful in food-related anaphylaxis than medication-related anaphylaxis

    C. Single measurement of tryptase has high sensitivity

    D. May be significantly elevated in septicaemia

    E. High tryptase may be due to mastocytosis

19. A 43-year-old woman presents with persistent itchy hives for 8 weeks. When asked, she says that each individual hive lasts for 2 or 3 days. Physical examination reveals multiple urticarial papules that do not blanch. Three days after initial consultation, she returns and some of the lesions are still present. What would be the next step in her work-up?

    A. Thyroid function tests

    B. An abdominal computed tomography to exclude an intra-abdominal malignancy

    C. Check hepatitis serology

    D. Check stool for ova and parasites

    E. Perform a biopsy of one of the lesions

20. A 25-year-old man presents with symptoms of nasal congestion, itchy eyes and a tickling sensation in his throat. He has been experiencing these symptoms for several years. Symptoms are present throughout the year and outdoor activities do not worsen the symptoms. He has a cat, which does not sleep in the same room as him. Allergy skin testing indicates a positive response to dust mites and cat dander. Which one of the following therapeutic interventions is the most effective for this patient's symptoms?

    A. Leucotriene receptor antagonists

    B. Removal of the allergen from the patient's environment

    C. Anti-histamines

    D. Intranasal corticosteroids

    E. Cromolyn sodium

21. A 28-year-old man who works in the timber industry has recently had an anaphylactic reaction to a yellow jacket (a type of wasp) sting. He has since been tested and found to be positive on venom skin test. What would be the most appropriate management plan for this man?

    A. Venom immunotherapy

    B. Commence leucotriene receptor antagonists

    C. Avoid outdoor activities

    D. Repeat skin test in 6 months

    E. Apply wasp repellent on the skin when at work

22. An Aboriginal patient with a history of rheumatic fever develops a sore throat from which Group A streptococci are cultured. The patient is started on treatment with penicillin and the sore throat resolves within a few days. However, on day 7 after initiation of penicillin therapy, the patient develops a fever of 38°C, a generalised maculopapular rash, arthralgia and malaise. The most likely explanation for this is:

    A. Development of subacute endocarditis

    B. Recurrence of rheumatic fever

    C. An IgG- and IgM-mediated response to penicillin

    D. A delayed lymphocyte-mediated hypersensitivity reaction to penicillin

    E. A delayed IgE-mediated response to penicillin

Theme: Primary immunodeficiency disease

(for Questions 23–25)

    A. X-linked hypogammaglobulinaemia

    B. Selective IgA deficiency

    C. Selective IgG deficiency

    D. Hereditary angio-oedema

    E. Chronic granulomatous disease

    F. Common variable immunodeficiency

    G. C3 deficiency

    H. Ataxia–telangiectasia

23. Which disease is caused by a defect in the ability of neutrophils to kill microorganisms?

24. Which disease is caused by a deficiency in an inhibitor of the C1 component of complement?

25. Which disease is characterised by an inability to synthesise immunoglobulin G (IgG) and other immunoglobulins, resulting in presentations of recurrent pyogenic bacterial infections?

Answers

BASIC SCIENCE

1. Answer C

MHC class II is normally expressed on antigen-presenting cells (APCs) and lymphocytes, while MHC class I is expressed on all nucleated cells except erythrocytes. While MHC is expressed in all vertebrates, the human form is called human leucocyte antigen (HLA) and is encoded on chromosome 6. The major role of MHC molecules is activation of T cells as, unlike antibodies which can bind to any class of molecule including carbohydrates, lipids and proteins, T-cell receptors can only recognise short peptides bound to MHC molecules.

An APC internalises a foreign protein, processes its antigens and then returns a peptide fraction to the surface, which can bind in the groove of specific MHC class II molecules. The APCs can migrate to lymph nodes and the epitope/MHC class II complex is recognised by the CD4 T-helper cells. MHC class II molecules are encoded by HLA-D and bind peptides that are usually 15–24 amino acids in length.

Class I MHC molecules bind peptides (8–10 amino acids in length) generated mainly from degradation of cytosolic proteins by the proteasome. The MHC–peptide complex is then inserted into the plasma membrane of the cell. The peptide is bound to the extracellular part of the class I MHC molecule, thereby displaying intracellular proteins to cytotoxic T cells (CTLs). A normal cell will display peptides from normal cellular protein turnover on its class I MHC, and CTLs will not be activated in response to them due to central and peripheral tolerance mechanisms. When a cell expresses foreign proteins, such as after viral infection, a fraction of the class I MHC will display these peptides on the cell surface. This enables CTLs specific for the MHC–peptide complex to recognise and kill the presenting cell. The genes encoding MHC class I are known as HLA-A, B and C and are highly polymorphic.

Matching of HLA antigens between donor and recipient can improve the outcome of solid organ transplants.

2. Answer E

Salient features of DiGeorge syndrome can be summarised using the mnemonic CATCH-22, with the 22 reminding one that the chromosomal abnormality is found on chromosome 22 (a deletion at 22q11.2, usually including the TBX1 gene):

- Cardiac abnormality (especially tetralogy of Fallot)
- Abnormal facies
- Thymic aplasia
- Cleft palate
- Hypocalcaemia/hypoparathyroidism (due to hypoplasia or absence of parathyroid glands).

Chronic granulomatous disease is the name for a genetically heterogeneous group of immunodeficiencies. The core defect is a failure of neutrophils to kill organisms that they have engulfed because of defects in a system of enzymes that produce free radicals and other toxic small molecules.

Severe combined immunodeficiency (SCID) is a genetic disorder in which both B cells and T cells of the adaptive immune system are impaired due to a defect in one of several possible genes. SCID is a severe form of heritable immunodeficiency and is the result of an immune system so highly compromised that it is considered almost absent (Riminton and Limaye, 2004).

 Riminton, D.S. and Limaye, S. (2004). Primary immunodeficiency diseases in adulthood. *Intern Med J* 34, 348–354.
http://www.ncbi.nlm.nih.gov/pubmed/15228396

3. Answer C
Toll-like receptors (TLRs) are a class of proteins that play a key role in the innate immune system. They are single, membrane-spanning, non-catalytic receptors that recognise structurally conserved molecules derived from microbes and subsequently activate immune cells. Lipopolysaccharide (LPS), which is the primary endotoxin found in Gram-negative bacteria, is considered to be the prototypical 'pathogen-associated molecular pattern' and TLR4 functions as an LPS-sensing receptor. Other types of non-self molecules recognised by TLRs include double-stranded RNA, DNA, peptidoglycan and lipopeptides.

4. Answer D
The following are a few of the advantages of killed viral vaccines:
- Contamination is less likely
- Do not revert to virulence
- Heat stable.
  In contrast, the advantages of live viral vaccines include:
- Virus multiplies in the host and produces a CD8 cytotoxic T-cell response
- Given by the natural route of infection and can induce an immunoglobulin G and A response
- Are contagious and may spread immunity to people who were never vaccinated
- Produce a response that is stronger and longer, and often confers lifelong protection.
  Most vaccines are given pre-exposure to disease-causing agents.

5. Answer A
Type II hypersensitivity is also known as cytotoxic hypersensitivity and may affect a variety of organs and tissues. The antigens are normally endogenous, although exogenous chemicals (haptens) which can attach to cell membranes can also lead to type II hypersensitivity. Drug-induced haemolytic anaemia and thrombocytope-

nia are examples. The reaction time is minutes to hours. Type II hypersensitivity is primarily mediated by antibodies of the IgM or IgG classes and complement. The lesion contains antibody, complement and neutrophils. Diagnostic tests include detection of circulating antibody against the tissues involved and the presence of antibody and complement in the lesion (biopsy) by immunofluorescence. The staining pattern is normally smooth and linear, such as that seen in Goodpasture nephritis (renal and lung basement membrane) and pemphigus (skin intercellular protein, desmosome).

Type III hypersensitivity is also known as immune complex hypersensitivity. The reaction may be general (e.g. serum sickness) or may involve individual organs, including the skin (e.g. systemic lupus erythematosus, Arthus reaction), kidneys (e.g. lupus nephritis), blood vessels (e.g. polyarteritis), joints (e.g. rheumatoid arthritis) or other organs. The reaction may take 3–10h after exposure to the antigen (as in Arthus reaction). It is mediated by soluble immune complexes, mostly of the IgG class, although IgM may be involved. The antigen may be exogenous (chronic bacterial, viral or parasitic infections), or endogenous (non–organ-specific autoimmunity, e.g. systemic lupus erythematosus) and is soluble. The immunofluorescent staining in type III hypersensitivity is usually granular. The presence of immune complexes in serum and depletion in the level of complement are also diagnostic.

6. Answer D

IgA is the major immunoglobulin isotype in humans, and its production exceeds that of all other immunoglobulin classes combined. In humans, IgA exists in two subclasses, IgA1 and IgA2, which differ in their heavy chains. The relative production of the two isotypes varies between different mucosal tissues. IgA1 predominates in the airways, whereas in the colon IgA2 is more abundant than IgA1. In the small intestine, both isoforms are produced in fairly equal amounts. IgA1 is the predominant subclass in the serum (Pabst, 2012).

In the gut lumen, secretory IgA (sIgA) acts as the first-line barrier limiting access of intestinal antigens to the blood circulation and controls the intestinal microbiota. These functions of sIgA are collectively referred to as 'immune exclusion'. Mechanistically, immune exclusion is still incompletely understood and comprises a range of activities. Interaction with sIgA can entrap antigens in the mucus and prevent them from binding to cell-surface receptors, as exemplified by the sIgA-mediated neutralisation of cholera toxin. Moreover, sIgA can affect bacterial virulence; for example, sIgA binding reduces the motility of *Salmonella* spp. and limits the invasiveness of *Shigella flexneri*. Collectively, the functions of IgA reinforce the integrity of the intestinal barrier, dampen pro-inflammatory immune responses and effectively contribute to intestinal homeostasis.

Pabst, O. (2012). New concepts in the generation and functions of IgA. *Nat Rev Immunol* 12, 821–832.
http://www.ncbi.nlm.nih.gov/pubmed/23103985

7. Answer C

Natural killer (NK) cells are part of the innate immune system. They destroy infected and malignant cells. Human NK cells comprise approximately 10% of all blood lymphocytes. NK cells are identified by the expression of the CD56 surface antigen and the lack of CD3. Functionally, NK cells are an important source of innate immunoregulatory cytokines, such as interferon (IFN)-gamma, tumour necrosis factor (TNF)-alpha, granulocyte–macrophage–colony stimulating factor (GM-CSF), which coordinate the early immune response and contribute to the delayed T-cell response following the infection.

NK cells also have direct or natural cytotoxic activity against some virus-infected and tumour cells. They also mediate antibody-dependent cellular cytotoxicity (ADCC) of targets through Fc RIII (CD16), a receptor that binds the Fc portion of antibody. NK cells can be found in the spleen, lung, bone marrow, lymph nodes, peripheral blood mononuclear cells and liver.

8. Answer B

Venom hypersensitivity may be mediated by immunological mechanisms (IgE-mediated or non-IgE-mediated venom allergy), but also by non-immunological mechanisms. Reactions to Hymenoptera stings are classified into normal local reactions, large local reactions, systemic toxic reactions, systemic anaphylactic reactions and unusual reactions. Systemic anaphylactic reactions are most often IgE mediated. Rarely, they may be due to short-term sensitising IgG antibodies or complement activation by IgG–venom complexes. The skin and gastrointestinal, respiratory and cardiovascular systems can be involved.

Risk factors influencing the outcome of an anaphylactic reaction include the time interval between stings, number of stings, severity of the preceding reaction, age, cardiovascular diseases and drug intake, insect type, elevated serum tryptase and mastocytosis. Diagnostic tests should be carried out in all patients with a history of a systemic sting reaction to detect sensitisation. They are not recommended in subjects with large local reaction or no history of a systemic reaction. Testing comprises skin tests with Hymenoptera venoms and analysis of the serum for Hymenoptera venom-specific IgE. Stepwise skin testing with incremental venom concentrations is recommended. If diagnostic tests are negative, they should be repeated several weeks later. Serum tryptase should be analysed in patients with a history of a severe sting reaction.

Bilo, B.M., Rueff, F., Mosbech, H., et al. (2005). Diagnosis of Hymenoptera venom allergy. *Allergy* 60, 1339–1349.
http://www.ncbi.nlm.nih.gov/pubmed/16197464

9. Answer E

Tolerance can be induced in immature lymphocytes either centrally (thymus for T cells, bone marrow for B cells) or in the periphery. If a T cell has a high affinity for a self-antigen in the thymus, it can undergo negative selection with activation-induced death (apoptosis). The most common mechanism of peripheral tolerance is the failure of T cells bearing low-affinity receptors to recognise an antigen. T cells bearing receptors with high affinity for an antigen can remain in an inactivated state if that antigen is sequestered from the immune effector cells. Another mechanism of peripheral tolerance involves the acquisition of anergy after ligation with the T-cell receptor complex. The most extensively characterised mechanism of anergy induction occurs when the T-cell receptor is ligated in the absence of co-stimulation. Another mechanism of tolerance is T-cell-mediated suppression, in which regulatory T cells actively inhibit an immune response to an antigen.

Kamradt, T. and Mitchison, N.A. (2001). Tolerance and autoimmunity. *N Engl J Med* 344, 655–664.
http://www.ncbi.nlm.nih.gov/pubmed/11228281

10. Answer C
Immunotherapy for allergic disorders is the administration of increasing amounts of specific allergen to which the patient is known to be allergic (O'Brien, 2003). Immunotherapy is used to reduce allergic reactivity in patients with severe reactions to specific inhaled or injected antigens. It is not indicated for patients with food allergies. Early researchers felt immunotherapy acted by reduction of the allergen-specific IgE or by induction of 'blocking' IgG antibodies. Although these effects were observed during immunotherapy, they do not happen for months or years. In addition, these changes in antibody concentration did not show any correlation with clinical efficacy. More recent findings suggested immunotherapy works by altering T-cell reactivity to the specific antigen, which in turn causes a reduction in the release of pro-allergic/inflammatory cytokines. Serious reactions to immunotherapy occur at a rate of approximately 1 in 500. Experienced staff familiar with the immunotherapy and resuscitation procedures should be present during the therapy.

O'Brien, R.M. (2003). Immunotherapy for allergic disorders. *Aust Prescr* 26, 91–93.
http://www.australianprescriber.com/magazine/26/4/91/3

11. Answer A
The two main populations of mature T cells are CD4+ (helper) T cells and CD8+ (cytotoxic or killer) T cells (Jiang and Chess, 2006). Antigen-induced activation of helper cells causes them to differentiate into subgroups of type 1 helper T (Th1) and type 2 helper T (Th2) cells. These subgroups produce distinctive cytokines, which constitute another level of control of CD4+ T cells. Th1 cells secrete interferon-gamma, which induces cellular immune responses and inhibits Th2 cells. Th2 cells secrete interleukin-4 (which participates in activating B cells) and transforming growth factor β (TGF-β) and interleukin-10 (which inhibit Th1 cells). Other cytokine-secreting subgroups of CD4+ cells, termed 'type 1 regulatory T

(Tr1)' or 'type 3 regulatory T (Tr3) cells', secrete the immunosuppressive cytokines interleukin-10, TGF-β or both.

Jiang, H. and Chess, L. (2006). Regulation of immune responses by T cells. *N Engl J Med* 354, 1166–1176.
http://www.ncbi.nlm.nih.gov/pubmed/16540617

12. Answer E
Macrophages perform the following functions:
- Phagocytosis
- Antigen presentation
- Cytokine production.

Macrophages produce several cytokines, the most important of which are interleukin-1 (IL-1) and tumour necrosis factor (TNF). IL-1 activates a wide variety of target cells, including T and B lymphocytes, neutrophils, epithelial cells and fibroblasts, to grow, differentiate or synthesise specific proteins. For example, IL-1 stimulates T lymphocytes to differentiate and produce IL-2. IL-1 also acts on the hypothalamus to cause fever associated with infections and other inflammatory reactions. In recent years, a recombinant form of human IL-1 receptor antagonist (e.g. Anakinra) has been used in the treatment of inflammatory disorders such as rheumatoid arthritis. This class of drug neutralises the activity of IL-1 and reduces the inflammatory response.

13. Answer D
Interleukin-2 (IL-2) is produced by helper T lymphocytes and stimulates both helper and cytotoxic T lymphocytes to grow. Resting helper T lymphocytes are stimulated by antigen or other stimulators to produce IL-2 and to form IL-2 receptors on their surface, thereby acquiring the capacity to respond to IL-2. Interaction of IL-2 with its receptor stimulates DNA synthesis. IL-2 also acts synergistically with IL-4 to stimulate the growth of B cells. Antibodies to the IL-2 receptor are in routine clinical use in solid organ transplantation to reduce the incidence of rejection (e.g. basiliximab, which is a chimeric mouse–human monoclonal antibody to the α chain (CD25) of the IL-2 receptor of T cells).

CLINICAL

14. Answer D

Fresh frozen plasma (FFP), which contains C1-inhibitor concentrate (C1 INH), can be used in the treatment of an acute episode of hereditary angio-oedema (HAE) if C1 INH is not available. Treatment with FFP has been shown to be as effective as C1 INH concentrate (Nagy et al., 2010). HAE is an autosomal dominant genetic disorder resulting from an inherited deficiency or dysfunction of the C1 inhibitor. It is characterised by recurrent episodes of angio-oedema, which most often affect the skin as well as the mucosal tissues of the upper respiratory and gastrointestinal tracts. Characteristically, there are no urticaria, wheals or pruritus.

Bradykinin, which is a potent vasodilator, is derived from high-molecular-weight kininogen by the action of kallikrein. C1 inhibitor, along with its actions on the complement system, is also an inhibitor of kallikrein. In HAE, deficient or defective C1 inhibitor leads to excess production of bradykinin.

In acute attacks, laryngeal swelling can occur in isolation or with swelling of the lips, tongue, uvula and soft palate, while gastrointestinal involvement can present with gastrointestinal colic, nausea, vomiting and/or diarrhoea. Diagnosis is by demonstration of low C1 inhibitor concentration and function in type I HAE, while type II HAE typically shows low function. The current treatments for acute episodes of HAE are replacement purified C1 INH (Berinert, Cinryze) or the bradykinin antagonist icatibant (Firazyr).

Nagy, N., Grattan, C.E., and McGrath, J.A. (2010). New insights into hereditary angio-oedema: Molecular diagnosis and therapy. *Australas J Dermatol* 51, 157–162.
http://onlinelibrary.wiley.com/doi/10.1111/j.1440-0960.2010.00649.x/abstract

Australasian Society of Clinical Immunology and Allergy (ASCIA)
http://www.allergy.org.au/health-professionals/papers/hereditary-angioedema

15. Answer C

This patient is at high risk for developing a more severe anaphylactic reaction in the future if she ingests shellfish. Risk factors for severe anaphylaxis include:
• A history of a previous anaphylactic reaction
• A history of asthma, especially if the asthma is poorly controlled
• Allergy to peanuts, nuts, fish or shellfish
• Possibly, female sex.

This patient had a type I or IgE-mediated, hypersensitivity reaction. Type II- and type IV-mediated hypersensitivity are usually antibody-mediated and T-lymphocyte-mediated, respectively. Allergies to foods, such as tree nuts, fish and seafood, are generally not outgrown, regardless of the age at which they develop. Persons with these allergies are likely to retain their allergic sensitivity throughout their lifetime.

Australasian Society of Clinical Immunology and Allergy (ASCIA)
http://www.allergy.org.au/patients/food-allergy/
allergic-and-toxic-reactions-to-seafood

16. Answer B

Annual influenza vaccination is recommended for Aboriginal and Torres Strait Islander adults over 50 years of age, because of the greatly increased risk of premature death from respiratory disease. For non-indigenous individuals, influenza vaccine should be given routinely on an annual basis to individuals over 65 years of age. The risk for the elderly is greatest if they also have chronic cardiac or lung disease, and is increased for residents of nursing homes and other chronic care facilities.

Pneumococcal vaccine should be given to the following:

- All individuals over the age of 65 years
- Aboriginal and Torrens Strait Islanders over 50 years of age
- Individuals with asplenia, either functional or anatomical, including sickle cell disease in persons older than 2 years of age; where possible, the vaccine should be given at least 14 days before splenectomy
- Immunocompromised patients at increased risk of pneumococcal disease (e.g. patients with HIV infection, nephrotic syndrome, multiple myeloma, lymphoma and organ transplant recipients)
- Immunocompetent persons at increased risk of complications from pneumococcal disease because of chronic illness (e.g. chronic cardiac, renal or pulmonary disease)
- Patients with cerebrospinal fluid leak.

Pneumococcal vaccine is strongly recommended for Aboriginal and Torrens Strait Islander adults because in some remote parts of Australia, the rates of pneumococcal infections remain high.

Torzillo, P.J., Hanna, J.N., Morey, F., et al. (1995). Invasive pneumococcal disease in central Australia. *Med J Aust* 162, 182–186.
http://www.ncbi.nlm.nih.gov/pubmed/7877538

Gracey, M. and King, M. (2009). Indigenous health part 1: determinants and disease patterns. *Lancet 374*, 65–75.
http://www.ncbi.nlm.nih.gov/pubmed/19577695

17. Answer B

Common variable immunodeficiency (CVID) is a rare immune deficiency, characterised by low levels of serum immunoglobulin G, A and/or M with loss of antibody production (Cunningham-Rundles, 2010). The diagnosis is most commonly made in adults between the ages of 20 and 40 years, but both children and older adults can be found to have this immune defect. The range of clinical manifestations is broad, including acute and chronic infections, inflammatory and autoimmune disease, and an increased incidence of cancer and lymphoma. The respiratory tract is most commonly involved, occurring in up to three-quarters of patients, with pneumonia attributable to *Streptococcus pneumonia*, *Haemophilus influenzae*, or *Mycoplasma* spp. appearing as the most prevalent condition before diagnosis. Other severe infections, such as empyema, meningitis or osteomyelitis, are less common but are observed in all studies. The primary treatment of CVID is replacement of antibody, achieved by either an intravenous or subcutaneous route of immunoglobulin. The goal of immunoglobin therapy is to prevent infection.

Cunningham-Rundles, C. (2010). How I treat common variable immune deficiency. *Blood* 116, 7–15.
http://www.ncbi.nlm.nih.gov/pmc/articles/PMC2904582/

18. Answer E

Getting the diagnosis of anaphylaxis right is important because then efforts at secondary prevention can be made. Further episodes and deaths can be prevented by identifying the likely cause(s) and thus appropriate avoidance strategies, and immunotherapy (for insect venom allergy), as well as provision of an epinephrine (adrenaline) auto-injector and an action plan for the patient to follow if another reaction occurs.

Measurement of mast cell tryptase may be useful in cases where the diagnosis of anaphylaxis is uncertain (Brown and Stone, 2011). Importantly, tryptase is more useful in insect venom and medication-related anaphylaxis compared to food-related anaphylaxis. Peak levels occur within 1–2 h of reaction onset. Single measurement of tryptase has low sensitivity because the peak may be missed or occur within the normal range. Serial measurements (presentation, 1 h later and then on discharge) improve sensitivity by up to 75%. High tryptase levels may be due to mastocytosis and it is important to follow an elevated result with a convalescent sample to rule out this diagnosis.

Circulating human tryptases consist mainly of the mature or active β-tryptases and inactive pro-tryptases (α and β). Baseline or 'constitutive' levels of immunoreactive tryptase in serum are thought to consist of the pro-α and pro-β tryptases, whereas mature β-tryptases are released by mast cell degranulation. Any detectable β-tryptase should be diagnostic of degranulation. A specific mature β-tryptase assay is not currently available for diagnostic use and a large-scale validation of sensitivity and specificity in a clinical setting is required.

Brown, S.G. and Stone, S.F. (2011). Laboratory diagnosis of acute anaphylaxis. *Clin Exp Allergy* 41, 1660–1662.
http://www.ncbi.nlm.nih.gov/pubmed/22107141

Australasian Society of Clinical Immunology and Allergy (ASCIA)
http://www.allergy.org.au/images/stories/anaphylaxis/ASCIA_HPIP_Anaphylaxis_2013.pdf

19. Answer E

Urticaria is a very common disorder, and an aetiology cannot be found in the majority of cases. The patient described here has urticarial lesions, each of which persists for more than 24 h. Generalised urticarial lesions that persist for longer than 24 h, produce a burning sensation or are not very pruritic may be a manifestation of vasculitis. Lesions associated with rheumatic illness usually do not blanch on diascopy and may result in ecchymosis and eventually hyperpigmentation. A biopsy should be performed on any urticaria that lasts for more than 24 h, is only mildly pruritic or non-pruritic, is associated with vesicles or bullae, or does not respond to appropriate therapy (Kanani et al., 2011).

Chronic urticaria is more common in adults and affects women more frequently than men. In general, chronic urticaria is classified as either chronic autoimmune urticaria or chronic idiopathic urticaria. The diagnosis of urticaria, with or without angio-oedema, is based primarily on a thorough clinical history and physical examination. The history and physical examination should include detailed information regarding: the frequency, timing, duration and pattern of recurrence of lesions; the shape, size, site and distribution of lesions; potential triggers (e.g. food, medications, physical stimuli, infections, insect stings); response to previous therapies used; and a personal or family history of atopy.

Many conditions can easily be confused with urticaria, particularly urticarial vasculitis and systemic mastocytosis. In urticarial vasculitis, the lesions are usually painful rather than pruritic, last longer than 48 h, and leave bruises or discolouration on the skin. Systemic mastocytosis (also called systemic mast cell disease) is a rare condition that involves the internal organs, in addition to the skin. In this disorder, atypical mast cells collect in various tissues that can affect the liver, spleen, lymph nodes, bone marrow and other organs.

Kanani, A., Schellenberg, R. and Warrington, R. (2011). Urticaria and angioedema. *Allergy Asthma Clin Immunol* 7 (Suppl 1), S9.
http://www.ncbi.nlm.nih.gov/pmc/articles/PMC3245442/

20. Answer B

Despite the advances in medications and pharmacological therapy for allergic illnesses, the most effective therapeutic intervention is still removal of the offending agent or allergen from the patient's environment (Plaut and Valentine, 2005). This includes appropriate linens for mattresses and pillows, adequate cleaning and lowering the ambient humidity in the house to minimise mould spores. Pets should be removed from the house or kept in a different room at all times. Patients sensitive to pollen should try to minimise the amount of time spent outdoors during those times of the year when the specific pollen is prevalent.

Plaut, M. and Valentine, M.D. (2005). Allergic rhinitis. *N Engl J Med* 353, 1934–1944.
http://www.ncbi.nlm.nih.gov/pubmed/16267324

21. Answer A

Venom immunotherapy is indicated in individuals of all ages with severe systemic reactions to stinging insects, as well as in adults who experience generalised reactions that are limited to the skin (Moote and Kim, 2011). Severe systemic reactions to Hymenoptera (classification of insects that includes bees and wasps) venom are relatively uncommon, but can be fatal. The purpose of venom immunotherapy is to reduce the severity of the reactions and the risk of fatality, and to improve patient quality of life.

Allergen-specific immunotherapy is contraindicated in patients with medical conditions that increase the patient's risk of dying from treatment-related systemic reactions, such as those with severe or poorly controlled asthma or significant cardiovascular diseases (e.g. unstable angina, recent myocardial infarction, significant arrhythmia and uncontrolled hypertension). Immunotherapy is also contraindicated in patients using beta-blockers since these agents can amplify the severity of the reaction and make the treatment of systemic reactions more difficult.

Venom immunotherapy provides rapid protection against Hymenoptera stings. There is a residual risk of systemic reactions of approximately 5–10% after completion of venom immunotherapy; however, when reactions to stings do occur following therapy, they are typically mild. Clinical features such as a notable history of very severe reactions to a sting, systemic reactions during immunotherapy and treatment duration of less than 5 years have been associated with a greater likelihood of relapse following the discontinuation of venom immunotherapy.

Typically, allergen-specific immunotherapy consists of two phases: a build-up phase (also known as up-dosing or induction) and a maintenance phase. During the build-up phase, the patient receives weekly injections, starting with a very low dose, with gradual increases in dose over the course of 5–8 months. After this period, the patient has usually built up sufficient tolerance to the allergen such that a maintenance (therapeutic) dose has been reached. During the maintenance phase, the patient receives injections of the maintenance dose every 3–4 weeks.

Moote, A. and Kim, H. (2011). Allergen-specific immunotherapy. *Allergy Asthma Clin Immunol* 7 (Suppl 1), S5.
http://www.ncbi.nlm.nih.gov/pmc/articles/PMC3245438/

22. Answer C

Penicillin, a beta-lactam antibiotic, and its semisynthetic chemical derivatives (such as ampicillin and amoxicillin) remain first-line or acceptable alternative treatments for many infections. Penicillin can cause all four types of immunological reactions proposed by Gell and Coombs:

- Type I: IgE-mediated – asthma, urticaria, angio-oedema, anaphylaxis
- Type II: Antibody-mediated – autoimmune haemolytic anaemia, thrombocytopenia

- Type III: Immune complex-mediated – serum sickness, vasculitis
- Type IV: T-lymphocyte-mediated – contact dermatitis.

The frequency of all adverse reactions to penicillin in the general population ranges from 0.7% to 10% (Arroliga and Pien, 2003). This wide variation in the frequency of adverse reactions to penicillin exists because of a number of variables, including exposure history, route of administration, duration of treatment, elapsed time between the reaction and diagnostic skin testing or re-exposure, and nature of the initial reaction. Most of these adverse reactions are maculopapular or urticarial rashes. Severe allergic reactions to penicillin such as anaphylaxis are less common, but can be potentially life threatening. Anaphylactic reactions occur in about 0.004–0.015% of penicillin courses and are most commonly seen in adults between the ages of 20 and 50 years.

Late penicillin hypersensitivity reactions are those that occur after 72 h of drug administration. These responses have been classified as types II, III or IV depending on the immune mechanism underlying the response. Because none of these reactions is IgE dependent, skin testing has no role in the evaluation of a patient with type II, III, IV or idiopathic responses to penicillin.

The scenario described in this vignette is indicative of a type III hypersensitivity reaction. This type of hypersensitivity occurs when antigen–antibody complexes induce an inflammatory response in target tissues such as blood vessels.

Arroliga, M.E. and Pien L. (2003). Penicillin allergy: Consider trying penicillin again? *Cleveland Clin J Med* 70, 313–326.
http://www.ccjm.org/content/70/4/313.long

23. Answer E

Chronic granulomatous disease (CGD) is an X-linked disease but it can be autosomal in inheritance in some patients. It is due to a defect in the intracellular microbicidal activity of neutrophils as a result of a lack of NADPH oxidase activity. This is caused by deletions or mutations in genes that encode subunits of the leucocyte– NADPH oxidase complex. These enzymes are required for the generation of peroxides and superoxides that kill the organisms. B- and T-cell functions are usually normal. CGD is characterised by recurrent life-threatening *Staphylococcus aureus, Proteus* or *Pseudomonas* infections, hypergammaglobulinaemia, and widespread chronic granulomatous infiltration. There are extreme differences in presentation between patients, varying from a relatively mild presentation late in life to fatal septicaemia in infancy. Treatment is based on anti-microbial drugs and interferon-gamma significantly reduces the frequency of recurrent infections.

24. Answer D

Hereditary angio-oedema (HAE) is an autosomal dominant disease due to deficiency of C1 esterase inhibitor (Gompels et al., 2005). In the absence of this inhibitor, C1 esterase continues to act on C4 to generate vasoactive kinin. This leads to capillary permeability and oedema in several organs. The diagnosis is confirmed by the presence of a low serum C4 and absent or greatly reduced C1 inhibitor level or function. The presentations of HAE are referrable to three prominent sites:

- Subcutaneous tissues (face, hands, arms, legs, genitals and buttocks), which manifest as oedema
- Abdominal organs (stomach, intestines, bladder and kidneys), which may manifest as vomiting, diarrhoea or paroxysmal colicky pain and mimic a surgical emergency
- Upper airway (larynx) and tongue, which may result in life-threatening laryngeal oedema and upper airway obstruction.

Attacks usually occur at a single site, but simultaneous involvement of subcutaneous tissue, viscera and the larynx is not uncommon. Attacks can be precipitated by trauma, infection and other stimulants.

Gompels, M.M., Lock, R.J., Abinun, M., et al. (2005). C1 inhibitor deficiency: consensus document. *Clin Exp Immunol* 139, 379–394.
http://onlinelibrary.wiley.com/doi/10.1111/j.1365-2249.2005.02726.x/full

ASCIA Position Paper – Hereditary Angioedema August 2012.
http://www.allergy.org.au/images/stories/pospapers/ASCIA_HAE_Position_Paper_August_2012.pdf

25. Answer F

Patients with common variable immunodeficiency (CVID) usually present with recurrent infections caused by pyogenic bacteria (Cunningham-Rundles, 2010). The number of B cells is normal but the ability to synthesise IgG and IgA is greatly reduced. About 50% of patients with CVID also have diminished serum immunoglobulin M (IgM) levels and T-lymphocyte dysfunction. About 20% of those with CVID develop an autoimmune disease. The primary treatment of CVID is replacement of antibody, achieved by either an intravenous or subcutaneous route of immunoglobulin. The goal of immunoglobulin therapy is to prevent infection.

Cunningham-Rundles, C. (2010). How I treat common variable immune deficiency. *Blood* 116, 7–15.
http://www.ncbi.nlm.nih.gov/pmc/articles/PMC2904582/

13 Clinical pharmacology

Questions

BASIC SCIENCE

Answers can be found in the Clinical pharmacology Answers section at the end of this chapter.

1. Which one of the following does NOT affect the bioavailability of an orally administered drug?
  A. First-pass metabolism
  B. Rate of gastrointestinal tract transit
  C. Presence of other drugs in the gastrointestinal tract
  D. Dose of the drug
  E. Lipid solubility of the drug

2. Acidic drugs, such as phenytoin, bind primarily to which one of the following plasma proteins?
  A. Alpha-fetoprotein (AFP)
  B. Lipoprotein
  C. Albumin
  D. Alpha$_1$-acid glycoprotein (AAG)
  E. Gamma globulin

3. Which one of the following does NOT interact with ligand-gated ion channels?
  A. Benzodiazepines
  B. Glutamate
  C. Glycine
  D. Insulin
  E. Serotonin

4. Which one of the following drugs is 100% renally cleared and has a narrow therapeutic index?
  A. Amoxicillin
  B. Oxypurinol
  C. Ceftriaxone

Passing the FRACP Written Examination: Questions and Answers, First Edition. Jonathan Gleadle, Tuck Yong, Jordan Li, Surjit Tarafdar, and Danielle Wu.
© 2013 John Wiley & Sons, Ltd. Published 2013 by John Wiley & Sons, Ltd.

D. Lithium
E. Atenolol

5. Which pharmacodynamic factor is the most important in determining the efficacy of lincosamides?
   A. Renal clearance
   B. Concentration above the minimum inhibitory concentration
   C. Maximum plasma drug concentration after dosing
   D. Tissue penetration
   E. Time the concentration is above the minimum inhibitory concentration

6. Which one of the following drugs is most likely to inhibit the metabolism of warfarin?
   A. Oral contraceptive
   B. Omeprazole
   C. Aspirin
   D. Rifampicin
   E. Amlodipine

7. The proportion of drug reabsorbed in the renal tubule depends on the:
   A. Volume of distribution
   B. Urine pH
   C. Glomerular filtration rate
   D. Extent of drug secretion into the renal tubule
   E. Serum creatinine

8. What is the mechanism of action of ivabradine in the treatment of stable angina?
   A. Coronary artery vasodilatation
   B. Blood pressure reduction
   C. Decreased cardiac contractility
   D. Reduction in heart rate
   E. Increased myocardial efficiency

9. During a constant rate of intravenous infusion of piperacillin/tazobactam, which one of the following factors determines the steady-state drug concentration?
   A. Bioavailability
   B. Dose rate
   C. Half-life
   D. Loading dose
   E. Volume of distribution

10. A 25-year-old man presents after intentionally taking a large dose of para-cetamol (in excess of 20 g) about 6 h prior to presentation. On the Rumack–Matthew nomogram, his plasma paracetamol level places him at risk of hepatic injury. He is commenced on N-acetylcysteine infusion after initial assessment. How does N-acetylcysteine prevent hepatic injury in paracetamol overdose?

A. Inhibits glucuronidation of paracetamol

B. Enhances sulphation of paracetamol

C. Inhibits cytochrome P450 2E1

D. Reduces paracetamol absorption in the gastrointestinal tract

E. Restores hepatic glutathione

11. Which one of the following pharmacodynamic factors is important in determining the efficacy of aminoglycosides?

A. Ratio of the maximum concentration over the minimum inhibitory concentration

B. Renal clearance

C. Total exposure of the body to the drug

D. Tissue penetration

E. Time the concentration is above the minimum inhibitory concentration

Theme: Pharmacology of diuretics (for Questions 12–15)

A. Amiloride

B. Acetazolamide

C. Chlorthalidone

D. Eplerenone

E. Frusemide

F. Indapamide

G. Mannitol

H. Spironolactone

For each of the following mechanisms of action, select the diuretic that is involved.

12. Which diuretic inhibits renal potassium secretion at the distal nephron by a mineralocorticoid-independent mechanism?

13. Which is an osmotic diuretic that is freely filtered by the glomeruli and remains in the tubular lumen?

14. Which diuretic inhibits the sodium–potassium–chloride transporter in the thick ascending limb of the loop of Henle?

15. Which diuretic inhibits the apical distal convoluted tubule epithelium sodium–chloride co-transporter and decreases peripheral vascular resistance?

CLINICAL

16. A woman with Liddle syndrome presents with severe symptomatic hypokalaemia and her medical practitioner starts her on 50 mg/day of spironolactone. Four days later, repeat potassium measurement shows persistent severe hypokalaemia. The persistence in severe hypokalaemia is best explained by:

    A. Underprescribing
    B. Poor compliance
    C. Prescription writing error
    D. Inappropriate prescribing
    E. Drug–drug interaction

17. Which one of the following describes correctly the pharmacological properties of azithromycin?

    A. Azithromycin is bactericidal
    B. Half-life of azithromycin is 12 h
    C. Azithromycin is a strong cytochrome P450 enzyme, CYP3A4 inhibitor
    D. Azithromycin inhibits formation of the bacterial cell wall
    E. Azithromycin is safe for use in pregnancy

18. Which one of the following factors increases the risk of liver toxicity from isoniazid therapy?

    A. Increasing age
    B. Use of a non-steroidal anti-inflammatory drug
    C. Co-administration of ethambutol
    D. Co-administration of phenytoin
    E. Co-administration of pyridoxine

19. Which one of the following best describes the mechanism of action of caspofungin?

    A. Forms artificial pores by binding to ergosterol in fungal membranes, thereby disrupting membrane permeability
    B. Prevents the synthesis of ergosterol from lanosterol by inhibiting cytochrome P450-dependent demethylation
    C. Inhibits the synthesis of glucan in fungal cell walls
    D. Deposits in newly formed keratin and disrupts microtubule structure
    E. Inhibits ergosterol synthesis by inhibiting squalene epoxidase

20. Which one of the following types of study for an investigational new drug involves each subject receiving a sequence of all the different treatments?

    A. Cross-over study
    B. Double-blind study
    C. Head-to-head study
    D. Placebo-controlled study
    E. Single-blind study

21. Which one of the following is true of the pharmacokinetics and metabolism of paracetamol?
  A. Rate of absorption from the gastrointestinal tract is age-dependent
  B. Volume of distribution of paracetamol increases with increasing age
  C. Total paracetamol clearance is not affected by age
  D. Metabolism in the liver involves conjugation to glucuronide and sulphate metabolites
  E. Metabolism in the liver involves N-demethylation

22. A 38-year-old man with epilepsy has been taking carbamazepine for the past 6 years and his seizures are well controlled. He commenced a new medication a week ago and presents with recurrent episodes of seizures. Which one of these drugs is most likely to be responsible?
  A. Amoxicillin
  B. Fusidic acid
  C. Rifampicin
  D. Tetracycline
  E. Voriconazole

23. A 54-year-old woman presents with pancytopenia for investigation. Her medical history is significant: a 2-year history of well-controlled autoimmune hepatitis for which she is on azathioprine 75 mg daily and prednisolone 2 mg daily. She developed a second episode of acute gout attack 3 months before this presentation. She was found to be hyperuricaemic and was started on allopurinol 300 mg daily upon resolution of the acute gout. What is the most likely explanation for this patient's pancytopenia?
  A. Idiosyncratic allopurinol toxicity
  B. Autoimmune pancytopenia
  C. Bone marrow suppression
  D. Cytomegalovirus infection
  E. Folate deficiency

24. Which one of the following is true about cytochrome P450 enzymes?
  A. Cytochrome P450 enzymes are not known to exhibit polymorphism
  B. Individuals with two copies of wild-type alleles for a cytochrome P450 enzyme are poor metabolisers
  C. Individuals with two copies of variant alleles for a cytochrome P450 enzyme are normal metabolisers
  D. Individuals with multiple copies of wild-type alleles for a cytochrome P450 enzyme will have severely reduced enzyme activity
  E. Cytochrome P450 enzymes are required for corticosteroid synthesis

25. Which receptor is involved in opioid-induced dysphoria, hallucination and psychosis?
  A. Gamma-aminobutyric acid (GABA) receptor
  B. Kappa receptor

C. Mu receptor
D. Nociceptin receptor
E. Sigma receptor

Theme: Immunosuppressive agents (for Questions 26–30)
    A. Anti-thymocyte globulin
    B. Azathioprine
    C. Basiliximab
    D. Ciclosporin
    E. Leflunomide
    F. Mycophenolate mofetil
    G. Sirolimus
    H. Tacrolimus
Select the immunosuppressive agent that best fits the following descriptions.

26. Which immunosuppressive drug binds FK506-binding protein 12 (FKBP12) to form a complex that inhibits T-cell activation?

27. The use of which immunosuppressive agent is associated with cytokine-release syndrome?

28. The use of which immunosuppressive agent is associated with pneumonitis?

29. Which immunosuppressive agent binds to and blocks CD25 antigen on activated T cells?

30. Which immunosuppressive agent can be used to treat BK-related polyoma-virus nephropathy?

Answers

BASIC SCIENCE

1. Answer D

The absolute bioavailability of a drug, when administered by an extravascular route, is the fraction of the dose that reaches the systemic circulation as intact drug, which is usually less than 1. It depends on both how well the drug is absorbed and how much drug is removed by the liver before reaching the systemic circulation. There are many factors affecting the bioavailability of drugs. Physical properties of the drug (e.g. hydrophobicity and lipid solubility) and drug formulation (e.g. manufacturing methods, modified release and sustained release) will have significant impact on the bioavailability of a drug. Whether a drug is taken with or without food will also affect absorption. Other drugs taken concurrently may alter absorption and first-pass metabolism, and intestinal motility alters the dissolution of the drug and may affect the degree of chemical degradation of the drug by intestinal microflora.

In pharmacology, relative bioavailability measures the bioavailability (estimated as the area under the curve, AUC) of a formulation (A) of a certain drug when compared with another formulation (B) of the same drug, usually an established standard, or compared with administration via a different route. Therefore, relative bioavailability is one of the measures used to assess bioequivalence between two drug products. Relative bioavailability is sensitive to drug formulation.

2. Answer C

Drug–protein binding is the reversible interaction of drugs with proteins in plasma. The major drug-binding proteins in plasma are albumin, alpha$_1$-acid glycoprotein and lipoproteins.

Phenytoin binds primarily to albumin in plasma, the bound fraction being 0.9 (0.69–0.95) under normal conditions. Protein binding may be greatly reduced in the presence of the following factors:

- Hypoalbuminaemia, e.g. due to severe hepatic or renal disease
- The last trimester of pregnancy, perhaps because of dilutional hypoalbuminaemia
- Renal failure because of a reduced affinity of albumin for phenytoin
- Displacement from protein-binding sites by salicylates, sodium valproate and sulphonylureas.

Albumin binds drugs and ligands, and therefore reduces the serum concentration of these compounds. An example is serum calcium, the free (ionised) concentration of which needs to be corrected for albumin. Competitive binding of drugs may occur at the same site or at different sites (conformational changes, e.g. warfarin and diazepam). The drugs that are important for albumin binding are warfarin, digoxin, non-steroidal anti-inflammatory drugs and benzodiazepines.

3. Answer D
Ligand-gated ion channels (LGICs) are a group of transmembrane ion channels that open or close in response to the binding of a chemical messenger (a ligand), such as a neurotransmitter (Mathie, 2010). The direct link between ligand binding and opening or closing of the ion channel, which is characteristic of LGICs, is contrasted with the indirect function of metabotropic receptors, which interact with G proteins and use second messengers and activating protein kinases. LGICs are also different from voltage-gated ion channels (which open and close depending on membrane potential), and stretch-activated ion channels (which open and close depending on mechanical deformation of the cell membrane).

Neurotransmitters activate LGIC receptors, such as glutamate, *gamma*-aminobutyric acid (GABA)$_A$, purinergic P2X, nicotinic acetylcholine (ACh) and 5-hydroxytryptamine (5-HT$_3$) receptors, and represent important therapeutic targets. Diazepam, varenicline, memantine and odansetron interact with GABA, nicotinic ACh, glutamate N-methyl-D-aspartic acid (NMDA) and 5-HT$_3$ receptors, respectively. Insulin binds to the extracellular portion of the alpha subunits of the insulin receptor. This, in turn, causes a conformational change in the insulin receptor that activates the kinase domain residing on the intracellular portion of the beta subunits. The activated kinase domain autophosphorylates tyrosine residues on the C-terminus of the receptor as well as tyrosine residues in the insulin receptor substrate 1 (IRS-1) protein.

Mathie, A. (2010). Ion channels as novel therapeutic targets in the treatment of pain. *J Pharm Pharmacol* 62, 1089–1095.
http://www.ncbi.nlm.nih.gov/pubmed/20796186

4. Answer D
Lithium is 100% renally cleared and has a narrow therapeutic index. Therefore, an estimate of renal function helps to select a starting dose for treatment. Subsequent dosing should be guided by measured drug concentrations and clinical response. Oxypurinol is the metabolite of allopurinol and it is 100% renally cleared, but has an intermediate therapeutic index. An estimate of renal function as an estimate of drug clearance provides useful guidance to dosing and can be used together with clinical and biochemical (e.g. serum urate concentration) measures of effect. Amoxicillin is 100% renally cleared, but has a wide therapeutic index. Most dosing guidelines for amoxicillin do not discriminate on the basis of renal clearance, except for patients with end-stage renal disease. A small change in the concentration of drugs with narrow therapeutic indices can cause toxicity or loss of efficacy (Doogue and Polasek, 2011).

Doogue, M.P. and Polasek, T.M. (2011). Drug dosing in renal disease.
Clin Biochem Rev 32, 69–73.
http://www.ncbi.nlm.nih.gov/pmc/articles/PMC3100283/

5. Answer E

The optimal route and dose of antibiotic administration will depend on the pharmacological properties of the drug, which can be separated into three categories: concentration-dependent killing, total exposure and time-dependent killing.

The lincosamide antibiotics include clindamycin and lincomycin. This lipophilic class of antibiotics achieves wide distribution throughout the body and therapeutic concentrations in most body compartments. The time the concentration is above the minimum inhibitory concentration (T > MIC) has been determined to be the pharmacodynamic factor correlated with efficacy. Free drug levels of lincosamides should exceed the MIC of the infective pathogen for at least 40–50% of the dosing interval. Beta-lactams (penicillins, cephalosporins and carbapenems) also display this property.

Drugs such as aminoglycosides and quinolones are dependent on the maximum plasma drug concentration at the binding site that eradicates the bacteria. These drugs are concentration-dependent in their eradication of bacteria. Vancomycin is an example of a drug that is dependent on the total exposure of the body to the antibiotic [as indicated by the ratio of the area under the concentration–time curve during a 24-h time period (AUC_{0-24})] to MIC.

6. Answer B

Warfarin has a complex metabolic pathway and can be metabolised by a number of cytochrome P450 enzymes, but notably CYP2C9 (Tadros and Shakib, 2010). The anti-coagulant effects of warfarin may be exacerbated through the inhibition of its metabolism by cytochrome P450. Omeprazole, metronidazole, cimetidine and amiodarone may all do this, so the international normalised ratio (INR) should be carefully monitored in people taking these drugs. Rifampicin induces cytochrome P450 and thus reduces the anti-coagulant effects of warfarin (as may other inducers of cytochrome P450, such as some anti-convulsants). Oestrogen may reduce the anti-coagulant effect independently of cytochrome P450.

Warfarin inhibits the vitamin K-dependent synthesis of biologically active forms of the calcium-dependent clotting factors II, VII, IX and X, as well as the regulatory factors protein C and protein S. Other proteins not involved in blood clotting, e.g. matrix Gla protein, may also be affected and this may contribute to the rare association of warfarin with calciphylaxis.

Warfarin activity is determined partially by genetic factors. Polymorphisms in two genes (VKORC1 and CYP2C9) are important. VKORC1 polymorphisms explain 30% of the dose variation between patients as well as why African–Americans are on average relatively resistant to warfarin while Asians are generally more sensitive. CYP2C9 polymorphisms explain 10% of the dose variation between patients.

Tadros, R. and Shakib, S. (2010). Warfarin – indications, risks and drug interactions. *Aust Fam Physician* 39, 476–479.
http://www.racgp.org.au/download/documents/AFP/2010/July/201007tadros_warfain.pdf

7. Answer B

Renal drug clearance is the net result of filtration clearance (at the glomerulus) plus clearance by active secretion (in the proximal tubule) minus reabsorption (which occurs all along the renal tubule). Passive tubular reabsorption is determined by the magnitude of the concentration gradient (which depends on the extent of water reabsorption) and the ease with which the drug can move through the membranes of the tubular cells. Only non-ionised drugs can pass through the lipid membrane readily and the ease with which this occurs depends on the lipid solubility of the non-ionised drug. The extent to which the drug is non-ionised depends on the pH of the urine and the acid dissociation constant (pK_a) of the drug. Therefore, for drugs that are lipid soluble enough to be reabsorbed, and can ionise to an anion or a cation, renal clearance varies with the urine pH.

8. Answer D

Ivabradine, unlike the traditional anti-anginal medications, has an anti-anginal effect by reducing heart rate but without any negative effect on left ventricular function (Marquis-Gravel and Tardif, 2008). Its anti-anginal and anti-ischaemic effects are not inferior to those of the beta-blocker atenolol and calcium-channel blocker amlodipine, and are superior to placebo. It acts on a specific channel, the f channel (I_f) in the sinus node, to reduce heart rate. Myocardial oxygen demand is reduced when the heart rate is decreased and oxygen supply is improved. Current guidelines recommend beta-blockers as first-line therapy, especially in post-myocardial infarction patients. Combination with calcium-channel blockers or long-acting nitrates may be indicated if the initial therapy fails. Ivabradine is indicated in patients with chronic stable angina who are in sinus rhythm and have a contraindication or an intolerance of beta-blockers. It is also a logical addition to the treatment of such patients when symptoms are not controlled by other anti-anginal medications.

Marquis-Gravel, G. and Tardif, J.C. (2008). Ivabradine: the evidence of its therapeutic impact in angina. *Core Evid* 3, 1–12.
http://www.ncbi.nlm.nih.gov/pmc/articles/PMC2899802

9. Answer B

Continuous intravenous infusion is an alternative way of administering drugs such as β-lactam and glycopeptide antibiotics. Given as a continuous infusion, the drug accumulates to a steady-state concentration determined only by the dose rate and clearance. The maintenance dose rate to achieve a target concentration can be calculated if the clearance is known. The time to reach steady-state is determined by the half-life, usually three to five half-lives.

It is well established that β-lactam and glycopeptide antibiotics exhibit time-dependent killing. The degree of anti-microbial killing correlates well with the amount of free drug remaining above the minimum inhibitory concentration (MIC) for a given amount of time over the dosing interval. Continuous infusion is a method of administration that allows for consistent steady-state concentrations and maximises the time above an organism's MIC. Studies have shown that continuous infusion of piperacillin/tazobactam or vancomycin is a safe and effective alternative to intermittent infusion for the treatment of appropriate infections. Continuous infusion of piperacillin/tazobactam should be considered for infections due to multidrug resistant organisms when sensitivities to piperacillin/tazobactam are reported as 'intermediate'. There is insufficient evidence to support the use of meropenem or cefepime administered as a continuous infusion.

10. Answer E
The primary pathways of paracetamol metabolism are glucuronidation and sulphation to non-toxic metabolites (>90% of a therapeutic dose), while approximately 5% is metabolised by cytochrome P450 2E1 to the electrophile N-acetyl-p-benzoquinone imine (NAPQI). NAPQI is extremely toxic to the liver. Ordinarily NAPQI is rapidly detoxified by interaction with glutathione to form cysteine and mercapturic acid conjugates. If glutathione is depleted, NAPQI interacts with various macromolecules, leading to hepatocyte injury and death. Glutathione is synthesised from the amino acids cysteine, glutamate and glycine. Glutamate and glycine are present in abundance in hepatocytes, but the availability of cysteine is the rate-limiting factor in glutathione synthesis. However, cysteine is not well absorbed after oral administration. In contrast, N-acetylcysteine is readily absorbed and rapidly enters cells, where it is hydrolysed to cysteine, thus providing the limiting substrate for glutathione synthesis.

The Rumack–Matthew nomogram, first published in 1975, estimates the likelihood of hepatic injury caused by paracetamol for patients with a single ingestion at a known time. To use the nomogram, the patient's plasma paracetamol concentration and the time since ingestion are plotted. If the resulting point is above and to the right of the sloping line, hepatic injury is likely and the use of N-acetylcysteine is indicated. Patients with repeated supratherapeutic ingestion or unknown time of ingestion cannot be evaluated with the use of this nomogram (Daly et al., 2008).

Daly, F.F., Murray, L., Graudins, A., and Buckley, N.A. (2008). Guidelines for the management of paracetamol poisoning in Australia and New Zealand – explanation and elaboration. *Med J Aust* 188, 296–301.
https://www.mja.com.au/journal/2008/188/5/guidelines-management-paracetamol-poisoning-australia-and-new-zealand-explanation

11. Answer A
Aminoglycosides are bactericidal. Their primary site of action is the 30S subunit of the prokaryotic ribosome as this interrupts bacterial protein synthesis. The three commonly used parenteral agents are gentamicin, tobramycin and amikacin. Other routes of administration include inhalation through a nebuliser (tobramy-

cin), and intraperitoneal and intraventricular administration (gentamicin). Two further agents, paromomycin and neomycin, are used orally for their bowel intraluminal activity, as they are not systemically absorbed.

There are two pharmacodynamic predictors of efficacy of aminoglycosides, namely the ratio of area under the curve over 24-h dosing (AUC_{0-24}) to minimum inhibitory concentration (MIC); and the ratio of maximal concentration (C_{max}) to MIC; dosing should aim to optimise these parameters. Target AUC values of 80–100 and C_{max} of 8–10, are reasonable based on animal and human pharmacodynamic studies. In clinical practice either or both of these parameters can be used, even though they are influenced differently by host factors. The C_{max}:MIC ratio is related exclusively to the volume of distribution, whereas the AUC_{0-24}:MIC ratio is influenced by both the volume of distribution and the clearance. It has been argued that the main aim of therapy against *Pseudomonas aeruginosa* infection is achieving high peaks to provide a satisfactory C_{max}:MIC ratio, because susceptible members of this species have median MIC values of less than 2 mg/L. However, for organisms with a MIC of 2 mg/L, a high C_{max} of at least 20 mg/L (10 times the MIC of 2 mg/L) is required. In theory, constant exposure to aminoglycosides is required when they are used in synergy with beta-lactams for endocarditis, and this is the basis for the recommendation for multiple daily dosing in many guidelines. However, clinical trials have demonstrated the efficacy of single daily doses for at least some pathogens.

Avent, M.L., Rogers, B.A., Cheng, A.C., and Paterson, D.L. (2011). Current use of aminoglycosides: indications, pharmacokinetics and monitoring of toxicity. *Intern Med J* 41, 110–119.
http://www.ncbi.nlm.nih.gov/pubmed/21309997

12. Answer A

Amiloride is a potassium-sparing diuretic that inhibits renal potassium secretion at the distal nephron by a mineralocorticoid-independent mechanism. It acts on the luminal side by blocking sodium entry at the luminal membrane, thereby decreasing the transmembrane potential difference and inhibiting hydrogen ion as well as potassium excretion.

13. Answer G

Osmotic diuretics are low-molecular-weight substances that are freely filtered by the glomeruli and remain in the tubular lumen because of limited reabsorption. By virtue of their size and high concentration, they contribute notably to the osmolality of the filtrate and this is responsible for their diuretic effect. Mannitol is a non-absorbable, non-metabolisable carbohydrate and it is the most commonly used osmotic diuretic. Most of the diuretic action of mannitol is due to an inhibition of sodium and water transport in the ascending loop of Henle. It is most often used intravenously to treat cerebral oedema.

14. Answer E

Loop diuretics, such as frusemide and bumetanide, inhibit the sodium–potassium–chloride transporter in the thick ascending limb of the loop of Henle, where up to 20% of the filtered load of sodium is reabsorbed. Frusemide also has a carbonic anhydrase inhibition activity. Frusemide also increases venous capacitance and enhances the interstitial-to-intravascular fluid movement, thereby reducing pulmonary oedema and maintaining blood volume during the diuresis.

15. Answer F

Similar to thiazide diuretics, indapamide is a diluting segment diuretic that inhibits the apical distal convoluted tubule epithelium sodium–chloride co-transporter where up to 10% of the filtered load of sodium is reabsorbed. Total peripheral resistance is significantly decreased and indapamide may also exert its anti-hypertensive effect by reducing vascular reactivity to various pressor stimuli by inhibiting the net inward flow of calcium and resultant phasic contractions in vascular smooth muscle. Indapamide differs from the thiazide diuretics in that it has comparatively high lipid solubility; it is also bound to blood proteins and elastin in vascular smooth muscle and little is eliminated in the urine.

For Question 12–15

Al Badarin, F.J., Abuannadi, M.A., Lavie, C.J., and O'Keefe, J.H. (2011). Evidence-based diuretic therapy for improving cardiovascular prognosis in systemic hypertension. *Am J Cardiol* 107, 1178–1184.
http://www.ncbi.nlm.nih.gov/pubmed/21316640

CLINICAL

16. Answer D

Errors in prescribing can be divided into irrational prescribing, inappropriate prescribing, ineffective prescribing, underprescribing, overprescribing and errors in writing the prescription (Aronson, 2009). One would expect rational prescribing to be appropriate, but that is not always the case. A rational approach can result in inappropriate prescribing if it is based on missing or incorrect information. This case is an example of such.

Liddle syndrome is a disorder that affects epithelial sodium channels. Therefore, a drug that has an action via sodium channel is preferred. Although spironolactone is a potassium-sparing drug, it acts via aldosterone receptors. Hence, amiloride, which acts via the sodium channels, is more appropriate in this setting.

Ineffective prescribing is prescribing a drug that is not effective for the indication in general or for the specific patient. Underprescribing is failure to prescribe a drug that is indicated and appropriate or the use of too low a dose of an appropriate drug. Overprescribing is prescribing a drug in too high a dose (too much, too often or for too long).

Aronson (2009) suggests that nine questions should be asked before writing a prescription:

- Indication: Is there an indication for the drug?
- Effectiveness: Is the medication effective for the condition?
- Diseases: Are there important co-morbidities that could affect the response to the drug?
- Other similar drugs: Is the patient already taking another drug with the same action?
- Interactions: Are there clinically important drug–drug interactions with other drugs that the patient is taking?
- Dosage: What is the correct dosage regimen (dose, frequency, route and formulation)?
- Orders: What are the correct directions for giving the drug and are they practical?
- Period: What is the appropriate duration of therapy?
- Economic: Is the drug cost-effective?
  The mnemonic for this list is 'i.e. do I dope?'

Aronson, J.K. (2009). Medication errors: what they are, how they happen, and how to avoid them. *QJM* 102, 513–521.
http://qjmed.oxfordjournals.org/content/102/8/513.full

17. Answer E

Azithromycin is an orally administered macrolide anti-microbial drug, structurally related to erythromycin but with an enhanced albeit similar spectrum of anti-microbial activity, more favourable pharmacokinetics and pharmacodynamics, once-daily administration and improved tolerability. It is commonly used for the treatment of respiratory tract infections, sexually transmitted diseases (e.g. chlamydia), trachoma, Mycobacterium avium complex (MAC). It binds to the bacterial 50S ribosomal subunit to inhibit translocation of peptide-tRNA from the acceptor to the donor site, thereby inhibiting bacterial protein synthesis. As a macrolide antibiotic, azithromycin is bacteriostatic. Its half-life is 60 h. An important feature is azithromycin's ability to achieve high tissue concentrations, with the agent being delivered to the sites of infection by direct uptake and by targeted delivery via phagocytes. High tissue concentrations are maintained for prolonged periods because of azithromycin's long half-life, allowing once-daily dosing for 3–5 days. Among the macrolide antibiotics, azithromycin is relatively free of drug–drug interactions. Azithromycin is generally considered safe for use in pregnancy, with observational studies not reporting any enhanced risk of fetal malformations.

18. Answer A

Isoniazid-related hepatitis may present insidiously at 4–6 months after initiation of therapy. Some patients experience flu-like symptoms (Chang and Schiano, 2007). Abnormal aspartate aminotransferase (AST) and alanine aminotransferase (ALT) elevations develop in up to 20% of patients taking isoniazid, but AST activity usually subsides to normal spontaneously. Risk of liver toxicity with isoniazid increases with age, especially in females older than 60 years.

Current recommendations for isoniazid therapy include screening patients for alcohol abuse and pre-existing liver and renal disease. The presence of chronic liver disease is not an absolute contraindication, but the indications for use should be reviewed and therapy monitored more closely in such patients. All patients older than 50 years should have serial monitoring of ALT and the use of isoniazid should be reconsidered when ALT elevations persist and remain greater than 100 U/L.

Paracetamol toxicity is increased by isoniazid because it induces cytochrome P450. Isoniazid inhibits hepatic metabolism of phenytoin and increases the risk of phenytoin toxicity. Pyridoxine is given concurrently with isoniazid to prevent peripheral neuropathy. There is no known drug–drug interaction between isoniazid and non-steroidal anti-inflammatory drugs or between isoniazid and ethambutol.

Chang, C.Y. and Schiano, T.D. (2007). Review article: drug hepatotoxicity. *Aliment Pharmacol Ther* 25, 1135–1151.
http://onlinelibrary.wiley.com/doi/10.1111/j.1365-2036.2007.03307.x/full

19. Answer C

Caspofungin is a member of the echinocandin class of anti-fungal agents. It non-competitively inhibits the synthesis of fungal cell wall β(1-3)-D-glucan. Caspofungin is an effective anti-fungal agent for severe infections and is better tolerated than amphotericin B. The cell wall of yeasts includes polymers of glucose, mannose and N-acetylglucosamine, forming the polysaccharides glucan, mannan and chitin, respectively. Glucan is a microfibril composed of three helically entwined polymers of glucose and the major component of the fungal cell wall.

Caspofungin has very limited oral bioavailability and is only available for intravenous administration. It is neither a significant substrate nor a potent inhibitor of P-glycoprotein or of hepatic cytochrome enzymes. Renal clearance is minimal. Caspofungin undergoes spontaneous peptide hydrolysis and N-acetylation. Amphotericin B forms artificial pores by binding to ergosterol in fungal membranes, thereby disrupting membrane permeability. Azole anti-fungals prevent the synthesis of ergosterol from lanosterol by inhibiting cytochrome P450-dependent 14α-demethylation. Griseofulvin is only active against dermatophytes by depositing in newly formed keratin and disrupting microtubule structure. Terbinafine prevents ergosterol synthesis by inhibiting squalene epoxidase.

20. Answer A

A cross-over study (also referred to as a cross-over trial) is a longitudinal study in which subjects receive a sequence of different treatments (or exposures). While cross-over studies can be observational studies, many important cross-over studies are controlled experiments. Randomised, controlled, cross-over experiments are especially important in obtaining high-quality evidence for the effects of interventions. In a randomised clinical trial, the subjects are randomly assigned to different arms of the study and receive different treatments. When the randomised clinical trial has a repeated measures design, the same measures are collected multiple times for each subject. A cross-over clinical trial has a repeated measures design in which each patient is randomly assigned to a sequence of at least two treatments (of which one 'treatment' may be a standard treatment or a placebo).

A cross-over study has two advantages over a non-cross-over longitudinal study. First, the influence of confounding co-variates is reduced because each cross-over patient serves as their own control. In a non-cross-over study, even when randomised, different treatment groups may be unbalanced in some co-variates. In a controlled, randomised cross-over design, such imbalances are unlikely (unless co-variates were to change systematically during the study). Second, optimal cross-over designs are statistically efficient and so require fewer subjects than do non-cross-over designs.

21. Answer D

Paracetamol is a simple analgesic recommended as the drug of choice for the management of mild-to-moderate pain and in combination with opioid analgesics in severe pain. Paracetamol is rapidly and completely absorbed from the gastrointestinal tract and neither the rate nor the extent of absorption appears to be age-dependent. Decreases in volume of distribution have been associated with increasing age and female sex.

A number of studies have identified a reduction in total paracetamol clearance in older people. The major pathways of paracetamol metabolism in the liver involve conjugation to glucuronide and sulphate metabolites. The intrinsic conjugative activity of the liver may be compromised in frail older people, but the significance of these changes is unclear given the wide safety margin of paracetamol.

Nikles, C.J., Yelland, M., Del Mar, C., and Wilkinson, D. (2005). The role of paracetamol in chronic pain: an evidence-based approach. *Am J Ther* 12, 80–91.
http://www.ncbi.nlm.nih.gov/pubmed/15662295

22. Answer C

Liver enzyme inducers can interact and increase the metabolism of carbamazepine. The enzyme inducers are phenytoin, carbamazepine, phenobarbitone (barbiturates), rifampicin, alcohol and sulphonamides. Clinically important interactions resulting in reduction of therapeutic effect have been demonstrated with oral contraceptives, hormone replacement therapy, corticosteroids, thyroid hormones, theophylline, doxycycline, ciclosporin, itraconazole, disopyramide, dihydropyridines, anti-convulsants and warfarin.

23. Answer C

Allopurinol is a xanthine oxidase inhibitor that blocks the synthesis of uric acid. It is effective in decreasing flares and tophi, particularly among patients in whom target urate levels are achieved.

Allopurinol reduces the metabolism of azathioprine and increases the risk of severe bone marrow toxicity. A similar drug interaction is also present with 6-mercaptopurine (6-MP). Azathioprine and 6-MP are both inactive pro-drugs. Azathioprine is converted to 6-MP, which is then further metabolised via three different routes. The balance of enzyme activities in the metabolic pathway determines the rate of production of each metabolite. The 6-thioguanine nucleotides (6-TGNs) are responsible for the majority of the immune suppressant activity of the thiopurines, but are also associated with bone marrow suppression at high concentrations. Inhibition of xanthine oxidase by allopurinol increases 6-TGN concentration by preferential metabolism along this pathway, resulting in greater immune suppression and greater risk of pancytopenia. The 6-methylmercaptopurine nucleotides (6-MMPs) are associated with hepatotoxicity in high concentration, although other metabolites probably also contribute to hepatotoxicity.

Gearry, R.B., Day, A.S., Barclay, M.L., Leong, R.W., Sparrow, M.P. (2010). Azathioprine and allopurinol: A two-edged interaction. *J Gastroenterol Hepatol* 25, 653–655.
http://onlinelibrary.wiley.com/doi/10.1111/j.1440-1746.2010.06254.x/full

24. Answer E

Cytochrome P450 (CYP450) enzymes are essential for the production of cholesterol, steroids, prostacyclins and thromboxane A_2. These enzymes also detoxify foreign chemicals and metabolise drugs. Drug metabolism through CYP450 enzymes exhibits polymorphism that influences a patient's response to a particular drug. A specific gene encodes each CYP450 enzyme. Every person inherits one genetic allele from each parent. Alleles are referred to as 'wild-type' or 'variant', with wild-type alleles occurring most commonly in the general population. A normal metaboliser has inherited two copies of wild-type alleles. Polymorphism occurs when a variant allele replaces one or both wild-type alleles. Variant alleles usually encode a CYP450 enzyme that has reduced or no activity. Individuals with two copies of variant alleles are 'poor' metabolisers, whereas those with one wild-type and one variant allele have reduced enzyme activity. Some individuals may inherit multiple copies of wild-type alleles, which results in excess enzyme activity. CYP450 enzyme polymorphism is responsible for variations observed in drug response among people of different ethnicity (Wilkinson, 2005).

Wilkinson, G.R. (2005). Drug metabolism and variability among patients in drug response. *N Engl J Med* 352, 2211–2221.
http://www.ncbi.nlm.nih.gov/pubmed/15917386

25. Answer E

Opioid receptors are a group of G protein-coupled receptors with opioids as ligands (Trescot et al., 2008). Activation of opioid receptors results in inhibition of synaptic neurotransmission in the central nervous system (CNS) and peripheral nervous system (PNS). Opioids bind to and enhance neurotransmission at four major classes of opioid receptors. It is also recognised that several poorly defined classes of opioid receptor exist with relatively minor effects. The physiological effects of opioids are mediated principally through mu and kappa receptors in the CNS and periphery. Mu receptor effects include analgesia, euphoria, respiratory depression and miosis. Kappa receptor effects include analgesia, miosis, respiratory depression and sedation. Two other opiate receptors that mediate the effects of certain opiates include sigma and delta receptors. Sigma receptors mediate dysphoria, hallucinations and psychosis; delta receptors are located largely in the brain and their effects are not well studied. They may be responsible for psychomimetic and dysphoric effects. They are also called OP1 and DOR (delta opioid receptors). The opiate antagonists (e.g. naloxone, nalmefene and naltrexone) antagonise the effects at all four opioid receptors.

Trescot, A.M., Datta, S., Lee, M., and Hansen, H. (2008). Opioid pharmacology. *Pain Physician* 11, S133–S153.
http://www.painphysicianjournal.com/2008/march/2008;11;S133-S153.pdf

26. Answer H

Tacrolimus engages FK506-binding protein 12 (FKBP12) and forms a complex that inhibits calcineurin phosphatase and T-cell activation. Ciclosporin is a cyclic peptide initially purified from a fungus that engages cyclophilin, an intracellular protein of the immunophilin family, forming a complex that engages calcineurin. Normally, calcineurin dephosphorylates the transcription nuclear factor of activated T cells (NFATc), which moves to the nucleus of the T cell and increases the activity of genes coding for interleukin 2 and related cytokines. Tacrolimus resembles ciclosporin in that it can result in nephrotoxicity and haemolytic–uraemic syndrome, but it is less likely to cause hyperlipidaemia, hypertension and cosmetic problems. However, tacrolimus is more likely to induce post-transplantation diabetes. Dose monitoring is important to optimise the therapeutic benefit and minimise side effects. Both ciclosporin and tacrolimus are metabolised in large part by cytochrome P450 3A4 and have a wide range of drug interactions.

27. Answer A

Cytokine-release syndrome is a symptom complex associated with the use of many monoclonal antibodies and polyclonal anti-thymocyte globulin (ATG). It results from the release of cytokines from cells targeted by the antibody, as well as immune effector cells recruited to the area. Features of this syndrome include fever, chills, tachycardia, dyspnoea and hypotension. In most patients, the symptoms are mild to moderate in severity and are manageable. However, some patients may experience severe, life-threatening reactions that result from massive release of cytokines. Severe reactions occur more commonly during the first infusion. Other complications that can arise from ATG include lymphopenia, thrombocytopenia and occasional serum sickness. ATG is produced by immunising horses or rabbits with human lymphoid cells, harvesting the IgG and absorbing out toxic antibodies (e.g. those against platelets and erythrocytes). Rabbit preparations are favoured over horse preparations because of their greater potency. As an induction agent, polyclonal ATG is usually used for 3–10 days to produce profound and durable lymphopenia that lasts beyond 1 year. It is often used in highly sensitised transplant recipients and in the treatment of acute severe cellular or vascular rejection.

28. Answer G

Sirolimus engages FK506-binding protein 12 (FKBP12) to create complexes that inhibit the target of rapamycin but cannot inhibit calcineurin. Inhibition of the target of rapamycin prevents cytokine receptors from activating the cell cycle. The principal non-immune toxic effects include hyperlipidaemia, anaemia, thrombocytopenia and impaired wound healing. Other adverse effects of sirolimus include delayed recovery from acute tubular necrosis in kidney transplants, aggravation of proteinuria, mouth ulcers, skin lesions and pneumonitis. Progressive interstitial pneumonitis has been observed in transplant recipients who are taking sirolimus with an incidence of 22% in one study. Increased risk factors for pneumonitis include a late switch to sirolimus and impaired renal function. Clinical symptoms consist of dyspnoea, dry cough, fever and fatigue. In one report of 24 patients, radiographic and broncho-alveolar lavage revealed bronchiolitis obliterans-organising pneumonia (BOOP) and lymphocytic alveolitis. Complete recovery was observed in all patients within 6 months of sirolimus withdrawal. Sirolimus also has anti-neoplastic and arterial protective effects. It has been incorporated into drug-eluting coronary stents to inhibit stent stenosis.

29. Answer C
Basiliximab is a chimeric monoclonal antibody against CD25 (interleukin-2-receptor α chain), which is widely used in kidney transplantation for induction in patients who have a low-to-moderate risk of rejection. Because expression of CD25 requires T-cell activation, anti-CD25 antibody causes little depletion of T cell. Anti-CD25 antibody is moderately effective because it reduces rejection by about one-third when used with calcineurin inhibitor and has minimal side effects.

30. Answer E
Leflunomide is a prodrug whose anti-metabolite, A77 1726, has both immuno-suppressive and anti-viral activity. Although approved for treatment of rheumatoid arthritis, it has also been used in kidney transplant recipients. Leflunomide exerts its anti-viral effect on CMV by disrupting virion assembly. Its mechanism of action against BK virus is unknown.

For Questions 26–30

Halloran, P.F. (2004). Immunosuppressive drugs for kidney transplantation. *N Engl J Med* 351, 2715–2729.
http://www.ncbi.nlm.nih.gov/pubmed/15616206

14 Clinical genetics

Questions

BASIC SCIENCE

Answers can be found in the Clinical genetics Answers section at the end of this chapter.

1. Which one of the following statements is correct regarding DNA?
   A. Consists of the nucleotides adenosine, cytosine, guanine and uracil
   B. Is translated to generate messenger RNA
   C. Topoisomerase generates a new copy from a template of DNA
   D. Gene expression is increased by DNA cytosine methylation
   E. Oxidative damage by ionising radiation can lead to double-strand DNA breaks

2. Wilson disease has a frequency of 1 in 8100 in a community. What is the carrier rate?
   A. 1 in 90
   B. 1 in 15
   C. 89 in 90
   D. 1 in 45
   E. 1 in 60

3. Which one of the following statements is FALSE regarding RNA?
   A. Human immunodeficiency virus (HIV) is a single-stranded RNA virus
   B. MicroRNAs are post-transcriptional regulators that target messenger RNA transcripts (mRNAs) for repression or degradation
   C. Viruses use reverse transcriptase to generate DNA molecules from RNA
   D. Transfer RNA (tRNA) is a small RNA chain that transfers a specific amino acid to a growing polypeptide chain during translation
   E. Ribosomes are the sites of RNA synthesis

4. Which one of the following processes is involved in the inactivation of the second X chromosome (Barr body) in females?
   A. DNA hypomethylation
   B. DNA hypermethylation
   C. Increased histone acetylation

Passing the FRACP Written Examination: Questions and Answers, First Edition. Jonathan Gleadle, Tuck Yong, Jordan Li, Surjit Tarafdar, and Danielle Wu.
© 2013 John Wiley & Sons, Ltd. Published 2013 by John Wiley & Sons, Ltd.

D. Chromosomal translocation
E. Decreased expression of non-coding RNAs

5. Which one of the following describes mature messenger RNAs (mRNAs) correctly?
  A. Mature mRNAs are created by post-transcriptional processing
  B. The production of protein from mature mRNA is called transcription
  C. Mature mRNAs are generated from introns
  D. Adenine, cytosine, guanine and thymine are the nucleotide bases found in mature mRNA
  E. Mature mRNA is degraded by ribosomes

6. Which one of the following is a feature of mitochondrial DNA disorder inheritance?
  A. Paternal transmission of gene mutation
  B. Autosomal dominant inheritance
  C. Point mutation is the type of defect identified in all mitochondrial gene mutations
  D. There is a single copy of mitochondrial DNA in each cell
  E. A mitochondrial gene mutation is present only in a proportion of the cell's mitochondrial genome copies

7. Which one of the following statements about single-nucleotide polymorphisms (SNPs) is correct?
  A. SNPs occur more frequently in coding regions than non-coding regions
  B. SNPs within a coding sequence always change the amino acid sequence of the protein that is produced
  C. SNPs that are not in protein-coding regions do not affect gene expression
  D. A SNP allele occurs at the same frequency across all human populations
  E. A SNP may cause a disease with Mendelian inheritance

8. What is the pattern of inheritance in the pedigree shown below?

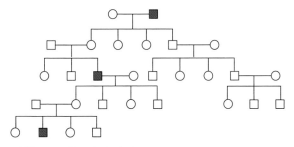

Solid figure = Affected individual
Open figure = Unaffected individual
Square = Male
Circle = Female

A. Autosomal dominant
B. Autosomal recessive
C. Autosomal dominant with sex limitation
D. X-linked dominant
E. X-linked recessive

CLINICAL

9. Which one of the following statements concerning familial adenomatous polyposis (FAP) is correct?

A. Testing of the adenomatous polyposis coli (APC) gene is cost-effective in identifying carriers of the APC gene mutation among at-risk relatives of individuals with FAP

B. First-degree relatives should be screened with DNA sequencing of p53

C. Persons with the APC gene mutation develop colorectal adenomas after the age of 30 years

D. FAP is an autosomal recessive disorder

E. Patients with an identified APC mutation should have a colonoscopy every 3 years

10. A 25-year-old Cambodian woman who is known to have mild and non-symptomatic anaemia associated with beta-thalassaemia trait presents for counselling regarding the inheritance risk for her children. She is about to marry a 28-year-old Cambodian man who has no symptoms but has recently been tested and also been found to have beta-thalassaemia trait. Which one of the following is the probability that they will have an unaffected child without either beta-thalassaemia or beta-thalassaemia trait?

A. 0.01

B. 0.1

C. 0.25

D. 0.5

E. 0.75

11. Which one of the following changes in genomic stability contributes to the development of colorectal cancer?

A. Chromosomal instability involves inactivation of genes required for repair of mismatches in DNA bases

B. Chromosomal instability causes the loss of a wild-type copy of APC, a tumour suppressor gene

C. Germline defect in mismatch-repair genes is the main explanation for familial adenomatous polyposis

D. Amplification of gene copy number occurs commonly in colorectal cancer

E. Gene rearrangement occurs commonly in colorectal cancer

12. Which one of the following statements is correct regarding Down syndrome?

A. Alzheimer-like changes in the brain develop in mid-life

B. Both males and females are infertile

C. Temporal lobe epilepsy occurs in 40% of individuals

D. The commonest chromosomal abnormality is translocation
E. Individuals have a higher risk of developing acute myeloid leukaemia but not acute lymphoblastic leukaemia

13. A 36-year-old man has parasthesiae in his hands and feet. On examination, he has diffuse cutaneous angiokeratomas, which are particularly predominant on the buttocks, upper thighs, lower abdomen and peri-umbilical area. He has a systolic murmur in the aortic area. Echocardiography reveals asymmetrical left ventricular hypertrophy and left ventricular outflow tract obstruction. What is the most likely diagnosis?
A. Fabry disease
B. Neurofibromatosis
C. Niemann–Pick disease
D. Tay–Sachs disease
E. Marfan syndrome

14. Which one of the following diseases exhibits genetic anticipation?
A. Familial hypercholesterolaemia
B. Friedreich ataxia
C. Myotonic dystrophy
D. Tuberous sclerosis
E. Von Willebrand disease

15. Which one of the following correctly describes the haemochromatosis (HFE) gene and iron-overload disease?
A. HFE gene mutation in hereditary haemochromatosis type I is inherited in an autosomal dominant manner
B. H63D mutation homozygotes are a common (>90%) finding in individuals with hereditary haemochromatosis
C. C282Y mutation homozygotes develop iron-overload disease before 30 years of age
D. HFE gene mutations can lead to impairment in the hepcidin–ferroportin axis
E. Disease penetration in homozygotes for C282Y mutation is high (>75%)

16. A 22-year-old woman is referred for review because her 50-year-old father has been diagnosed with Huntington disease. She wants to know what this means for her. What is the most appropriate information for this patient?
A. She may have inherited the gene for Huntington disease, but it usually manifests in men only
B. There is a 50% chance that she has inherited the gene for Huntington disease; if she has, she is likely to show symptoms at a younger age than her father
C. There is a 50% chance that she has inherited the gene for Huntington disease, but if she has, she is likely to develop symptoms at an older age than her father

    D. There is a 50% chance that she has inherited the gene for Huntington disease, but fewer than half of the people with the gene develop the disease

    E. She is a carrier of the gene for Huntington disease, but she is unlikely to get the disease herself unless it runs in her mother's family also

17. Which one of the following occurs in Klinefelter syndrome?

    A. Normal fertility

    B. Decreased testosterone concentrations

    C. Hirsutism

    D. Small stature

    E. Reduced gonadotrophin concentrations

18. A 23-year-old man with a family history of acute intermittent porphyria (AIP) presents with abdominal pain and constipation. What is the best initial screening test for AIP in this man?

    A. Spot urinary porphobilinogen (PBG) excretion during an attack

    B. Erythrocyte porphobilinogen deaminase (PBGD)

    C. DNA testing for ferrochelatase mutations

    D. Faecal haem levels

    E. Provocation test with phenobarbitone

19. A 39-year-old woman presents with a significant pneumothorax needing intercostal chest drain. She is known to have had epilepsy since the age of 16 years and mild cognitive impairment. She complained of left-sided loin pain and had a computed tomography (CT) abdomen which showed multiple, predominantly fat-density renal lesions suggestive of angiomyolipomas in both kidneys. An image from her previous chest CT is shown below. What is the most likely diagnosis?

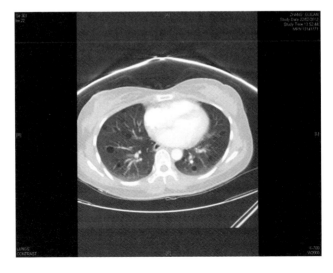

A. Von Hippel–Lindau syndrome
B. Birtt–Hogg–Dubé syndrome
C. Tuberous sclerosis
D. Prader–Willi syndrome
E. Marfan syndrome

20. Which one of the following diseases involves genomic imprinting?
A. Angelman syndrome
B. Down syndrome
C. Fragile X syndrome
D. Huntington disease
E. Motor neurone disease

21. Which one of the following conditions is often found in female patients with a 45, X karyotype?
A. Hypertrophic cardiomyopathy
B. Hyperthyroidism
C. Carcinoma
D. Spontaneous fertility
E. Sensorineural hearing loss

Theme: Genetic inheritance (for Questions 22–25)
A. Autosomal dominant
B. Autosomal recessive
C. X-linked dominant
D. X-linked recessive
E. Y-linked
F. Co-dominant
G. Mitochondrial inheritance
H. Genomic imprinting
For each of the following conditions, select the correct mode of genetic inheritance from the options above.

22. What is the pattern of inheritance for type 1 von Willebrand disease?

23. What is the pattern of inheritance for alpha-1-anti-trypsin deficiency?

24. What is the pattern of inheritance for Leber hereditary optic neuropathy?

25. What is the pattern of inheritance for Duchenne muscular dystrophy?

Answers

BASIC SCIENCE

1. Answer E

The DNA nucleotides are the purines adenine and guanine, and the pyrimidines cytosine and thymine. Uracil is the base that takes the place of thymidine in RNA. Transcription is carried out by a DNA-dependent RNA polymerase that copies the sequence of a DNA strand into RNA. Translation is the generation of protein from mRNA.

Topoisomerase is an enzyme involved in changing the amount of supercoiling of DNA and is required for many processes involving DNA, such as DNA replication and transcription. Fluoroquinolone antibiotics act by disrupting the function of bacterial topoisomerases, whilst several chemotherapeutic agents involved in cancer treatment are mammalian topoisomerase inhibitors, including topotecan and doxorubicin.

Base and histone modifications are involved in DNA gene expression, with regions that have low or no gene expression usually containing high levels of methylation of cytosine bases.

Ionising radiation can produce oxidative lesions in DNA, the most dangerous of which are double-strand breaks, as these are difficult to repair and can produce point mutations, insertions and deletions and chromosomal translocations.

2. Answer D

Wilson disease is an autosomal recessive disease. Patients with an autosomal disease are represented using 'aa' " or 'a^2' as shown in the table below. In this case, a^2 = 1/8100 (a = 1/90). The sum of frequencies of the dominant and recessive genes equals 1 (A + a = 1). As a result, A = 1 − a = (1 − 1/90) = 89/90. The carrier rate = 2 × A × a = 2 × 89/90 × 1/90. To simplify the calculation, 89/90 approximates to 1. As a result, the carrier rate equals 2 × A × a = 2 × 1 × 1/90 = 1/45.

	A	a
A	AA (normal gene)	Aa (carrier)
a	Aa (carrier)	aa (diseased)

These calculations assume that the population is at Hardy–Weinberg equilibrium and, for example, there is no survival advantage or disadvantage in utero. It can be expressed as a^2 + A^2 + 2Aa = 1

3. Answer E

HIV is a single-stranded RNA virus. Such viruses use reverse transcriptase to generate double-stranded DNA. The viral DNA is then integrated into the host chromosomal DNA, which then allows host processes, such as transcription and translation, to reproduce the virus. Reverse transcriptase enzymes are inhibited by anti-retroviral drugs such as zidovudine and tenofovir.

MicroRNAs are short (20–22 nucleotides) RNA molecules that bind to complementary sequences in the downstream region of multiple target mRNAs, usually resulting in their decreased expression or translation. Their importance in the control of gene expression is being increasingly recognised.

Transfer RNA (tRNA) is a small RNA chain of about 80 nucleotides that transfers a specific amino acid to a growing polypeptide chain at the ribosomal site of protein synthesis during translation. It has sites for amino acid attachment and an anti-codon region for codon recognition that binds to a specific sequence on the messenger RNA chain through hydrogen bonding.

Ribosomes are the sites of protein biosynthesis, the process of translating mRNA into protein. Certain antibiotics such as chloramphenicol and aminoglycosides exert their anti-bacterial effects by binding to and inhibiting bacterial ribosomes.

4. Answer B

Epigenetics is defined as heritable changes in gene expression that are not attributable to alterations in the sequence of DNA (Hamilton, 2011). The predominant epigenetic mechanisms are DNA methylation, modifications to chromatin structure, loss of imprinting and non-coding RNA. An important feature of epigenetic modifications is that they are heritable between mother and daughter cells (mitotic inheritance) and between generations (meiotic inheritance). Epigenetics is one of the explanations for how cells and organisms with identical DNA can have such dramatic phenotypic differences (such as caterpillars and butterflies).

DNA methylation is the covalent addition or subtraction of a methyl group to a cytosine nucleotide in a sequence of DNA. Hypermethylation also occurs as a normal physiological process, e.g. during inactivation of the second X chromosome (Barr body) in females (lyonisation). The inactive X chromosome (Xi) is characterised by high levels of DNA methylation, low levels of histone acetylation, low levels of histone H3 lysine-4 methylation and high levels of histone H3 lysine-9 methylation, all of which are associated with gene silencing. These processes are guided by the X-inactive specific transcript (Xist) gene, which encodes a large non-coding RNA that is responsible for mediating the specific silencing of the X chromosome from which it is transcribed. The inactive X chromosome is coated by Xist RNA, whereas the active X chromosome (Xa) is not. In addition, hypermethylation is a physiological process associated with ageing and methylation-induced transcriptional repression of repetitive DNA elements helps to prevent chromosomal instability.

Hamilton, J.P. (2011). Epigenetics: principles and practice. *Dig Dis 29*, 130–135.
http://www.karger.com/Article/FullText/323874

5. Answer A

The human genome is made up of DNA which consists of a long sequence of nucleotide bases of four types: adenine (A), cytosine (C), guanine (G) and thymine (T). RNA is similar to DNA in terms of nucleotide bases, except T is replaced by uracil (U). In certain regions of DNA, which encode proteins and are called genes, there are alternating segments called exons and introns. Exons are segments of a gene that are represented in the mature RNA product and introns are spliced out during processing. Individual exons typically include protein-coding sequences. Introns are non-coding DNA sequences that separate neighbouring exons in a gene.

RNA is transcribed from genes and then undergo post-transcriptional processing, and the resultant mature mRNA is used as the template for the translation process that results in synthesis of a protein. mRNA that has been processed and transported to the cytoplasm (i.e. mature mRNA) can then be translated by the ribosome. It is mainly through altered protein function that changes in the sequence in the DNA affect health and disease. The stability of mRNAs may be controlled by the 5′ untranslated region (UTR) and/or 3′ UTR due to varying affinity for RNA-binding proteins that can promote or inhibit RNA degradation.

6. Answer E

Mitochondria have their own chromosomes and these are passed on from a mother to all of her children, but not from the father. These chromosomes contain only 37 genes that have a high and variable number of DNA copies and very little non-coding DNA and no introns. Many different mitochondrial mutations, including point mutations, deletions and duplications, alone or in combination, can result in a variety of different disorders. Moreover, the relationship between genotype and phenotype is not straightforward, in part due to heteroplasmy, the tendency for a mitochondrial mutation to be present in only a proportion of the cell's mitochondrial genome copies.

Schapira, A.H. (2012).Mitochondrial diseases. *Lancet* 379, 1825–1834.
http://www.ncbi.nlm.nih.gov/pubmed/22482939

Koopman, W.J., Willems, J.H., and Smeitink, J.A. (2012). Monogenic mitochondrial disorders. *N Engl J Med* 366, 1132–1141.
http://www.ncbi.nlm.nih.gov/pubmed/22435372

7. Answer E

Single-nucleotide polymorphism (SNP) is a DNA sequence variation occurring when a single nucleotide – A, T, C or G – in the genome differs between paired chromosomes in human. Almost all common SNPs have only two alleles. SNPs usually occur in non-coding regions more frequently than in coding regions. SNPs within a coding sequence do not necessarily change the amino acid sequence of the protein that is produced, due to degeneracy of the genetic code. SNPs that are not in protein-coding regions may still affect gene splicing, transcription factor binding, messenger RNA degradation or the sequence of non-coding RNA. Gene expression affected by this type of SNP is referred to as an eSNP (expression SNP). A SNP may cause a Mendelian disease. For multifactorial diseases, SNPs do not usually function individually; rather, they work in coordination with other SNPs to manifest a disease condition, as has been seen in hypertension and diabetes.

Within a population, SNPs can be assigned a minor allele frequency – the lowest allele frequency at a locus that is observed in a particular population. There are variations between human populations, so a SNP allele that is common in one geographical or ethnic group may be much rarer in another. The greatest importance of detection of millions of SNPs is for comparing regions of the genome between matched cohorts with and without a disease in genome-wide association studies that lead to the identification of gene variants associated with disease.

8. Answer E

X-linked recessive inheritance is characterised by a higher incidence of the trait in males than females. The genetic trait is passed from a male through all of his daughters to, on average, half of their sons. The trait is never transmitted directly from father to son, but may be transmitted through a series of carrier females. Examples of X-linked recessive disorders include haemophilia A and B, Duchenne muscular dystrophy and X-linked agammaglobulinaemia.

CLINICAL

9. Answer A

Familial adenomatous polyposis (FAP) is an autosomal dominant disorder and one of many inherited predispositions to cancer (Foulkes, 2008; Lynch and de la Chapelle, 2003). Persons with a causative APC (adenomatous polyposis coli) gene mutation develop adenomas in the colon and rectum, starting at around 16 years; in these individuals, the number of adenomas increases to hundreds or thousands, and colorectal cancer develops at about the age of 40 years. The mean age at death is 42 years in those who go untreated. Testing for the APC gene has been shown to be cost-effective when used to identify carriers of the disease-causing APC gene mutation among at-risk relatives of individuals with FAP. Early diagnosis via pre-symptomatic testing reduces morbidity and increases life expectancy through improved surveillance and timely prophylactic colectomy.

Patients who have an APC mutation or who have one or more first-degree relatives who have FAP or an identified APC mutation (or both) are at high risk and should be screened with flexible sigmoidoscopy by the age of 12 years. Patients with colonic polyps, a verified APC germline mutation or both require annual colonoscopy. However, as the disease advances, as often occurs in the late teens and early 20s, too many colonic polyps may be present for adequate and safe colonoscopic polypectomy; when this occurs, prophylactic subtotal colectomy followed by annual endoscopy of the remaining rectum is recommended. Upper endoscopy is also necessary because of the potential for adenomas, which increase the risk of stomach cancer.

Foulkes, W.D. (2008). Inherited susceptibility to common cancers. *N Engl J Med* 359, 2143–2153.
http://www.ncbi.nlm.nih.gov/pubmed/19005198

Lynch, H.T. and de la Chapelle, A. (2003). Hereditary colorectal cancer. *N Engl J Med* 348, 919–932.
http://www.ncbi.nlm.nih.gov/pubmed/12621137

10. Answer C

Beta-thalassaemia is an autosomal recessive condition. As described in this vignette, when two partners each have the recessive gene mutation, there is classically a one in four chance of an affected offspring, two in four chance of carriers of the recessive gene and one in four chance of a normal unaffected offspring. Therefore, the probability of a normal (unaffected) child is 0.25. The probability of an offspring who is a carrier of the beta-thalassaemia trait is 0.5.

11. Answer B

The loss of genomic stability can drive the development of colorectal cancer by facilitating the acquisition of multiple tumour-associated mutations (Markowitz and Bertagnolli, 2009). In this disease, genomic instability takes several forms. The most common type of genomic instability in colorectal cancer is chromosomal instability, which causes numerous changes in chromosomal copy number and structure. Chromosomal instability is an efficient mechanism for causing the physical loss of a wild-type copy of a tumour-suppressor gene, such as adenomatous polyposis coli (APC), p53 and SMAD family member 4 (*SMAD4*), whose normal activities oppose the malignant phenotype. In colorectal cancer, there are numerous rare inactivating mutations of genes whose normal function is to maintain chromosomal stability during replication, and in the aggregate, these mutations account for most of the chromosomal instability in such tumours. In contrast to some other cancers, colorectal cancer does not commonly involve amplification of gene copy number or gene rearrangement.

In a subgroup of patients with colorectal cancer, there is inactivation of genes required for repair of base–base mismatches in DNA, collectively referred to as mismatch-repair genes. The inactivation can be inherited, as in hereditary non-polyposis colorectal cancer (HNPCC), also known as the Lynch syndrome, or acquired, as in tumours with methylation-associated silencing of a gene that encodes a DNA mismatch-repair protein. In patients with HNPCC, germline defects in mismatch-repair genes (primarily MLH1 and MSH2) confer a lifetime risk of colorectal cancer of about 80%, with cancers evident by the age of 45 years, on average. The loss of mismatch-repair function in patients with HNPCC is due not only to the mutant germline mismatch-repair gene, but also to somatic inactivation of the wild-type parental allele. Genomic instability arising from mismatch-repair deficiency dramatically accelerates the development of cancer in patients with HNPCC.

Markowitz, S.D. and Bertagnolli, M.M. (2009). Molecular basis of colorectal cancer. *N Engl J Med* 361, 2449–2460.
http://www.ncbi.nlm.nih.gov/pmc/articles/PMC2843693

12. Answer A

The major chromosomal abnormality in 95% of patients with Down syndrome (DS) is a trisomy of chromosome 21. The frequency of trisomy 21 in the population is 1 in 650–1000 live births. These cases are due to the failure of disjunction during meiosis and are associated with increased maternal age (risk of having a live birth with DS at maternal age 30 is 1 in 1000 and at maternal age 40 is 9 in 1000). The risk of recurrence in subsequent pregnancies is approximately 1%. The remaining 5% of patients with DS have either a translocation involving chromosome 21 or mosaicism.

Previously, infant mortality was high but with improved management of cardiac and gastrointestinal defects, survival into adult life is more common with a significant percentage of individuals now living beyond 50 years. Individuals with DS often have specific congenital malformations such as cardiac (up to 30%), particularly atrioventricular septal defect (AVSD), and gastrointestinal, such as duodenal stenosis or atresia, imperforate anus and Hirschsprung disease. Signs of premature ageing and Alzheimer-like changes in the brain commonly develop in the fourth or fifth decades. Senile plaques and neurofibrillary tangles are present in the brain of all individuals with DS over the age of 40 years and the triplication of the amyloid precursor protein gene may causative. There is no association between temporal lobe epilepsy and DS. Women with DS are fertile and may become pregnant. Nearly all males with DS are infertile because of impairment of spermatogenesis. The majority of individuals have a hearing loss, commonly conductive in aetiology.

The risk of developing acute lymphoblastic leukaemia is approximately 10–20 times higher in DS compared to children without DS. Transient leukaemia, also known as transient myeloproliferative disease (TMD) or transient abnormal myelopoiesis (TAM), is a form of leukaemia that almost exclusively affects newborns with DS.

13. Answer A

Fabry's disease is an X-linked lysosomal storage disorder (Zarate and Hopkin, 2008). It is the second most prevalent lysosomal storage disorder after Gaucher disease. It is caused by a deficiency of alpha-galactosidase A, which leads to accumulation of globotriaosyl ceramide (Gb3) within lysosomes in a wide variety of cells. The accumulation of Gb3 is particularly prominent in the vascular endothelium (at levels up to 460-fold higher than normal), vascular smooth muscle cells and pericytes. The deposition of glycosphingolipid in these cells may lead to vascular occlusion, ischaemia and infarction. Accumulation of Gb3 in autonomic ganglia, dorsal root ganglia, renal glomerular, tubular and interstitial cells, cardiac muscle cells, vascular smooth muscle cells, valvular fibrocytes and cardiac conduction fibres can lead to the other manifestations of the disease.

Approximately 80% of males have neurological, dermatological and cardiac manifestations by the second, third and fifth decades of life, respectively. Renal manifestations occur in approximately 50% of affected patients by the age of 35 years, and the incidence increases significantly with age. The skin lesion is known as angiokeratoma corporis diffusum.

Zarate, Y.A, and Hopkin, R.J. (2008). Fabry's disease. *Lancet* 372, 1427–1435. http://www.ncbi.nlm.nih.gov/pubmed/18940466

14. Answer C

Genetic anticipation refers to the increasing severity and earlier age of onset of certain genetic diseases in successive generations. The common molecular feature is the presence of a tract of trinucleotide repeat units that lies within or adjacent to a disease-associated gene. There is a tendency for the tract to become progressively larger by expansion at meiosis once it becomes unstable by reaching a certain threshold size. Although the trinucleotide repeat may not be harmful initially, the expansion of the tract beyond a certain size results in it becoming a pathogenic mutation. The diseases associated with genetic anticipation all have neurological symptoms. These diseases include Huntington disease, fragile X syndrome, spinocerebellar ataxia types 1, 2, 3, 6, 7, 8, 12 and 17, and myotonic dystrophy.

15. Answer D

The most common disorder of the hepcidin–ferroportin axis is haemochromatosis (HFE) gene-associated hereditary haemochromatosis (Fleming and Ponka, 2012). Nearly 10% of the white population carries the most prevalent C282Y HFE mutation. HFE gene mutation is inherited in an autosomal recessive manner with variable expressibility. Although biochemical penetrance of homozygosity for this mutation is substantial (36–76%), disease penetrance is lower; 2–38% among men and 1–10% among women. Polymorphisms in modifier genes, environmental factors or both influence the risk of overt disease. Compound heterozygotes, C282Y/H63D mutations and homozygotes for H63D mutations are rare causes of iron overload. Mutations in the HFE gene uncommonly lead to iron-overload disease before the age of 30 years.

Fleming, R.E. and Ponka, P. (2012). Iron overload in human disease. *N Engl J Med* 366, 348–359.
http://www.ncbi.nlm.nih.gov/pubmed/22276824

16. Answer B

Huntington disease is an autosomal dominant, fully penetrant, progressive and fatal neurodegenerative disease (Ross and Tabrizi, 2011). Onset of Huntington disease is typically in middle age (mean, approximately 40 years); however, the age span includes both the young and old. Disease duration, typically from diagnosis to death, is approximately 17 years. Adult-onset disease is characterised by a triad of progressive motor, cognitive and psychiatric symptoms.

Normal chromosomes possess cytosine–adenine–guanine (CAG) alleles ranging from six to 34 units. People with the adult-onset form of Huntington disease typically have 40–50 CAG repeats in the huntingtin (HTT) gene, while people with the early-onset form of the disorder tend to have more than 60 CAG repeats. Repeat expansion of 40 units or more are fully penetrant, leading to onset of overt clinical symptoms of Huntington disease. Those with repeats of 36–39 units may exhibit reduced penetrance. Each child of an affected parent has a 50% chance of inheriting the defective gene and developing the disease. The repeats show somatic and germline instability. As a result of this, there can be expansion of the CAG repeat number over successive generations. This may cause earlier disease onset and a progressive worsening of the phenotype in subsequent generations, a phenomenon termed anticipation. Anticipation is more common following paternal transmission of the disease allele.

Ross, C.A. and Tabrizi, S.J. (2011). Huntington's disease: from molecular pathogenesis to clinical treatment. *Lancet Neurol* 10, 83–98.
http://www.ncbi.nlm.nih.gov/pubmed/21163446

17. Answer B

Klinefelter syndrome is the clinical result of an additional X chromosome in males (47, XXY), although other chromosome abnormalities (such as 46, XY/47, XXY mosaicism; 48, XXXY; 49, XXXXY) account for 10–20% of cases (Blevins and Wilson, 2012). Classical clinical findings include infertility, small testes, hypergonadotropic hypogonadism (elevated luteinising hormone and follicle-stimulating hormone concentrations with low or low-to-normal testosterone concentrations), decreased facial and body hair, gynaecomastia, tall stature with eunuchoid features and psychosocial morbidity.

Estimated frequencies of clinical features of Klinefelter syndrome are:

Clinical finding	Frequency (%)
Infertility	99–100
Small testes (<4 mL)	98
Increased gonadotropin concentrations*	90–100
Decreased testosterone concentrations	79
Decreased facial hair	77
Decreased pubic hair	61
Abdominal adiposity	50
Crypto-orchidism	27–37
Gynaecomastia	50–75

*Luteinising hormone and follicle-stimulating hormone.

Klinefelter syndrome has been associated with several complications, many of which are secondary to chronic untreated hypogonadism. Early recognition of hypogonadism can lead to appropriate management and prevention of associated outcomes. Complications such as cardiovascular disease, diabetes, pulmonary embolism and peripheral vascular disease have been associated with increased mortality rates in patients with Klinefelter syndrome. In addition, early recognition of psychosocial morbidity can facilitate speech therapy and educational support, which improve scholastic performance.

If there is clinical evidence of androgen deficiency, testosterone replacement should be considered at puberty. In patients with Klinefelter syndrome, testosterone replacement therapy improves mood, muscle strength, libido, self-esteem and behavioural difficulties; increases body hair; reduces fatigue; and has been associated with improved cardiovascular outcomes and increased bone mineral density.

Blevins, C.H. and Wilson, M.E. (2012). Klinefelter's syndrome. *BMJ* 345, e7558.
http://www.ncbi.nlm.nih.gov/pubmed/23207502

18. Answer A

Testing for urinary porphobilinogen (PBG) is the screening test of choice for acute intermittent porphyria (AIP).

Porphyrias are metabolic disorders caused by enzymatic defects in the haem synthetic pathway (Puy et al., 2010). The three most common porphyrias are porphyria cutanea tarda (PCT), erythropoietic porphyria (EPP) and AIP. PCT is characterised by bullae, blisters and a variety of skin lesions on sun-exposed parts of the body, with abnormal liver enzyme levels but rarely advanced liver disease. EPP is characterised by photosensitivity, usually starting in infancy or early child-hood, and hepatobiliary manifestations, e.g. gall stones and cholestatic liver disease.

AIP is an autosomal dominant disorder resulting from partial deficiency of porphobilinogen deaminase (PBGD), which is the third enzyme in the haem bio-synthetic pathway. This leads to accumulation of δ-aminolevulinic acid (ALA) and PBG.

Most people affected with AIP are asymptomatic and symptomatic disease may skip generations. The presentation is highly variable with abdominal pain (com-monest presentation), constipation/ileus, vomiting, hypertension, tachycardia, neuropsychiatric symptoms and peripheral neuropathy. Provocations may include specific drugs, alcohol and infection, but deliberate provocation can be danger-ous. In an acute attack of porphyria, provoking agents should be stopped, infec-tion treated and hypertension, pain and electrolyte disturbances corrected. Intravenous glucose and/or hemin therapy may be required.

First-line screening is with urinary PBG when the patient is symptomatic. Eryth-rocyte PBGD activity is not a very reliable initial test, although it is used as a second-line test to confirm the diagnosis. Patients should have DNA testing to identify the underlying PBGD mutation. This establishes the diagnosis firmly and also helps identify affected family members.

Puy, H., Gouya, L., and Deybach, J.C. (2010). Porphyrias. *Lancet* 375, 924–937.
http://www.ncbi.nlm.nih.gov/pubmed/20226990

19. Answer C

The computed tomography scan shows multiple thin-walled pulmonary cysts suggestive of lymphangioleiomyomatosis. The combination of renal angiomyol-ipomas, lymphangioleiomyomatosis, cognitive impairment and epilepsy are sug-gestive of tuberous sclerosis (Crino et al., 2006).

Tuberous sclerosis a multisystem, autosomal dominant disorder resulting from mutations in one of two genes, *TSC1* (encoding hamartin) or *TSC2* (encoding tuberin). Though no single feature is diagnostic, there is usually involvement of the skin, central nervous system (CNS), kidneys and lungs.

The characteristic renal lesions are multiple angiomyolipomas, which are benign tumours composed of abnormal vessels, immature smooth-muscle cells and fat cells, but which can cause significant haemorrhages. Lungs show lymphangioleio-myomatosis, which affects women almost exclusively and is characterised by widespread cystic changes within the lung parenchyma with pneumothorax as a potential complication. The neurological manifestations include epilepsy and cognitive disability. CNS lesions may be glioneuronal hamartomas, also called cortical tubers, subependymal giant cell tumours and nodules. Characteristic skin lesions consist of hypopigmented macules (formerly known as ash-leaf spots), adenoma sebaceum, shagreen patch and ungual fibromas.

Von Hippel–Lindau (VHL) syndrome is characterised by multiple renal cysts and renal cell carcinomas of clear-cell type, haemangioblastomas in the cerebellum and retina, and phaeochromocytomas. The mutation of the VHL gene leads to uncontrolled activation of the transcription factor hypoxia-inducible factor (HIF), which is normally central to coordinating the cellular responses to hypoxia.

Birt–Hogg–Dubé syndrome is characterised by multiple pulmonary cysts, skin lesions called fibrofolliculomas, which are benign hamartomatous tumours of hair follicles, and multiple renal cell carcinomas, which are either chromophobic tumours or a hybrid of chromophobic tumours and oncocytomas.

Prader–Willi syndrome is the most common syndromic form of obesity, with most patients presenting early with features of hypothalamic and pituitary dysfunction manifested as short stature, central obesity, hypogonadism and osteoporosis.

Crino, P.B., Nathanson, K.L., and Henske, E.P. (2006). The tuberous sclerosis complex. *N Engl J Med* 355, 1345–1356.
http://www.ncbi.nlm.nih.gov/pubmed/17005952

20. Answer A

Genomic imprinting is a genetic phenomenon by which certain genes are expressed in a parent-of-origin-specific manner. It is an inheritance process independent of the classical Mendelian inheritance. Imprinted alleles are silenced such that the genes are either expressed only from the non-imprinted allele inherited from the mother or, in other instances, from the non-imprinted allele inherited from the father. Genomic imprinting is an epigenetic process that involves methylation and histone modifications in order to achieve monoallelic gene expression without altering the genetic sequence. These epigenetic marks are established in the germline and are maintained throughout all the somatic cells of an organism. Appropriate expression of imprinted genes is important for normal development, with numerous genetic diseases associated with imprinting defects, including Beckwith–Wiedemann syndrome, Silver–Russell syndrome, Angelman syndrome and Prader–Willi syndrome.

Angelman syndrome is a neuro-genetic disorder characterised by intellectual and developmental disability, sleep disturbance, seizures, jerky movements (especially hand-flapping), frequent laughter or smiling, and usually a happy demeanour.

21. Answer E

Turner syndrome is a disorder in females characterised by the absence of all or part of a normal second sex chromosome (Sybert and McCauley, 2004). This leads to physical findings that often include congenital lympho-oedema, short stature and gonadal dysgenesis. Approximately 50% of women with Turner syndrome have monosomy X (45, X). Progressive sensorineural hearing loss is a major feature of Turner syndrome in adults. In one study, 90% had sensorineural hearing loss with clinically significant loss in two-thirds.

Congenital heart disease is reported in 17–45% of patients with Turner syndrome. Coarctation of the aorta and bicuspid aortic valve are the most common malformations. Structural renal malformations, including horseshoe kidney and duplication of the collecting system, are found in up to 40% of patients. Hypothyroidism occurs in 15–20% of patients with Turner syndrome. Ophthalmologic conditions, such as strabismus, cataracts and nystagmus, also occur more commonly in Turner syndrome. Recurrent otitis media is also a major problem in childhood. Turner syndrome is also characterised by skeletal dysplasia, with short stature, mild epiphyseal dysplasia and bone alterations. There is no evidence that the neoplasia rate is higher in Turner syndrome. Spontaneous fertility is rare and is most likely in women with mosaicism. About 70% of patients with Turner syndrome have learning disabilities affecting non-verbal perceptual motor and visuospatial skills. These deficits appear to be more common among patients with 45, X karyotype. Patients with Turner syndrome have a decreased life expectancy, primarily related to complications of heart disease and diabetes. Growth hormone and oestrogen treatments may be considered (Ross et al., 2011).

Ross, J.L., Quigley, C.A., Cao, D., et al. (2011). Growth hormone plus childhood low-dose estrogen in Turner's syndrome. *N Engl J Med* 364, 1230–1242.
http://www.ncbi.nlm.nih.gov/pmc/articles/PMC3083123/

Sybert, V.P. and McCauley, E. (2004). Turner's syndrome. *N Engl J Med* 351, 1227–1238.
http://www.ncbi.nlm.nih.gov/pubmed/15371580

22. Answer A

von Willebrand disease (vWD) is due to mutations that lead to an impairment in the synthesis or function of von Willebrand factor (vWF). vWD has been classified into 3 types. Type 1 and 2 are inherited as autosomal dominant while type 3 is autosomal recessive. vWF plays an important role in primary haemostasis by binding to both platelets and endothelial components, forming an adhesive bridge between platelets and vascular subendothelial structures. It also contributes to fibrin clot formation by acting as a carrier protein for factor VIII, which has a greatly shortened half-life and abnormally low concentration unless it is bound to vWF. Although decreased levels of vWF are relatively common, only some of these cases will have bleeding symptoms. This low incidence of bleeding is due to the mild nature of the disease in many patients and to the lack of bleeding challenges.

The usual clinical manifestations of vWD are similar to those seen in platelet disorders. These include easy bruising, skin bleeding and prolonged bleeding from mucosal surfaces, such as gastrointestinal and uterine mucosal surfaces. Patients with vWD can become symptomatic at any age. A typical history in a patient with mild-to-moderate disease includes epistaxis lasting longer than 10 min in childhood, lifelong easy bruising, and bleeding with or following dental extractions or other forms of surgery. Women with vWD usually have a history of heavy menstrual bleeding. Bleeding from the gastrointestinal tract can be serious, but is less common. In patients with mild vWD, the ingestion of aspirin or non-steroidal anti-inflammatory drugs can precipitate bleeding that may not have occurred otherwise.

Rodeghiero, F., Castaman, G., and Tosetto, A. (2009). How I treat von Willebrand disease. *Blood* 114, 1158.
http://bloodjournal.hematologylibrary.org/content/114/6/1158.long

23. Answer F

Alpha-1-anti-trypsin deficiency (A1AD) is a genetic disorder that causes defective production of alpha-1-anti-trypsin (A1AT), leading to decreased A1AT activity in the blood and lungs, and deposition of excessive abnormal A1AT protein in liver cells (Silverman and Sandhaus, 2009). There are several forms and degrees of deficiency, principally depending on whether the sufferer has one or two copies of the affected gene because it is a co-dominant trait. Severe A1AT deficiency causes pan-acinar emphysema or chronic obstructive pulmonary disease in adult life in many people with the condition (especially those who smoke cigarettes), as well as various liver diseases in a minority of children and adults, and occasionally other unusual problems as well. With co-dominant inheritance, two different alleles of a gene can be expressed and determine the phenotypic characteristics of the condition.

Silverman, E.K. and Sandhaus, R.A. (2009). Clinical practice. Alpha1-antitrypsin deficiency. *N Engl J Med* 360, 2749–2757.
http://www.ncbi.nlm.nih.gov/pubmed/19553648

Stoller, J. and Aboussouan, L. (2005). Alpha1-antitrypsin deficiency. *Lancet* 365, 2225–2236.
http://www.ncbi.nlm.nih.gov/pubmed/15978931

24. Answer G

Leber hereditary optic neuropathy (LHON) is degeneration of retinal ganglion cells (RGCs) and their axons, leading to an acute or subacute loss of central vision. This disorder results from mutations in the mitochondrial DNA. Monogenic mitochondrial disorders, such as LHON, have a maternal inheritance, i.e. only females pass on mitochondrial mutations to their children and can potentially appear in every generation of a family, affecting both males and females. However, fathers do not pass these disorders to their children.

Newman, N.J. (2005). Hereditary optic neuropathies: from the mitochondria to the optic nerve. *Am J Ophthalmol* 140, 517–523.
http://www.ncbi.nlm.nih.gov/pubmed/16083845

25. Answer D

The Duchenne and Becker muscular dystrophies (DMD and BMD), as well as a third intermediate form, are caused by mutations of the dystrophin gene and are therefore named dystrophinopathies. Weakness is the principal symptom as muscle fibre degeneration is the primary pathological process. The dystrophinopathies are inherited in an X-linked recessive pattern and have varying clinical characteristics:

- DMD is associated with the most severe clinical symptoms
- BMD has a similar presentation to DMD, but typically has a later onset and a milder clinical course
- Patients with an intermediate phenotype (outliers) may be classified clinically as having either mild DMD or severe BMD.

DMD is caused by a defective gene located on the X chromosome that is responsible for the production of dystrophin. The dystrophin gene is the largest gene yet identified in humans, spanning approximately 2.3 megabases at chromosome Xp21.2. The protein product is also extremely large (427 kDa). Weakness selectively affects the proximal before the distal limb muscles, and the lower before the upper extremities. Patients are usually wheelchair bound by the age of 12 years. DMD also causes a primary dilated cardiomyopathy (DCM) and conduction abnormalities, especially intra-atrial and inter-atrial, but also involving the AV node, and a variety of arrhythmias, primarily supraventricular.

Compared with DMD, the age of onset of symptoms in those with BMD is usually later and the symptoms are milder. Patients typically remain ambulatory at least until age 15 years and commonly well into adult life. This retained strength permits the clinical distinction between BMD and DMD. Mental retardation and contractures are also not as common or severe and there is relative preservation of neck flexor muscle strength in BMD. Although muscle involvement is less severe than in DMD, cardiac involvement in BMD is often more evident. In one report, echocardiography revealed evidence of cardiac involvement in 60–70% of patients (mean age 18 years) with subclinical or benign BMD.

Ferlini, A., Neri, M., and Gualandi, F. (2013). The medical genetics of dystrophinopathies: Molecular genetic diagnosis and its impact on clinical practice. *Neuromuscul Disord* 23, 4–14.
http://www.ncbi.nlm.nih.gov/pubmed/23116935

15 General medicine, geriatric medicine and other topics

Questions

BASIC SCIENCE

Answers can be found in the General medicine, geriatric medicine and other topics Answers section at the end of this chapter.

1. Which one of the following features can be observed with vasovagal syncope?
  A. Increase in heart rate
  B. Increase in cardiac output
  C. Reduction in heart rate
  D. Increase in blood pressure
  E. Pulsus paradoxus

2. Which one of the following describes the physiological function and regulation of magnesium?
  A. Extracellular magnesium accounts for most (>90%) of the total body magnesium
  B. In muscle contraction, magnesium stimulates calcium re-uptake by the calcium-activated ATPase
  C. Magnesium is mainly absorbed in the colon by an active paracellular mechanism
  D. Renal reabsorption of magnesium occurs mainly in the proximal tubule
  E. Parathyroid hormone is a major regulator of renal reabsorption of magnesium

3. Which one of the following drugs inhibits reuptake of dopamine, norepine-phrine (noradrenaline) and serotonin at neuronal synapses?
  A. Alcohol
  B. Cocaine
  C. Lysergic acid diethylamide (LSD)
  D. Cannabis
  E. Nicotine

Passing the FRACP Written Examination: Questions and Answers, First Edition. Jonathan Gleadle, Tuck Yong, Jordan Li, Surjit Tarafdar, and Danielle Wu.
© 2013 John Wiley & Sons, Ltd. Published 2013 by John Wiley & Sons, Ltd.

4. What is the mechanism of action of ezetimibe?
   A. Modulates lipoprotein synthesis and catabolism by activating peroxisome proliferator-activated nuclear receptors
   B. Reduces cholesterol synthesis by inhibiting 3-hydroxy-3-methylglutaryl coenzyme A reductase
   C. Inhibits the transport of dietary and biliary cholesterol across the intestinal wall
   D. Increases the demand for cholesterol for bile acid synthesis
   E. Suppresses fatty acid release from adipose tissue

Theme: Monogenic forms of arterial hypertension

(for Questions 5 and 6)
   A. Hydroxysteroid dehydrogenase
   B. Sodium–chloride co-transporter
   C. Sympathetic nervous system
   D. Epithelial sodium channel
   E. Endothelin
   F. Aldosterone
   G. Angiotensin II
   H. Prostacyclin

Select the factor above that has a gene mutation contributing to the hypertensive disorder described.

5. Which of the above has a gene mutation resulting in Liddle syndrome, which is characterised by hypertension, hypokalaemia and metabolic alkalosis?

6. Which of the above has increased expression in Gordon syndrome (pseudohypoaldosteronism type IIA), which is characterised by hypertension, hyperkalaemia and metabolic acidosis?

CLINICAL

7. Which one of the following features of alcohol withdrawal usually has an onset at about 48–72 h after cessation of alcohol intake in a patient with alcohol dependence?
   A. Delirium tremens
   B. Headache
   C. Insomnia
   D. Korsakoff psychosis
   E. Tremor

8. Technetium-99m bone scan is LEAST useful in which of the following conditions?
   A. Evaluation of bone viability in avascular necrosis
   B. Evaluation of prosthetic joint for infection
   C. Evaluation of fractures difficult to assess on X-ray
   D. Evaluation of vertebral insufficiency fracture
   E. Evaluation of osteolytic lesions in multiple myeloma

9. Which one of the following statements is true about the treatment of patients with metastatic breast cancer?
   A. Bone is a rare site of metastasis of breast cancer
   B. Denosumab can reduce the incidence of pathological fracture due to metastatic breast cancer
   C. Fluoxetine is a suitable anti-depressant for patients taking tamoxifen
   D. Symptomatic hypercalcaemia should be treated with increased oral fluids and oral bisphosphonate
   E. Neuropathic pain usually responds quickly to opioid analgesics

10. A 47-year-old man presents for management of his chronic low back pain, which started 4 months ago. The pain is located in his lower back and does not radiate. The patient denies having any weakness or sensory deficits. The pain is worse when he walks or when he lifts weights and it is interfering with his work as a brick-layer. The patient's medical history and review of systems are non-contributory. He has tried over-the-counter paracetamol and ibuprofen as required but without relief. He had a magnetic resonance imaging (MRI) of his lumbosacral spine 5 years ago which showed disc protrusion at L3–4 with no signs of spinal cord compression. On physical examination, there is diffuse tenderness in his lower back, and a leg-raising test is normal. His neurological examination, including sphincter tone, is normal. How would you manage this patient?
   A. Order a lumbosacral plain X-ray
   B. Order a repeat MRI
   C. Recommend that the patient apply for a disability pension because of his chronic pain

D. Prescribe regular paracetamol up to a maximum of 4 g/day, educate the patient about low back pain and recommend physiotherapy
E. Refer to a neurosurgeon for discectomy

11. Which one of the following treatments is beneficial for producing sustainable sleep improvements in patients with chronic insomnia?
A. Temazepam
B. Zolpidem
C. Amitriptyline
D. Cognitive-behavioural therapy
E. Psychotherapy

12. A 75-year-old widow was diagnosed with Alzheimer disease 3 years ago but has remained relatively independent since. Her daughter is concerned about her driving a car. Her mini-mental state examination score is 23 out of 30. The rest of her examination did not reveal any abnormalities. What recommendation should be given to this patient?
A. A driving co-pilot is required because this practice reduces car accidents
B. An occupational therapy on-road driving test
C. Neuropsychological assessment for further evaluation
D. Suspend her driving licence
E. The patient is fit to continue driving

13. A 28-year-old man sustained bilateral femoral fractures and a fractured pelvis after a motor vehicle accident. Four days after open reduction and fixation of his fractures, he becomes acutely breathless. His chest X-ray reveals a diffuse pulmonary infiltrate bilaterally. He suddenly becomes disoriented and paranoid. Which one of the following is the most likely explanation for his acute deterioration?
A. Pulmonary embolism
B. Fat embolism syndrome
C. Aspiration pneumonia
D. Extradural haematoma
E. Subarachnoid haemorrhage

14. A 50-year-old homeless man was found collapsed in the street in winter. When the ambulance crew brought him to an Acute Medical Unit, he was unresponsive with a Glasgow Coma Score of 8 and temperature of 31°C. A 12-lead electrocardiography (ECG) was recorded on admission. Which one of the following ECG findings is consistent with his temperature reading?
A. Second-degree heart block
B. Prominent P waves
C. Short PR interval
D. J waves
E. U waves

15. A 54-year-old man has been diagnosed with motor neurone disease. While discussing the current management and future palliative care plan, you will advise:
   A. Riluzole will relieve the symptoms related to respiratory failure, but does not slow the disease progression
   B. Stem cell transplant is an effective treatment
   C. Non-invasive ventilation relieves symptoms related to respiratory failure and also prolongs survival
   D. Benzodiazepine is contraindicated because of the concern for respiratory failure
   E. Baclofen can be used to relieve fasciculations

16. Which one of the following conditions is usually NOT associated with hypomagnesaemia?
   A. Usage of aminoglycosides
   B. Primary hyperaldosteronism
   C. Hungry bone syndrome
   D. Chronic alcohol abuse
   E. Chronic kidney disease

17. A 55-year-old woman who has diabetic nephropathy and neuropathy involving her lower extremities complains of paraesthesia and chronic 'electric shock-like' pains in the feet. For the past 6 months she has been taking a combination of paracetamol and codeine. Despite this, she has persistent symptoms. Her pain has limited her ability to perform her job, which involves long periods of standing. Which one of the following is the most appropriate option for treating this patient's chronic pain?
   A. Add pregabalin as an adjuvant analgesic agent
   B. Add high-dose ibuprofen three times a day
   C. Discontinue current medications and refer to physiotherapy
   D. Substitute her current analgesic agents with celecoxib
   E. Substitute her current analgesic agents with oxycodone

18. A 27-year-old woman who is in her 20th week of gestation presents with pleuritic chest pain and dyspnoea. A spiral chest computed tomogram (CT) is performed and reveals multiple bilateral pulmonary emboli. Which one of the following is appropriate management for this patient?
   A. Patient should be started on low-molecular-weight heparin (LMWH) twice a day or once-daily regimen
   B. LMWH should not be stopped with the rupture of the membranes as the risk of venous thromboembolism is very high during this period
   C. There is no need to monitor anti-Xa level if LMWH is used
   D. LMWH can be stopped 1 week after delivery provided the patient is mobilising
   E. Direct thrombin inhibitor can be used routinely in the treatment of pregnancy-related venous thromboembolism

19. An 86-year-old resident of a long-term care facility with a history of multiple strokes is noted to have an ulcer measuring 2×2 cm over the sacrum. On examination, the wound appears to be a stage II ulcer, extending partially through the dermis but not to the fascial plane. There is minimal surrounding erythema and no apparent eschar formation or undermining. Which one of the following interventions is most likely to prevent progression and promote healing of the ulcer?
   A. Surgical debridement followed by wet-to-dry dressings
   B. Daily topical antibiotic therapy with silver sulphadiazine
   C. Dressings with povidone-iodine–soaked gauze applied daily
   D. Frequent turning and use of a low-air-loss mattress to reduce pressure under bony prominences
   E. Initiation of tube feeding to improve nutrition

20. A 35-year-old man who works in the automobile industry and had been depressed and threatening to kill himself for several days is brought to the emergency department by his wife. He is haemodynamically stable and mildly disoriented. Apart from a bicarbonate level of 13 mmol/L (22–26 mmol/L), blood tests show a normal electrolyte profile, glucose, liver function tests, coagulation and undetectable alcohol levels. Urine does not show any ketones and arterial blood gas shows a pH of 7.26 (7.35–7.45) with a raised anion gap and normal lactate level. The patient's calculated serum osmolality is 310 mOsm/kg, and his measured serum osmolality 355 mOsm/kg. What is the likely cause of this presentation?
   A. Diabetic ketoacidosis
   B. Paracetamol overdose
   C. Tricyclic anti-depressant overdose
   D. Carbon monoxide poisoning
   E. Methanol poisoning

21. Which of the following finding is most suggestive of refeeding syndrome?
   A. Hypocalcaemia
   B. Hyperkalemia
   C. Hypoglycaemia
   D. Hypophosphatemia
   E. Hypermagnesaemia

22. A 72-year-old man is admitted to hospital because of non-ST elevation myocardial infarction. He is a current smoker but is keen to quit. Which one of the following is the correct information to give this patient?
   A. Smoking cessation is most effective during hospitalisation
   B. Most current smokers are simply addicted to nicotine
   C. Low-tar cigarettes are a useful tool for smoking cessation
   D. A smoking cessation medication should be used in the first attempt to quit
   E. Varenicline achieves superior quit rates to bupropion

23. Which one of the following features of encephalopathy in thiamine (vitamin B_1) deficiency reverses most rapidly with thiamine replacement therapy?
   A. Ocular palsies
   B. Ataxia
   C. Apathy
   D. Confusion
   E. Psychosis

24. Several different approaches have been taken to allocate the scarce availability of donated solid organs. Which one of the following describes the rationale for allocation of donated allografts according to a utility-based policy?
   A. Allocates allograft according to the age of potential recipients
   B. Allocates allograft according to the likelihood of graft survival
   C. Allocates allograft according to the recipient who will have the maximum benefit
   D. Allocates allograft on a first-come, first-served basis
   E. Allocates allograft to patients at the lowest risk of death

25. A 55-year-old Aboriginal man has had multiple medical problems, which include ischaemic heart disease, hypertension, type 2 diabetes, chronic atrial fibrillation, stage 4 chronic kidney disease (CKD) due to diabetic nephropathy, diverticulosis and a seizure due to previous ischaemic stroke. He is taking warfarin. His health-care worker is concerned that he is not taking warfarin regularly. He is reluctant to have a blood test. He would like you to consider changing his warfarin to dabigatran. Which one of the following is correct about dabigatran?
   A. Dabigatran can be used in patients with stage 4 CKD provided the dose is halved
   B. Lower gastrointestinal tract bleeding is decreased with dabigatran compared with warfarin
   C. Patients with documented poor adherence to warfarin are good candidates to switch to dabigatran
   D. Dabigatran cannot be used concomitantly with anti-platelet agents in patients with ischaemic heart disease
   E. Dabigatran can interact with drugs inhibiting transporter P-glycoprotein

26. A 65-year-old life-long smoker with no prior medical history is diagnosed to have essential hypertension. Any of the following could be used as first-line therapy EXCEPT:
   A. Beta-blocker
   B. Calcium-channel blocker
   C. Angiotensin-receptor blocker
   D. Angiotensin-converting enzyme inhibitor
   E. Thiazide diuretic

27. A 42-year-old man presented with a 2-day history of decreased consciousness, nausea and vomiting. He is known to have a long-standing history of epilepsy which is well controlled. His medications included phenytoin 300 mg twice daily and sodium valproate 1500 mg twice daily. Findings on admission included a normal physical examination, electrolytes, liver function tests and full blood count. Serum ammonia level is 240 μmol/L (reference range: <50 μmol/L). What is the most likely cause for this presentation?

A. Non-convulsive status epilepticus
B. Valproate-induced hyperammonemic encephalopathy
C. Phenytoin-induced hepatic failure
D. Acute alcoholic hepatitis
E. Urea cycle disorder

28. A 78-year-old man is brought to the Acute Medical Unit from a high-level residential care facility for evaluation after a fall. He has a history of hypertension, benign prostatic hypertrophy and Parkinson disease. His medications include prazosin, hydrochlorothiazide, aspirin, carbidopa–levodopa and temazepam. On physical examination, the patient appears frail; he has an unsteady shuffling gait and uses a walking stick for support. Which of the following statements regarding falls in nursing home residents receiving long-term care is true?

A. There is a consistent association between falling and the use of psychotropic medications
B. Widespread use of physical restraints has been shown to reduce the rate of falls in long-term care facilities
C. Community-dwelling elderly are more prone to falling than those living in residential care facilities
D. Hip protectors are the most effective way of preventing falls in elderly people living in residential care facilities
E. Patients who have a fear of falling after previous falls have a reduced rate of falls in the long-term

29. A 75-year-old man who is a retired fireman is referred to a memory clinic by his general practitioner. He has been noted to have increasing forgetfulness in the past 2 years by his wife. His physical examination is normal but he has difficulties recalling and doing sequential subtraction. He scored 24 out of 30 on the Mini-Mental State Examination. Laboratory investigations and magnetic resonance imaging of the brain were all normal. What treatment should be initiated?

A. Vitamin E
B. Sertraline
C. Risperidone
D. Donepezil
E. Memantine

30. A 45-year-old man presents with stage 3 chronic kidney disease (creatinine 145 μmol/L; reference range: 80–120 μmol/L), a painful peripheral neuropathy and left ventricular hypertrophy on echocardiography. Which one of the following inherited disorders is the most plausible cause?
  A. Fabry disease
  B. Autosomal dominant polycystic kidney disease
  C. Autosomal recessive polycystic kidney disease
  D. Familial hypertrophic cardiomyopathy
  E. Alport syndrome

Theme: Secondary hypertension (for Questions 31–34)
  A. Autosomal dominant polycystic kidney disease
  B. Acromegaly
  C. Coarctation of the aorta
  D. Cushing syndrome
  E. Primary hyperaldosteronism
  F. Phaeochromocytoma
  G. Renal artery stenosis
  H. Systemic sclerosis

For each of the following scenarios, select the most likely diagnosis from the options above.

31. A 38-year-old man presents with recurrent episodes of panic attacks. On various occasions, his blood pressure has been measured to be high with systolic measurements in excess of 210 mmHg when he has these attacks. Focused questioning reveals he is very anxious that this may be cancer as his family have a history of 'renal and pancreatic growths'. Which diagnosis should be evaluated for?

32. A 35-year-old woman presents to your clinic with a history of headaches, weakness, fatigue and polyuria. Her blood pressure is 170/94 mm Hg. The results of laboratory tests are given below. Which is the most likely diagnosis?

	Value	Reference range
Arterial pH	7.50	7.35–7.45
Sodium (mmol/L)	146	137–145
Potassium (mmol/L)	2.7	3.2–4.5
Bicarbonate (mmol/L)	37	26–35
Creatinine (μmol/L)	97	50–100
C-reactive protein (mg/L)	2.1	<10
Plasma renin (μIU/mL)	2.1	7.0–50.0

33. A 48-year-old woman presents with headache, blurred vision and palpitations. She has been having more frequent headaches that are associated with blurring of her vision. Her past medical history is unremarkable. Her family history includes a mother who died suddenly at 35 years from a cerebral haemorrhage and her maternal grandfather died from renal failure. Routine observations record a blood pressure reading of 168/100 mmHg with a pulse of 115 beats/min. The results of laboratory investigations are shown below. Which is the most likely diagnosis?

	Value	Reference range
Arterial pH	7.35	7.35–7.45
Sodium (mmol/L)	144	137–145
Potassium (mmol/L)	3.1	3.2–4.5
Bicarbonate (mmol/L)	18	26–35
Creatinine (μmol/L)	278	50–100
C-reactive protein (mg/L)	8	<10
Plasma renin (μIU/mL)	37	7.0–50.0

34. A 57-year-old woman presents with sudden severe breathlessness. She was diagnosed with hypertension about a year before this presentation. Her blood pressure remains poorly controlled despite compliance with a combination of hydrochlorothiazide, amlodipine, perindopril and metoprolol. Her other medical problems include hyperlipidaemia and type 2 diabetes. She denies having headaches, palpitations or chest pain. Her blood pressure is 200/100 mmHg. The results of laboratory investigations and chest X-ray are shown below. What is the most likely diagnosis?

	Value	Reference range
Arterial pH	7.25	7.35–7.45
PaO$_2$ (on 6 L/min of oxygen) (mmHg)	63	>80
Sodium (mmol/L)	132	137–145
Potassium (mmol/L)	5.4	3.2–4.5
Bicarbonate (mmol/L)	18	26–35
Creatinine (μmol/L)	137	50–100
C-reactive protein (mg/L)	22	<10
Plasma renin (μIU/mL)	57.0	7.0–50.0

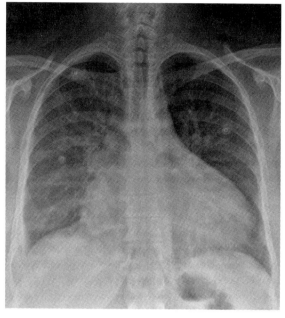

Chest X-Ray

Answers

BASIC SCIENCE

1. Answer C

Vasovagal syncope can follow prolonged standing, standing quickly or other upsetting and unpleasant stimuli (Sutton et al., 2012). Vasovagal syncope involves a massive parasympathetic response, associated with pooling of blood in the peripheries and leading to reduced cerebral perfusion. The patient generally has cold, clammy, pale skin but blood is pooled in deeper vasodilated muscle vessels. Mechanoreceptors in the left ventricle are not only innervated by stretch but also by vigorous and forceful systolic contraction. In patients with vasovagal syncope, overzealous left ventricular contraction occurs in response to reduced venous return. Hence, the afferent signals from the left ventricle override the baroreceptor responses, leading to an inappropriate decrease in sympathetic tone and an increase in parasympathetic (vagal) tone. The peripheral pulses are weak and a reflex vagal bradycardia is accompanied by a reduced cardiac output and fall in blood pressure. In distinction to most forms of shock, the heart rate in vasovagal syncope decreases rather than increases. This can be a helpful sign to distinguish vasovagal syncope from other more serious causes.

Sutton, R., Brignole, M., and Benditt, D.G. (2012). Key challenges in the current management of syncope. *Nat Rev Cardiol 9*, 590–598.
http://www.ncbi.nlm.nih.gov/pubmed/22805641

2. Answer B

Magnesium is integral to the function of adenosine triphosphate (ATP) and plays a role in many enzymatic reactions and transport processes, as well as the synthesis of protein, DNA and RNA. About 99% of total body magnesium is intracellular and located in bone, muscles and non-muscular soft tissue. Extracellular magnesium is primarily found in serum and red blood cells (Jahnen-Dechent and Ketteler, 2012).

In muscle contraction, magnesium stimulates calcium reuptake by the calcium-activated ATPase of the sarcoplasmic reticulum. Magnesium homeostasis is maintained by the intestine, bone and kidneys. Magnesium is mainly absorbed in the small intestine by a passive paracellular mechanism, which is driven by an electrochemical gradient and solvent. Intestinal absorption of magnesium is dependent on magnesium status rather than the intake.

The kidneys are an important regulator of magnesium because its concentration is mainly controlled by excretion in urine. Of the filtered load, about 95% is immediately reabsorbed and only 3–5% is excreted in the urine. The major reabsorption site is the thick ascending limb of the loop of Henle where 60–70% of magnesium is reabsorbed.

Jahnen-Dechent, W. and Ketteler, M. (2012). Magnesium basics. *Clin Kidney J* 5 (Suppl 1), i3–i14.
http://ckj.oxfordjournals.org/content/5/Suppl_1/i3.full

3. Answer B

Cocaine acts by blocking the reuptake of three neurotransmitters – dopamine, norepinephrine (noradrenaline) and serotonin. By binding to the transporters that normally remove the excess of these neurotransmitters from the synaptic gap, cocaine prevents them from being reabsorbed by the neurones that released them and thus increases their concentration in the synapses. The group of neurones thus modified produces the euphoria (from dopamine), feelings of confidence (from serotonin) and energy (from norepinephrine) typically experienced by people who take cocaine.

4. Answer C

Ezetimibe reduces absorption of dietary and biliary cholesterol by inhibiting its transport across the intestinal wall. This leads to an upregulation of low-density lipoprotein (LDL) receptors on the surface of cells and an increased LDL–cholesterol uptake into cells, thus decreasing levels of LDL in the blood plasma, which contributes to atherosclerosis and cardiovascular events.

Statins competitively inhibit 3-hydroxy-3-methylglutaryl co-enzyme A (HMG-CoA) reductase (a rate-limiting enzyme in cholesterol synthesis). Statins increase hepatic cholesterol uptake from blood, reduce concentrations of total cholesterol, LDL and triglyceride (modest), and produce a small increase in high-density lipoprotein (HDL) concentrations.

Fibrates activate peroxisome proliferator-activated nuclear receptors and modulate lipoprotein synthesis and catabolism. They reduce plasma triglyceride, moderately increase HDL and have a variable effect on LDL concentrations.

Bile acid-binding resins bind bile acids in intestinal lumen, preventing reabsorption and increasing bile acid excretion in the faeces. Increased demand for cholesterol for bile acid synthesis results in an increase in LDL uptake and removal from plasma.

Nicotinic acid probably suppresses fatty acid release from peripheral tissue, especially adipose tissue. In doses of greater than 1 g daily, nicotinic acid reduces LDL and triglycerides, increases HDL and lowers potentially atherogenic lipoprotein.

5. Answer D

Liddle syndrome is characterised by hypokalaemia, metabolic acidosis, low renin activity and low aldosterone levels. It is caused by an autosomal dominant gain-of-function mutation in the epithelial sodium channel (ENaC) expressed at the apical surface of cells of the collecting duct. Serum levels of potassium and bicarbonate may remain normal in this group of patients if salt intake is limited.

Hypokalaemia and metabolic alkalosis only manifest after oral sodium intake increases.

6. Answer B

Gordon syndrome or pseudohypoaldosteronism type IIA is an autosomal dominant disorder characterised by hyperkalaemia, metabolic acidosis, low plasma renin activity and normal aldosterone levels. The normal plasma aldosterone level is a remarkable feature as hyperkalaemia should stimulate aldosterone secretion. All the abnormalities of Gordon syndrome are corrected after administration of a thiazide diuretic. Genetic studies indicate that a mutation in WNK4, a kinase that regulates the activity of the thiazide-sensitive sodium–chloride co-transporter (NCCT), leads to increased expression of the NCCT and thus increased sodium absorption. These monogenic inherited forms of hypertension demonstrate a number of renal mechanisms involved in arterial hypertension.

Renal mechanisms involved in arterial hypertension include:

- Reduced glomerular filtration rate
- Impaired renal tubular sodium handling
- Reduced nephron mass
- Activation of the sympathetic nervous system
- Activation of the renin–angiotensin–aldosterone system
- Endothelin and prostaglandin release.

CLINICAL

7. Answer A

Chronic alcohol ingestion enhances the effect of gamma-aminobutyric acid (GABA) on brain neuroreceptors, resulting in decreased brain excitability (Kosten and O'Connor, 2003; Welch, 2011). With abrupt cessation of alcohol, brain hyperexcitability results in symptoms of withdrawal. Early symptoms of withdrawal include tremor, insomnia, anxiety, palpitations, sweating, anxiety, agitation, nausea and vomiting. Approximately 24 h after alcohol withdrawal, generalised seizures may develop but these can occur as early as 2 h after cessation of alcohol. Alcohol withdrawal seizures are more common in those with multiple prior alcohol withdrawal episodes. At 48–72 h following withdrawal, hallucinations, tachycardia, low-grade fever, delirium tremens and agitation typically occur and these symptoms peak at 5 days. Delirium tremens is characterised by fluctuating disturbance of consciousness, changes in cognition, exacerbation of autonomic symptoms (sweating, nausea, palpitations and tremor), fear or terror, and may include hallucinations, delusions, seizures, cardiac arrhythmias and even circulatory collapse. Korsakoff is an amnesic syndrome with impaired recent memory and relatively intact intellectual function and is seen in patients with chronic alcohol abuse. Patients may confabulate to fill gaps in their memory. In many patients there is overlap with Wernicke encephalopathy.

 Kosten, T.R. and O'Connor, P.G. (2003). Management of drug and alcohol withdrawal. *N Engl J Med* 348, 1786–1795.
http://www.ncbi.nlm.nih.gov/pubmed/12724485
http://www.nejm.org/doi/full/10.1056/NEJMra020617

 Welch, K.A. (2011). Neurological complications of alcohol and misuse of drugs. *Pract Neurol* 11, 206–219.
http://www.ncbi.nlm.nih.gov/pubmed/21746706

8. Answer E

Bone scan provides a sensitive, non-invasive modality for diagnosing a number of skeletal conditions (Lee et al., 2012). It uses technetium-99m-labelled bisphosphonates [e.g. technetium (^{99m}Tc) medronic acid]. Like their therapeutic counterparts, these radiolabelled bisphosphonates bind to hydroxyapatite at sites of active bone formation (osteogenesis). Osteogenesis is a non-specific response of bone to a range of stimuli, such as physiological growth/turnover, mechanical stress or injury, fractures, infection and involvement by tumour.

Bone scan is indicated in the following situations:

- Diagnosis and follow-up of metastatic cancer
- To differentiate between soft-tissue infection and osteomyelitis
- To evaluate fractures difficult to assess on X-ray, especially stress fracture and fractures of complex structures
- To evaluate prosthetic joints for infection, loosening or fracture

- To determine a bone biopsy site
- The evaluation of bone pain when X-ray is normal.

Bone scan has low sensitivity for tumours that are confined to the marrow, such as myeloma, and those that are predominantly osteolytic with little osteogenic reaction, such as metastasis from renal cell carcinoma. Bone scan is also not helpful for the diagnosis of osteoporosis.

 Lee, J.C., Hennessy, A.D. and Khafagi, F.A. (2012). Bone scans. *Aust Fam Physician* 41, 689–692.
http://www.racgp.org.au/afp/2012/september/bone-scans/

9. Answer B

Bone is among the most common sites of breast cancer metastasis, and metastasis can result in pain, hypercalcaemia, pathological fracture, loss of mobility and spinal cord compression (Irvin et al., 2011). Patients with symptomatic hypercalcaemia of malignancy or severe hypercalcaemia usually require immediate treatment with intravenous hydration with isotonic saline and intravenous bisphosphonates. Pain caused by bone metastasis should be treated as necessary with non-steroidal anti-inflammatory drugs, opioid and non-opioid analgesics, corticosteroids, adjuvant agents, interventional procedures, local radiation therapy and surgery. Spinal cord compression (manifesting as leg weakness) is an emergency that requires prompt neurosurgical and radiation oncology consultation, and the use of corticosteroids, usually in the form of intravenous dexamethasone.

Denosumab, a monoclonal antibody to receptor activator of nuclear factor κ-B ligand, is effective for prolonging the time to skeletal-related events and inhibiting the onset of pain via the suppression of osteoclast activation. Denosumab has been shown to have a greater effect compared with zoledronic acid in patients with breast or prostate cancer.

For those with advanced breast cancer, mood disorders, such as major depression, and anxiety disorders, are common. Anti-depressants and anxiolytics can be effective, but monitoring for drug interactions is essential. Women taking tamoxifen for breast cancer should avoid taking cytochrome P450 (CYP450) 2D6 strong inhibitors, such as fluoxetine, paroxetine and bupropion. Tamoxifen metabolism is complex, but it is known that CYP2D6 is necessary to form its two most important active metabolites.

For neuropathic pain related to metastases, adjuvant analgesics such as anti-depressants (e.g. amitriptyline, imipramine, duloxetine or venlafaxine) and anti-convulsants (i.e. gabapentin or pregabalin) are first-line therapies in conjunction with opioids, with the recommendation to start with a low dose and increase every 3–14 days as tolerated.

 Irvin, W., Jr., Muss, H.B., and Mayer, D.K. (2011). Symptom management in metastatic breast cancer. *Oncologist* 16, 1203–1214.
http://theoncologist.alphamedpress.org/content/16/9/1203.long

10. Answer D

Non-specific low back pain is a major health problem (Balague et al., 2012). Non-specific low back pain is defined as low back pain not attributable to a recognisable, known specific pathology, such as infection, tumour, fracture, structural deformity, inflammatory disorder, radicular syndrome or cauda equina syndrome. A herniated lumbar disc should be considered in patients with back pain who have symptoms of radiculopathy, as suggested by pain radiating down the leg with symptoms reproduced by straight-leg raising. Magnetic resonance imaging (MRI) may be necessary to confirm a herniated disc, but should be interpreted with caution, because many asymptomatic persons have disc abnormalities. This patient has no signs of radiculopathy. Also, the MRI reports a bulging disc with no signs of compression: a finding that is frequently seen in healthy persons. Surgery would be considered if there were signs of radiculopathy and the MRI showed a herniated disc with evidence of spinal or nerve root compression; however, this is not the situation in this case. A repeat MRI is not indicated, because it is unlikely that a herniated disc is the cause of this patient's symptoms.

The management of chronic back pain in this patient should include physiotherapy and an exercise programme. Regular paracetamol initially and judicious use of non-steroidal anti-inflammatory drugs (NSAIDs) may improve patient function and outcome. Anti-depressants are recommended as second-line treatment for patients with persistent low back pain in some guidelines as they have shown a small-to-moderate benefit. The place for surgery in chronic non-specific low back pain is very limited (if any) and its overuse has been criticised.

Balague, F., Mannion, A.F., Pellise, F., and Cedraschi, C. (2012). Non-specific low back pain. *Lancet* 379, 482–491.
http://www.ncbi.nlm.nih.gov/pubmed/21982256

11. Answer D

Insomnia is a prevalent complaint in clinical practice that can present independently or co-morbidly with other medical or psychiatric disorders (Morin and Benca, 2012). Of the different therapeutic options available, benzodiazepine and cognitive-behavioural therapy (CBT) are supported by the best evidence. Benzodiazepines are readily available and effective in the short-term management of insomnia, but evidence of long-term efficacy is scarce and most hypnotic drugs are associated with potential adverse effects. CBT is an effective alternative for chronic insomnia. The most common approach includes a behavioural (stimulus control, sleep restriction, relaxation) component combined with a cognitive and an educational (sleep hygiene) component. The objective of CBT is to change factors that perpetuate insomnia, including behavioural factors (poor sleep habits, irregular sleep schedules), psychological factors (unrealistic expectations, worry, unhelpful beliefs), and physiological factors (mental and somatic tension, hyperarousal). The main indications for CBT are persistent insomnia, primary or co-morbid, and insomnia in young and older adults. Caution is advised for use of sleep restriction, which could produce daytime sleepiness or exacerbate mania in a bipolar patient.

Morin, C.M. and Benca, R. (2012). Chronic insomnia. *Lancet* 379, 1129–1141.
http://www.ncbi.nlm.nih.gov/pubmed/22265700

12. Answer B

Some people with mild dementia may drive safely. Therefore, it is unreasonable to suspend a patient's licence based solely on a diagnosis of mild dementia. Regular review (at least every 6 months) of safe driving capacity is required in patients who retain a driving licence in early dementia.

A driving co-pilot is not a recognised safe practice for reducing safety risk in dementia. An occupational therapy on-road driving test is accepted as a 'gold standard' assessment. Neuropsychological results generally do not sufficiently or consistently correlate with on-road driving performance.

Australian and New Zealand Society for Geriatric Medicine. Position statement number 11: Driving and dementia. Revised 2009.
http://www.anzsgm.org/documents/PS11DrivingandDementiaapproved6Sep09.pdf

13. Answer B

The most likely explanation for this man's change in clinical state is fat embolism syndrome (Akhtar, 2009). Minute globules of fat can often be demonstrated in the circulation following fractures of long bones which have fatty marrows. Less commonly, it is also associated with extensive burns, rapid decompression syndrome, cardiopulmonary bypass, organ transplantations and neoplasms. Some features are reminiscent of those that occur in atherosclerotic or cholesterol emboli.

Characteristic clinical features include the sudden onset of fever, tachycardia, respiratory distress, delirium, restlessness, stupor and, most seriously, coma. It usually develops in the 12–72-h period or more after the injury. Focal or generalised seizures, aphasia and hemiparesis in association with more severe disturbances of consciousness may develop. Hypoxaemia is very common and an evolving anaemia and thrombocytopenia may occur. Fine petechiae may be observed in the conjunctiva, retina or axillary folds. The most common findings on computed tomography of the head are diffuse oedema, small infarcts after a week and cerebral atrophy later. Treatment includes supplementary oxygen, supportive care, corticosteroids and haloperidol for disruptive behaviour. Restoration of normal arterial oxygen levels may not relieve the central nervous system abnormalities, which usually resolve a day or two after the pulmonary manifestations. Mortality can be as high as 40% and as many as 25% of patients have irreversible neurological deficits.

Akhtar, S. (2009). Fat embolism. *Anesthesiol Clin* 27, 533–550.
http://www.ncbi.nlm.nih.gov/pubmed/19825491

14. Answer D

The most characteristic and recognisable electrocardiography feature of hypothermia is the J wave (Aslam et al., 2006). This is the convex positive deflection at the junction of the QRS complex and the early part of the ST segment. The pathophysiology of the J wave is not well understood, but it is theorised that the hypothermic state causes an increased repolarisation response in phase 1 of the epicardial action potential due to effects on voltage-gated potassium channels. It also has been suggested to be the result of anoxia, a response to injury and delayed ventricular depolarisation. J waves are seen in 80% of hypothermic patients. They are not, however, considered pathognomonic as they have also been reported in normothermic patients. They may also be seen in some patients with cerebral injuries and in others with myocardial ischaemia.

The other ECG findings in hypothermia may include absent P waves, PR interval prolongation and prolonged QRS complex and QT interval. ECG features are reversible with rewarming, but ventricular and atrial fibrillation can occur.

Aslam, A.F., Aslam, A.K., Vasavada, B.C., and Khan, I.A. (2006). Hypothermia: evaluation, electrocardiographic manifestations, and management. *Am J Med* 119, 297–301.
http://www.ncbi.nlm.nih.gov/pubmed/16564768

15. Answer C

Motor neurone disease (MND) is a progressive neurodegenerative disease involving both upper and lower motor neurones (Zoing and Kiernan, 2011). It is characterised by motor system failure due to the death of neurones responsible for all voluntary movements, leading to limb paralysis, weakness of the muscles of speech and swallowing, and ultimately respiratory failure. MND usually strikes in the fifth to sixth decades, and it has a short trajectory from diagnosis to death with an average life expectancy of less than 3 years.

Riluzole, an inhibitor of glutamate release, has a modest effect in MND, increasing survival by 3–6 months. A recent advance in the treatment of MND has been the discovery of the benefits of non-invasive ventilatory support, which may relieve symptoms related to respiratory insufficiency, prolong survival by up to 12 months and improve quality of life. Stem cell transplant is not an established treatment for MND. A short-acting benzodiazepine is used in relieving dyspnoea on exertion, whilst a long-acting benzodiazepine can be used in dyspnoea at rest. Baclofen is usually used to relieve muscle spasm/spasticity. Carbamazepine and gabapentin is helpful in relieving fasciculations.

Zoing, M. and Kiernan, M. (2011). Motor neurone disease – caring for the patient in general practice. *Aust Fam Physician* 40, 962–966.
http://www.racgp.org.au/afp/2011/december/motor-neurone-disease/

16. Answer E

Hypomagnesaemia is common in hospitalised patients with a prevalence of 9–12%. Many nephrotoxic medications, such as aminoglycosides, cisplatin, tacrolimus and ciclosporin, can cause urinary magnesium wasting. Persistent mineralocorticoid excess is also associated with hypomagnesaemia. The ascending limb of the loop of Henle is the primary site of tubular magnesium reabsorption. Inhibition of sodium transport in this segment during aldosterone escape may be associated with a parallel decline in magnesium reabsorption. Hypomagnesaemia can occur as part of the 'hungry bone' syndrome in which there is increased magnesium uptake by renewing bone following parathyroidectomy for hyperparathyroidism. Hypomagnesaemia is common in alcoholic patients. Alcohol can cause renal tubular dysfunction, leading to excessive urinary excretion of magnesium. Because magnesium is predominately excreted by the kidney, chronic renal failure is usually associated with hypermagnesaemia, rather than hypomagnesaemia.

17. Answer A

Neuropathic pain is common in patients with diabetic neuropathy and in those who have had shingles (post-herpetic neuralgia) (Turk et al., 2011). Several studies have demonstrated the efficacy of tricyclic anti-depressants, carbamazepine and gabapentin in the treatment of neuropathic pain related to these conditions. Carbamazepine was one of the first anti-convulsant drugs to be tested in neuropathic pain, but recent reviews suggest that the evidence for its efficacy is mixed. Gabapentin and pregabalin act as neuromodulators by selectively binding to the $\alpha2\delta$ subunit protein of calcium channels in various regions of the brain and the superficial dorsal horn of the spinal cord. This process inhibits the release of excitatory neurotransmitters, which are important in the production of pain. Pregabalin and duloxetine [a selective serotonin and norepinephrine (noradrenaline) reuptake inhibitor (SNRI)], are recommended by the UK National Institute of Health and Clinical Excellence (NICE) as the two first-line treatments for patients with neuropathic pain.

Chronic use of opioids should not be abruptly discontinued because of the potential for withdrawal symptoms. The administration of high-dose non-steroidal anti-inflammatory drugs or cyclooxygenase-2 inhibitors would be inappropriate in this patient with diabetic nephropathy, given their effects on renal blood flow.

Turk, D.C., Wilson, H.D., and Cahana, A. (2011). Treatment of chronic non-cancer pain. *Lancet* 377, 2226–2235.
http://www.ncbi.nlm.nih.gov/pubmed/21704872

18. Answer A

Venous thromboembolism (VTE) complicates 0.1–0.2% of pregnancies, with pulmonary embolism being a leading cause of maternal mortality and deep vein thrombosis an important cause of maternal morbidity. Low-molecular-weight heparin (LMWH) in therapeutic dose is the treatment of choice during pregnancy, and anti-coagulation (LMWH or vitamin K antagonists post-partum if the patient is not breast-feeding or after careful consultation) should be continued until 6 weeks after delivery with a minimum total duration of 3 months.

Most clinicians monitor anti-factor Xa levels 4h after injection, target to an anti-Xa level of 0.8–1.6 with a once-daily regimen of LMWH at infrequent intervals, and combine this with the platelet monitoring.

There are currently no data on the use of new oral anti-coagulants (i.e. direct thrombin inhibitors and anti-Xa inhibitors) or parenteral thrombin inhibitors in pregnancy.

 Middeldorp S. (2011). How I treat pregnancy-related venous thromboembolism. *Blood* 118, 5394–5400.
http://www.ncbi.nlm.nih.gov/pubmed/21921048

19. Answer D

Pressure is the most important factor in the development and progression of pressure ulcers. Other aetiological factors include shearing forces, moisture and injury from friction. The first step in managing ulcers of all stages is pressure reduction. This patient does not have evidence of full-thickness ulcer or eschar that would require surgical debridement. Topical antibiotics are appropriate for use in clean ulcers that are not healing with pressure relief and dressings, but their use alone is unlikely to result in healing. It is also important to optimise nutrition to promote wound healing, but it would be inappropriate to initiate tube feeding without first attempting local measures, such as pressure relief and use of wet-to-dry dressings with saline-soaked gauze. Povidone-iodine should not be applied to open wounds because of its toxic local effects.

20. Answer E

The history, raised serum osmolar gap, and high anion gap metabolic acidosis is suggestive of methanol poisoning (Brent, 2009).

The normal serum osmolar gap is calculated with the following formula:

$$(2 \times \text{serum[sodium]}) + [\text{glucose}] + [\text{urea}](\text{a in mmol/L})$$

The serum osmolal gap represents the difference between the measured and calculated serum osmolality. A high serum osmolal gap (greater than 10 mOsm/kg) in a patient with an otherwise unexplained high anion gap metabolic acidosis may be an important clue to the presence of methanol or ethylene glycol poisoning. Methanol and ethylene glycol are frequently found in high concentration in automotive anti-freeze and de-icing solutions, windshield wiper fluid, solvents, cleaners, fuels, and other industrial products. While methanol and ethylene glycol are relatively non-toxic, and cause mainly central nervous system (CNS) sedation, profound toxicity can ensue when these parent alcohols are oxidised primarily by alcohol dehydrogenase and aldehyde dehydrogenase. Methanol is metabolised to formaldehyde and subsequently formic acid, which causes retinal and optic nerve damage. Ethylene glycol is metabolised to glycolic acid, which is responsible for metabolic acidosis, and oxalic acid, which may combine with ionised calcium in the plasma to form calcium oxalate and this in turn may precipitate in the renal tubules, causing acute kidney injury. In severe cases, calcium oxalate crystals deposit diffusely in multiple organs.

Treatment consists of inhibition of alcohol dehydrogenase as that blocks conversion of both methanol and ethylene glycol to their toxic acid metabolites. This can be achieved with fomepizole, which is a competitive inhibitor of alcohol dehydrogenase. In patients with strong suspicion of methanol or ethylene glycol toxicity, fomepizole therapy should begin immediately, without waiting for the result of a measured methanol or ethylene glycol concentration. In urgent cases, one could use intravenous ethanol because alcohol dehydrogenase has greater affinity for ethanol than for methanol or ethylene glycol.

Brent, J. (2009). Fomepizole for ethylene glycol and methanol poisoning. *N Engl J Med* 360, 2216–2223.
http://www.ncbi.nlm.nih.gov/pubmed/19458366

21. Answer D

Hypophosphatemia is the hallmark of the refeeding syndrome (Mehanna et al., 2008). Refeeding syndrome can be defined as the potentially fatal shifts in fluids and electrolytes that may occur in malnourished patients receiving artificial refeeding (whether enterally or parenterally). Apart from hypophosphatemia, refeeding syndrome is associated with hypokalaemia, hypomagnesaemia, vitamin (e.g. thiamine) and trace mineral deficiencies, fluid overload and oedema.

The following groups of patients are at higher risk of refeeding syndrome:

- Patients with anorexia nervosa
- Patients with chronic alcoholism
- Oncology patients
- Postoperative patients
- Elderly patients
- Patients with uncontrolled diabetes mellitus (electrolyte depletion, diuresis)
- Long-term users of diuretics (loss of electrolytes)
- Long-term users of antacids (magnesium and aluminium salts bind phosphate)
- Patients with chronic malnutrition:
  - Morbid obesity with profound weight loss
  - Malabsorptive syndromes (such as inflammatory bowel disease, chronic pancreatitis, cystic fibrosis, short bowel syndrome).

Refeeding should be started at a reduced level of energy replacement. Vitamin supplementation should be started with refeeding and continued for at least 10 days. Correction of electrolyte and fluid imbalances is essential.

 Mehanna, H.M., Moledina, J., and Travis, J. (2008). Refeeding syndrome: what it is, and how to prevent and treat it. *BMJ* 336, 1495–1498.
http://www.ncbi.nlm.nih.gov/pmc/articles/PMC2440847/

22. Answer E

Most people who are regular smokers are dependent on cigarettes and the smoking process, rather than being addicted to nicotine. The elements of this dependence include the context of smoking, as well as certain smoking-related rituals, sensory stimulation and the reinforcing effects of nicotine (Rigotti, 2012).

Even people who smoke relatively small numbers of cigarettes have increased cardiovascular risk. So-called light or low-tar cigarettes are a marketing tool, and have no role in smoking cessation. The aim should be complete cessation rather than smoking reduction.

With the exception of smokers with features of high dependency, there is a reasonable case that the first attempt at cessation should be undertaken without a smoking cessation medication. If one or more attempts to quit have been unsuccessful, particularly if cravings were a problem, a smoking cessation medication should be recommended.

The use of nicotine replacement therapy (NRT) increases the chance of successful cessation by 70%. Both bupropion and varenicline are as effective as NRT, with some evidence for varenicline achieving superior quit rates compared to bupropion.

 Rigotti, N.A. (2012). Strategies to help a smoker who is struggling to quit. *JAMA* 308, 1573–1580.
http://www.ncbi.nlm.nih.gov/pubmed/23073954

23. Answer A

Thiamine deficiency can lead to Wernicke encephalopathy (Sechi and Serra, 2007). While commonly observed in patients with chronic heavy alcohol intake, thiamine deficiency can also occur after some types of bariatric surgery. While most patients present with some form of abnormal mental functioning, the classic triad of ophthalmoplegia, confusion and ataxia is rarely encountered. Thiamine will commonly relieve the ocular palsies within hours, but improvement in ataxia, apathy and confusion takes longer. Many of those who recover from the acute encephalopathy may experience memory and learning impairment, known as Korsakoff psychosis.

Sechi, G. and Serra, A. (2007). Wernicke's encephalopathy: new clinical settings and recent advances in diagnosis and management. *Lancet Neurol* 6, 442–455. http://www.ncbi.nlm.nih.gov/pubmed/17434099

24. Answer B

Solid organ transplantation is often a life-saving procedure. Because of the short-fall between the number of people who could benefit from a transplant and the availability of organs, this life-saving procedure must be rationed. Therefore, there needs to be clear criteria for selection (who gets on to the transplant list) and allocation (who receives a donated organ) (Neuberger, 2012).

There are several different approaches to organ allocation. A needs-based policy prioritises those at greatest risk of death. While the impact of such a policy has had varying success, in general it has been successful, but is associated with increased cost and denies access to transplantation to those with good organ function but an unacceptable quality of life that could be corrected by transplantation.

Outcomes-based allocation can be considered in various ways: from listing or transplantation, for patient or graft, absolute or adjusted for quality of life; choice of outcomes will impact on criteria and may be difficult to predict. Allocation according to utility, in effect, places the survival of the graft as the priority. Alloca-tion according to benefit will give the graft to that recipient who will have the maximum benefit when survival without and with transplant are estimated. Because the recipient with the shortest anticipated survival without transplanta-tion may well be the sickest, the post-transplant survival may be reduced com-pared with a less sick recipient and so the utility reduced and health-care costs increased. To avoid futility, the concept of minimum benefit is generally accepted.

Equity of access may mean that every person in need of a transplant will have a similar opportunity, regardless of other factors such as age, gender, co-morbidities and expected survival with or without a transplant. Organs could be allocated on a first-come, first-served basis; however, this approach would have to be modified to include those factors that significantly affect outcome, such as blood group or donor-recipient size match. Equity of access may mean that those with similar characteristics will all be treated in the same way. Geographical equity implies patients awaiting a graft will have the same chance of getting a graft irrespective of where they live or receive treatment.

Neuberger, J. (2012). Rationing life-saving resources – how should allocation policies be assessed in solid organ transplantation. *Transplant Int* 25, 3–6. http://onlinelibrary.wiley.com/doi/10.1111/j.1432-2277.2011.01327.x/full

25. Answer E

Dabigatran is a direct thrombin inhibitor and the Randomized Evaluation of Long-Term Anticoagulant Therapy (RE-LY) study provided good evidence that, when administered at a dose of 150 mg twice daily, dabigatran produces a reduced risk of stroke and a similar bleeding risk as warfarin targeted to an international normalised ratio (INR) of 2.0–3.0.

Dabigatran is mainly eliminated via the kidneys (80%) and accumulation occurs in severe renal failure. The current recommendation is that warfarin remains the treatment of choice for patients with a calculated creatinine clearance close to or less than 30 mL/min/1.73 m². Dabigatran has not been evaluated in patients with mechanical heart valves.

Lower gastrointestinal bleeding is significantly increased with dabigatran compared with warfarin. This is probably because low bioavailability results in high concentrations of active drug in the faeces. Therefore, patients with intestinal angiodysplasia, inflammatory bowel disease or diverticulosis, or those with a history of gastrointestinal bleeding may experience gut bleeding on treatment with dabigatran.

Dabigatran has to be administered twice daily for patients with atrial fibrillation, which suggests that it should not be seen as an alternative to warfarin in patients who have been poorly compliant with warfarin. The inability to monitor dabigatran, coupled with its short half-life (14–17 h), suggests that patients who are poorly compliant are at high risk of stroke, because failure to take medication will quickly lead to a loss of anti-thrombotic efficacy. For patients treated with warfarin and who undergo international normalised ratio (INR) monitoring, the clinician is at least aware of inadequate anti-coagulation, suggesting that aggressive measures to increase compliance can be put in place.

 Schulman, S. and Crowther, M.A. (2012). How I treat with anticoagulants in 2012: new and old anticoagulants, and when and how to switch. *Blood* 119, 3016–3023.
http://bloodjournal.hematologylibrary.org/content/119/13/3016.full.pdf+html

26. Answer A

Beta-blockers are not recommended as initial monotherapy for the treatment of hypertension, especially in the elderly, on account of increased incidence of stroke (particularly among smokers) and an increased risk of developing diabetes. Both the LIFE study (Losartan Intervention for Endpoint Reduction in Hypertension) and the ASCOT-BPLA trial (Anglo-Scandinavian Cardiac Outcomes Trial—Blood Pressure Lowering Arm) showed a higher incidence of stroke in patients treated with a beta-blocker for hypertension.

As per the 2010 update of the European Society of Hypertension and European Society of Cardiology guidelines, and the Australian Heart Foundation guidelines, beta-blockers should not be used as first-line anti-hypertensive therapy, particularly in those over the age of 60 years, unless there is a compelling reason such as heart failure or ischaemic heart disease.

All the other anti-hypertensive agents mentioned in the question have equal efficacy as first-line agents.

National Heart Foundation of Australia. Guide to management of hypertension 2008. Updated December 2010.
http://www.heartfoundation.org.au/SiteCollectionDocuments/
HypertensionGuidelines2008to2010Update.pdf

27. Answer B

Valproate-induced hyperammonemic encephalopathy (VHE) should be suspected when a patient on valproate presents with unexplained impairment in consciousness and raised ammonia with normal liver function tests and serum valproate levels (Tarafdar et al, 2011). An asymptomatic increase in serum ammonia is seen in 16–52% of patients receiving valproate therapy. The typical presentation of VHE is with impaired consciousness and lethargy with or without focal neurological symptoms.

Tarafdar, S., Slee, M., Doogue, M., and Ameer, F. (2011). A case of valproate induced hyperammonemic encephalopathy. *Case Rep Med* 2011, 969505.
http://www.ncbi.nlm.nih.gov/pmc/articles/PMC3099231/

28. Answer A

Accidental falls are a common and serious problem in elderly patients. Multiple studies have identified risk factors for falling; these risk factors are either intrinsic (e.g. muscular weakness, poor balance) or extrinsic (e.g. poor lighting, polypharmacy). Among the most important are muscle weakness, a history of falls, gait and balance deficits, visual deficits, cognitive impairment and age older than 80 years. In studies both of patients receiving care in the home and in long-term residential care facilities (RCF), an association between psychotropic medications and falls has been demonstrated. It is recommended that all older persons be asked at least once a year about falls, and any patient who reports a single fall should be observed performing 'get up and go' manoeuvres. Patients demonstrating difficulty with this test should undergo further assessment, including review of the circumstances associated with the fall, medications, and directed assessment of vision and neurological and cardiac function, as indicated. There is no evidence to support the routine use of restraints for the prevention of falls, given their significant drawbacks, which include deconditioning, depression, and development of pressure sores.

There is evidence that multifactorial interventions reduce falls and risk of falling in hospitals and may do so in RCFs as well. Vitamin D supplementation is effective in reducing the rate of falls in RCFs. Exercise in subacute hospital settings appears effective, but its effectiveness in nursing care facilities remains uncertain (Cameron et al., 2010).

Cameron, I.D., Murray, G.R., Gillespie, L.D., et al. (2010). Interventions for preventing falls in older people in nursing care facilities and hospitals. *Cochrane Database Syst Rev* CD005465.
http://www.ncbi.nlm.nih.gov/pubmed/20091578

29. Answer D

The patient in the vignette most likely has Alzheimer disease with mild-to-moderate cognitive impairment. Of the options given, initiating treatment with one of the cholinesterase inhibitors, probably donepezil, starting at 5 mg each night at bedtime, is potentially beneficial. Randomised, placebo-controlled clinical trials of cholinesterase inhibitors have shown significant but clinically marginal benefits with respect to cognition, daily function and behaviour in patients with mild-to-moderate Alzheimer dementia (Mayeux, 2010). The condition of patients who are taking these drugs often remains stable for a year or more and then may decline, though at a rate that is slower than that among untreated patients.

Memantine is an N-methyl-D-aspartate receptor antagonist, which can be used as an adjunct to cholinesterase inhibitors. However, it is currently not recommended alone for treatment of early Alzheimer disease and recent trials have indicated greater benefits with donepezil than memantine (Howard et al., 2012). Behavioural and psychiatric symptoms typically increase with disease progression. In patients with co-existing depression, selective serotonin-reuptake inhibitors are commonly used. Psychosis may occur infrequently and treatment with conventional or atypical anti-psychotic agents may be helpful in this instance.

Vitamin E is a dietary compound that functions as an anti-oxidant scavenging toxic free radicals. Evidence that free radicals may contribute to the pathological processes of cognitive impairment, including Alzheimer disease, has led to interest in the use of vitamin E in the treatment of Alzheimer disease and mild cognitive impairment (MCI). However, there is no evidence of efficacy of vitamin E in the prevention or treatment of patient with Alzheimer disease or MCI.

Howard, R., McShane, R., Lindesay, J., et al. (2012). Donepezil and memantine for moderate-to-severe Alzheimer's disease. *N Engl J Med* 366, 893–903.
http://www.ncbi.nlm.nih.gov/pubmed/22397651

Mayeux, R. (2010). Clinical practice. Early Alzheimer's disease. *N Engl J Med* 362, 2194–2201.
http://www.ncbi.nlm.nih.gov/pubmed/20558370

30. Answer A

Fabry disease or Andersen–Fabry disease is an X-linked lysosomal storage disorder of glycosphingolipid (GL) metabolism, caused by a deficiency in alpha-galactosidase A (alpha-gal A). The progressive accumulation of glycosphingolipid in tissues results in the clinical manifestations of the disease, which are more evident in hemizygous males and include characteristic skin lesions (angiokeratomas), neurological symptoms (acroparesthesia due to a painful small-fibre neuropathy), cardiac involvement (left ventricular enlargement, conduction abnormalities), cerebrovascular manifestations (thromboses, haemorrhage, etc.) and kidney involvement with progression to end-stage renal failure (ESRF). Alpha-gal A enzyme replacement therapy may slow disease progression and symptoms, but is very expensive (Schiffmann, 2007).

Autosomal dominant polycystic kidney disease and Alport syndrome could cause renal impairment and associated hypertension might lead to left ventricular enlargement, but a neuropathy would be unusual at this level of renal function. Autosomal recessive polycystic kidney disease presents in infancy or early childhood. A hypertrophic cardiomyopathy might produce the echo findings, but not renal failure or neuropathy.

Schiffmann, R. (2007). Enzyme replacement in Fabry disease: the essence is in the kidney. *Ann Intern Med* 146, 142–144.
http://annals.org/article.aspx?articleid=732156

31. Answer F

Phaeochromocytoma is a rare tumour of the sympathetic nervous system notable for the production of catecholamines (Pacak et al., 2007). Tumours may be adrenal or extra-adrenal and occur in both children and adults. The 'rule of 10' mnemonic is a helpful way of remembering that phaeochromocytomas are 10% ectopic, 10% malignant and 10% multiple. Symptoms may often be mistaken for anxiety attacks or be cardiac in origin with palpitations, tremors, severe anxiety and chest pain. Severe hypertension is commonly associated (though hypotension can occur). Plasma metanephrines (metabolic products of the catecholamine pathways) is the most sensitive investigation. The negative predictive value is extremely high, and normal plasma fractionated metanephrines exclude phaeochromocytoma, except in patients with early preclinical disease and those with strictly dopamine-secreting neoplasms, but the specificity is poor at 85–89%; the specificity falls to 77% in patients older than 60 years. Another useful screening tool is the 24-h urine collection for metanephrines and catecholamines.

Imaging modalities should be used only on the basis of a strong clinical suspicion and/or biochemical evidence of a catecholamine disturbance as the incidence of an adrenal mass (a so-called incidentaloma) found on imaging is 7% in the elderly population.

32. Answer E

Primary hyperaldosteronism is an underdiagnosed cause of hypertension (Rossi, 2011). It is characterised by hypertension, hypokalaemia (an inconsistent finding), mild hypernatraemia, metabolic alkalosis and a low plasma renin level (as seen in this patient). Secondary hyperaldosteronism is not usually associated with hypokalaemia or metabolic alkalosis; it is usually associated with a high plasma renin level.

There are many subtypes of primary aldosteronism described, including aldosterone-producing adenomas, bilateral idiopathic hyperaldosteronism, unilateral hyperplasia or primary adrenal hyperplasia (caused by micronodular or macronodular hyperplasia of the zona glomerulosa of predominantly one adrenal gland), familial hyperaldosteronism type I (glucocorticoid-remediable aldosteronism), type II (the familial occurrence of aldosterone-producing adenoma or bilateral idiopathic hyperplasia or both) and type III due to KCNJ5 potassium-channel mutations.

The treatment goal is to prevent the morbidity and mortality associated with hypertension, hypokalaemia, renal toxicity and cardiovascular damage. Normalisation of blood pressure is not the only goal. Therefore, normalisation of circulating aldosterone or mineralocorticoid receptor blockade should be part of the management plan for all patients with primary aldosteronism.

33. Answer A

Elevated blood pressure, significant renal impairment and a family history of renal failure complicated by cerebral haemorrhage should prompt consideration of a diagnosis of autosomal dominant polycystic kidney disease (ADPKD) (Grantham, 2008). ADPKD is associated with cerebral (Berry) aneurysms, cysts in other organs, such as the liver, pancreas and spleen, and cardiac valvular defects. Renal failure is progressive and may lead to end-stage renal disease (ESRD). Renal ultrasound scan is a very sensitive and specific tool in detecting cystic abnormalities of the kidneys and may well confirm the suspected diagnosis. Patients with ADPKD and a family history of premature stroke should have high-resolution CT angiography (CTA) or magnetic resonance angiography (MRA) screening for intracerebral aneurysms. However, routine screening is not recommended because the risk-to-benefit ratio of screening asymptomatic patients is uncertain.

34. Answer G

This patient's presentation is consistent with flash pulmonary oedema with significantly elevated blood pressure. Flash pulmonary oedema is a term that is used to describe a dramatic form of acute decompensated heart failure in which acute increases in left ventricular diastolic pressure cause rapid fluid accumulation in the pulmonary interstitium and alveolar spaces. There is a greater degree of urgency to the implementation of initial therapies and the search for triggering causes. Patients with bilateral renal artery stenosis are at increased risk for developing flash pulmonary oedema. Flash pulmonary oedema may be an indication for renal artery revascularisation.

Renal artery stenosis is a relatively common cause of hypertension (Baumgartner and Lerman, 2011). The incidence of this disorder is probably less than 1% in patients with mild hypertension, but rises to as high as 10–40% in patients with acute, severe or refractory hypertension. There are two major causes of the renal arterial stenosis:

- Atherosclerosis, which usually affects patients over the age of 50 years and usually involves the aortic orifice or the proximal main renal artery
- Fibromuscular dysplasia (FMD), which most often affects women under the age of 50 years and typically involves the distal main renal artery or the intrarenal branches.

References for Questions 31–34

Baumgartner, I. and Lerman, L.O. (2011). Renovascular hypertension: screening and modern management. *Eur Heart J* 32, 1590–1598.
http://eurheartj.oxfordjournals.org/content/32/13/1590.long

Grantham, J.J. (2008). Clinical practice. Autosomal dominant polycystic kidney disease. *N Engl J Med* 359, 1477–1485.
http://www.ncbi.nlm.nih.gov/pubmed/18832246

Pacak, K., Eisenhofer, G., Ahlman, H., et al. (2007). Pheochromocytoma: recommendations for clinical practice from the First International Symposium. October 2005. *Nat Clin Pract Endocrinol Metab* 3, 92–102.
http://www.ncbi.nlm.nih.gov/pubmed/17237836

Rossi, G.P. (2011). Diagnosis and treatment of primary aldosteronism. *Endocrinol Metab Clin North Am* 40, 313–332, vii–viii.
http://www.ncbi.nlm.nih.gov/pubmed/21565669

16 Psychiatry

Questions

BASIC SCIENCE

Answers can be found in the Psychiatry Answers section at the end of this chapter.

1. Which one of the following statements is correct regarding clozapine?
  A. Smoking cessation may lead to enhanced drug levels
  B. Ciprofloxacin may lead to reduced drug levels
  C. The risk of developing agranulocytosis is highest after a year of treatment
  D. Clozapine is indicated for severe bipolar disorder
  E. A full blood count should be undertaken once at 4 weeks after initiation

2. If a patient taking a first-generation monoamine oxidase inhibitor ingests red wine containing tyramine, which one of the following acute responses is most likely?
  A. Stimulation of norepinephrine (noradrenaline) release
  B. Inhibition of norepinephrine release
  C. Stimulation of acetylcholine release
  D. Inhibition of acetylcholine release
  E. No dopaminergic response due to the monoamine inhibitor

3. Which receptor is antagonised by atypical anti-psychotics such as olanzapine and risperidone, but not by conventional anti-psychotics such as haloperidol and pericyazine?
  A. Dopamine (D_2)
  B. Serotonin ($5\text{-}HT_2$)
  C. Alpha$_1$-adrenergic
  D. Alpha$_2$-adrenergic
  E. Beta-adrenergic

Passing the FRACP Written Examination: Questions and Answers, First Edition. Jonathan Gleadle,
Tuck Yong, Jordan Li, Surjit Tarafdar, and Danielle Wu.
© 2013 John Wiley & Sons, Ltd. Published 2013 by John Wiley & Sons, Ltd.

CLINICAL

4. Which one of the following is a feature of serotonin syndrome?
   A. Clonus
   B. High serum serotonin concentration
   C. Hypotonia
   D. Erythroderma
   E. Hypothermia

5. Which one of the following abnormalities is commonly observed in patients with anorexia nervosa?
   A. Tachycardia
   B. Leucocytosis
   C. Hyperphosphatemia
   D. Reduced serum cortisol
   E. Osteoporosis

6. A 36-year-old woman is brought in 6h after an overdose of lithium carbonate. Her two serum lithium levels taken 1h apart were 4.0mmol/L and 3.9mmol/L, respectively (normal therapeutic range is 0.5–1.2mmol/L). She has an episode of convulsions 2h after presentation. Which one of the following is essential for this patient's recovery?
   A. Haemodialysis
   B. Hydration with normal saline
   C. Alkaline diuresis with sodium bicarbonate
   D. Oral charcoal
   E. Intravenous diuretics

7. A 38-year-old man is diagnosed to have schizophrenia and was commenced on an anti-psychotic agent 5 days ago. His nurse reports that he is more confused, sweaty and tremulous. Which one of the following features concerning neuroleptic malignant syndrome (NMS) is correct?
   A. NMS occurs most commonly more than 4 weeks after commencing anti-psychotics
   B. The dose of the anti-psychotic agent should be reduced
   C. NMS is not associated with depot anti-psychotics
   D. Labile blood pressure is a feature of NMS
   E. Serum creatine kinase (CK) is elevated in all patients with NMS

8. An over-worked consultant physician in an Acute Medical Unit presents after self-harm, having consumed a bottle of vodka and a variety of pain killing tablets. Which one of the following is a risk factor for suicide after self-harm?
   A. Disclosure of intention at time of self-harm
   B. Female sex

C. First episode of self-harm
D. Alcohol misuse
E. Good physical health

9. A 55-year-old woman is admitted after being found next to an empty bottle of medicine by her daughter. She is confused and unable to provide a history. On examination, her heart rate is 110 beats/min and blood pressure is 90/60 mmHg, but with warm peripheries. Her temperature is 37.6°C. Her pupils are dilated. Her electrocardiography shows a prolonged QT interval. Which medication is the patient most likely to have taken an overdose of?
A. Fluoxetine
B. Sodium valproate
C. Sertraline
D. Citalopram
E. Doxepine

Answers

BASIC SCIENCE

1. Answer A

Cytochrome P450 1A2 (CYP1A2) is primarily responsible for clozapine metabolism. Agents that induce cytochrome CYP1A2, such as tobacco cigarette smoke, will increase the metabolism of clozapine. Tobacco smokers may require twice the dose of clozapine compared to non-smokers to achieve similar blood levels. Agents that inhibit CYP1A2 (e.g. theophylline, ciprofloxacin, fluvoxamine) and smoking cessation can decrease the metabolism of clozapine and may produce clinical toxicity. Clozapine plasma concentrations can rise 1.5 times in the 2–4 weeks following smoking cessation and in some instances by 50–70% within 2–4 days. If baseline plasma concentrations are higher – particularly over 1 mg/L – the plasma concentration may rise dramatically due to non-linear kinetics. If patients smoking more than 7–12 cigarettes/day while taking clozapine decide to quit, the dose may need to be reduced by 50%.

Agranulocytosis occurs in about 1% of patients who take clozapine during the first few months of treatment and the risk of developing it is highest about 3 months into treatment. Patients who have agranulocytosis with clozapine should not receive it again. Patients taking clozapine should be enrolled in a monitoring programme. This requires weekly blood tests for 18 weeks and then monthly blood tests while on clozapine. Clozapine is indicated for schizophrenia in patients who are non-responsive to other neuroleptic agents.

2. Answer A

Tyramine is physiologically metabolised by monoamine oxidase A (MAO-A) (Flockhart, 2012). In humans, if monoamine metabolism is compromised by the use of monoamine oxidase inhibitors (MAOIs) and foods high in tyramine are ingested, a hypertensive crisis can result, as tyramine can cause the release of stored monoamines, such as dopamine, norepinephrine (noradrenaline) and epinephrine (adrenaline). The physiological effects of tyramine include peripheral vasoconstriction, increased cardiac output, increased respiration, elevated blood glucose and release of norepinephrine. MAO-A deaminates serotonin in the central nervous system and dietary monoamines in the gastrointestinal system. MAO-B is found predominantly in liver and muscle and deaminates dopamine and phenylethylamine. The first generation of MAOI drugs are non-specific, inhibit both isoforms of MAO and this inhibition is considered irreversible. The second generation drugs, termed RIMA for reversible inhibitor monoamine (such as selegiline), are selective in inhibition, reversible and carry little risk of a hypertensive effect in low dosage, as in the treatment of Parkinson disease.

Flockhart, D.A. (2012). Dietary restrictions and drug interactions with monoamine oxidase inhibitors: an update. *J Clin Psychiatry* 73 Suppl 1, 17–24. http://www.ncbi.nlm.nih.gov/pubmed/22951238

3. Answer B

All currently available effective anti-psychotics block dopamine (D_2) receptors. Atypical anti-psychotics, such as clozapine, olanzapine, risperidone and quetiapine, also antagonise serotonin ($5\text{-}HT_2$) receptors, which influences the drug activity. There is also some evidence to suggest that differential blockade of other dopamine receptors (such as D_1) may influence therapeutic and adverse effects.

Tricyclic anti-depressants, in addition to inhibiting reuptake of norepinephrine (noradrenaline) and serotonin, also block alpha$_1$-adrenergic, serotonergic, histaminergic and cholinergic receptors.

CLINICAL

4. Answer A

Excess serotonin in the central nervous system leads to a condition commonly referred to as the serotonin syndrome, but is better described as a spectrum of toxicity – serotonin toxicity (Isbister et al., 2007). It can occur from an overdose, drug interaction or adverse drug effect involving serotonergic agents.

Serotonin toxicity is characterised by neuromuscular excitation (hyper-reflexia, clonus, myoclonus, rigidity), autonomic stimulation (hyperthermia, tachycardia, sweating, tremor, flushing) and changed mental state (anxiety, agitation, confusion). Serotonin toxicity can be mild (serotonergic features that may or may not concern the patient); moderate (toxicity that causes significant distress and deserves treatment, but is not life-threatening); or severe (a medical emergency characterised by rapid onset of severe hyperthermia, muscle rigidity and multiple organ failure).

There are several drug mechanisms that cause excess serotonin, but severe serotonin toxicity only occurs with combinations of drugs acting at different sites, most commonly including a monoamine oxidase inhibitor and a serotonin reuptake inhibitor. Less severe toxicity occurs with other combinations, overdoses and even single-drug therapy in susceptible individuals. Serotonin syndrome is a clinical diagnosis; serum serotonin concentrations do not correlate with clinical findings and severity, and no laboratory test confirms the diagnosis. Treatment should focus on cessation of the serotonergic medication and supportive care. Some anti-serotonergic agents have been used in clinical practice, but the preferred agent, dose and indications are not well defined.

Isbister, G.K., Buckley, N.A., and Whyte, I.M. (2007). Serotonin toxicity: a practical approach to diagnosis and treatment. *Med J Aust* 187, 361–365.
http://www.ncbi.nlm.nih.gov/pubmed/17874986

5. Answer E

For reasons that are unclear, patients with anorexia nervosa commonly have bradycardia and may have hypotension (Mitchell and Crow, 2006). Cytopenias and hypoplastic bone marrow changes occur and leucopenia is a common finding. Cortisol levels are usually elevated. The combination of decreased sex steroids and elevated cortisol, and nutritional deficiencies, can lead to severe osteoporosis. Important electrolyte abnormalities include hypokalaemia, hypophosphatemia and hypomagnesaemia. Dermatological manifestations are common and include xerosis, lanugo-like body hair, telogen effluvium, carotenoderma, acne and hyperpigmentation.

Mitchell, J.E. and Crow, S. (2006). Medical complications of anorexia nervosa and bulimia nervosa. *Curr Opin Psychiatry* 19, 438–443.
http://www.ncbi.nlm.nih.gov/pubmed/16721178

6. Answer A

In acute overdose of lithium, initial elevation of concentration can be misleading because tissue distribution occurs over several hours. An initial high level can fall to 1 mmol/L with final distribution, so repeated measurement of serum lithium levels and serial mental status examination are essential in the assessment of toxicity.

Symptoms of lithium toxicity include apathy, lethargy, tremor, slurred speech, ataxia and muscle fasciculation, which may progress to choreoathetosis, convulsions, coma and death. There may be residual neurological sequelae in the long-term.

In addition to intensive supportive care, the treatment of choice for serious intoxication is haemodialysis. Dialysis must be considered in any patient with convulsions or coma with lithium concentrations above 2.5 mmol/L, or when serum lithium levels at equilibrium are 4 mmol/L and above. Dialysis is the only route of elimination for patients with renal failure.

Sodium and water depletion and dehydration lead to marked increases in renal reabsorption of lithium, resulting in raised serum concentrations. Diuretics should not be used in the treatment of lithium overdosage. Administration of intravenous normal saline may promote lithium excretion, but the value of forced saline diuresis is unclear and it is not recommended. Alkalinisation is of no value and activated charcoal does not absorb lithium and is also useless.

7. Answer D

Neuroleptic malignant syndrome (NMS) is a potentially life-threatening complication of treatment with anti-psychotic drugs and is characterised by fever, severe muscle rigidity and autonomic and mental status changes (Strawn et al., 2007). About 16% of cases of NMS develop within 24 h after initiation of anti-psychotic treatment, 66% within the first week and virtually all cases within 30 days. Once NMS is diagnosed, oral anti-psychotic drugs should be stopped. NMS is self-limiting in most cases though intensive supportive care may be required. The mean recovery time after drug discontinuation is in the range of 7–10 days. The duration of NMS episodes may be prolonged when long-acting depot anti-psychotics are causative. Importantly, although NMS is striking in its classical form, the condition is heterogeneous in onset, presentation, progression and outcome. Labile blood pressure may occur due to autonomic dysfunction and patients with NMS usually have tachycardia. Creatine kinase (CK) is often markedly elevated but a normal CK can be seen if rigidity is not well developed, particularly early in the syndrome.

Restarting anti-psychotic treatment after resolution of an NMS episode has been associated with an estimated likelihood of developing NMS again as high as 30%. Nevertheless, most patients who require anti-psychotic treatment can be safely treated, provided precautions are taken.

 Strawn, J.R., Kerk, P.E. Jr, and Caroff, S.N. (2007). Neuroleptic malignant syndrome. *Am J Psychiatry* 164, 870–876.
http://ajp.psychiatryonline.org/data/Journals/AJP/3818/07aj0870.PDF

8. Answer D

Self-harm is a strong predictor of suicide, with the risk being at its highest in the first 6 months after a harming episode, but it persists for many decades (Hawton and van Heeringen, 2009; Skegg, 2005). Once a person has self-harmed, the likelihood that he or she will die by suicide increases 50–100 times, with one in 15 dying by suicide within 9 years of the index episode. In studies of risk factors for suicide, a history of self-harm or suicide attempts is the strongest factor, present in at least 40% of cases. Male sex, older age and multiple episodes of self-harm have been identified as epidemiological associations with later suicide, but such risk factors are poor predictors for an individual's suicide risk. It is important to carefully enquire about each individual's current suicidality. This can inform likely suicide risk. If significant risk for suicide is identified, a clearly articulated plan should be formed with management that might include planned engagement with health professionals, environmental interventions to reduce risk (e.g. restricting access to lethal means, increased supervision, detention), psychotherapeutic or medication interventions, and facilitating access to community services.

Other risk factors for suicide after self-harm include:

- Past psychiatric care
- Psychiatric disorder such as depression, anxiety disorder and personality disorder
- Substance misuse (especially in young people)
- Social isolation
- Repeated self-harm
- Medically severe self-harm
- Strong suicidal intent
- Avoiding discovery at time of self-harm
- Hopelessness
- Poor physical health.

Psychiatric disorders are present in up to 90% of people who kill themselves, with increased risk in those suffering from depression, bipolar disorder, alcohol misuse, anorexia and schizophrenia. Of patients with bipolar disorder, 10–15% die by suicide. Risk of suicide is increased in health-care professionals, including nurses, physicians, dentists and pharmacists, and may relate in part to ready access to medicinal drugs.

Hawton, K. and van Heeringen, K. (2009). Suicide. *Lancet* 373, 1372–1381.
http://www.ncbi.nlm.nih.gov/pubmed/19376453

Skegg, K. (2005). Self-harm. *Lancet* 366, 1471–1483.
http://www.ncbi.nlm.nih.gov/pubmed/16243093

9. Answer E

Doxepine is a tricyclic anti-depressant (TCA)-like drug. The peripheral autonomic nervous system, central nervous system and heart are affected following overdose (Body et al., 2011). Initial symptoms typically develop within 2 h and include tachycardia, drowsiness, a dry mouth, nausea and vomiting, urinary retention, confusion, agitation and headache. More severe complications include hypotension, cardiac rhythm disturbances, hallucinations and seizures. Electrocardiogram (ECG) abnormalities are frequent and cardiac dysrhythmias can occur, the most common being sinus tachycardia, prolonged QT intervals and intraventricular conduction delay resulting in prolongation of the QRS complex.

Tricyclics have a narrow therapeutic index and the toxic effects of TCAs are caused by four major pharmacological actions: anti-cholinergic effects, excessive blockade of norepinephrine (noradrenaline) reuptake at the preganglionic synapse, direct alpha-adrenergic blockade and, importantly, blockade of sodium membrane channels with slowing of membrane depolarisation, thus having quinidine-like effects on the myocardium.

Initial treatment of an acute overdose includes gastric decontamination by activated charcoal lavage, which absorbs the drug in the gastrointestinal tract, either orally or via a nasogastric tube. Activated charcoal is most useful if given within 1–2 h of ingestion. Symptomatic patients are usually monitored in an intensive care or high-dependency unit for a minimum of 12 h, with close attention paid to the airway, blood pressure monitoring, arterial pH and continuous ECG monitoring. Supportive therapy is given if necessary, including respiratory assistance, maintenance of body temperature and administration of intravenous sodium bicarbonate, which has been shown to be an effective treatment for resolving the metabolic acidosis and cardiovascular complications of TCA poisoning. If sodium bicarbonate therapy fails to improve cardiac complications, conventional anti-dysrhythmic drugs such as magnesium can be used to reverse any cardiac abnormalities.

Fluoxetine and citalopram are selective serotonin reuptake inhibitor (SSRI), which do not cause severe anti-cholinergic side effects or cardiac arrhythmias in overdose. Sodium valproate can cause encephalopathy, respiratory depression and heart block in overdose, but not the severity of anti-cholinergic side effects or hypotension.

Body, R., Bartram, T., Azam, F., and Mackway-Jones, K. (2011). Guidelines in Emergency Medicine Network (GEMNet): guideline for the management of tricyclic antidepressant overdose. *Emerg Med J* 28, 347–368.
http://www.ncbi.nlm.nih.gov/pubmed/21436332

17 Statistics, epidemiology and research

Questions

BASIC SCIENCE

Answers can be found in the Statistics, epidemiology and research Answers section at the end of this chapter.

1. In a study of 100 people with hypertension screened for hyperlipidaemia, 40 were found to have hyperlipidaemia. Of those with hyperlipidaemia, 10 subsequently had myocardial infarction and of those who did not, three had a myocardial infarction. What can be concluded from this study?
- **A.** The relative risk of myocardial infarction in those with hyperlipidaemia is 5
- **B.** The attributable risk of hyperlipidaemia in myocardial infarction is 20%
- **C.** The attributable risk of hyperlipidaemia in myocardial infarction is 5%
- **D.** Hyperlipidaemia is not a risk factor for myocardial infarction
- **E.** A relative risk greater than 1 implies hyperlipidaemia is a cause of myocardial infarction

2. Range, standard deviation and variance are common measures of dispersion. Which one of the following is a correct description about measures of dispersion?
- **A.** Variance is the standard deviation squared
- **B.** Range is the most commonly used measure of dispersion of a mean value
- **C.** In a normal distribution, 80% of the values will fall between one standard deviation above and below the mean value
- **D.** The range gives the width of the entire distribution and the pattern of the distribution
- **E.** In a skewed distribution, the extreme values will affect the median to a larger degree than the mean

3. Which one of the following definitions for data interpretation of diseases is used correctly?
- **A.** Prevalence is identical to incidence
- **B.** Cumulative incidence rate is an alternative measure of prevalence

---

Passing the FRACP Written Examination: Questions and Answers, First Edition. Jonathan Gleadle, Tuck Yong, Jordan Li, Surjit Tarafdar, and Danielle Wu.
© 2013 John Wiley & Sons, Ltd. Published 2013 by John Wiley & Sons, Ltd.

C. Incidence is the number of newly affected individuals in a study population over a given time period

D. Prevalence is the incidence multiplied by the population number

E. Lifetime incidence is the proportion of a population experiencing the disease at some point in their life

4. A study has been testing a new drug 'DONTCLOT' compared to warfarin for treating deep venous thrombosis. The study shows that there was no statistical significant difference between the two treatments. A statistician examined the study and suggested that there was a type II error. What does this mean?

A. DONTCLOT should have been compared with placebo

B. Warfarin is better than DONTCLOT

C. The P value is incorrect

D. The study suggests that there is no difference but the trial was too small to detect the real difference existing between the treatment groups

E. The absence of statistical difference is not true

5. A randomised controlled trial was undertaken to compare a new endoscopic procedure with a conventional method. The main finding is that the new procedure reduces the risk of persistent peptic ulcer bleeding from 8% to 4%. What does this study show regarding the new endoscopic technique?

A. Statistical significance

B. Successful trial

C. Incomplete response

D. Effectiveness of new procedure

E. Efficacy of new procedure

CLINICAL

6. A study investigated whether drug X is better as a single agent or in combination with a new drug Y for hyperglycaemia treatment. After randomisation of recruited subjects with type 2 diabetes, a few patients on both drugs (X + Y) dropped out of the study because of adverse effects; there were also several deaths. How should the data be analysed?
  A. Exclude analysis of those subjects who died
  B. Exclude the subjects who dropped out from statistical analysis
  C. Recruit more subjects to the X + Y cohort
  D. Analyse the two comparison groups separately
  E. Include the outcomes of subjects who dropped out in the drug X + Y group

7. A new drug for the treatment of cirrhosis has been evaluated in a randomised controlled trial. The 5-year mortality rate with the drug is 45% and without the drug is 50%. How many patients with cirrhosis have to be treated with this new drug to prevent one extra death over a 5-year period?
  A. 2
  B. 5
  C. 10
  D. 20
  E. 50

8. Rofecoxib (Vioxx), a cyclooxygenase-2 inhibitor, was approved by the Food and Drug Administration (FDA) in May 1999 but was then voluntarily withdrawn from the market in September 2004 due to concerns about twice the risk of myocardial infarction and stroke associated with long-term and high-dosage use. In which clinical phase was rofecoxib withdrawn?
  A. Phase I
  B. Phase II
  C. Phase III
  D. Phase IV
  E. Phase V

9. In order to evaluate a new test for hepatitis C, a cohort of 2000 subjects is investigated. This test is positive in 76 of the 2000 subjects. Hepatitis C infection defined by conventional 'gold standard' hepatitis C RNA testing, was present in 40 of the 2000 subjects. Of the 76 patients with a positive result from the new test, 36 were shown to have hepatitis C by conventional testing and 40 were false positives who did not have the disease. The new test was negative in 1924 of the 2000 subjects;.four of the 1924 were false negatives who were shown subsequently to have hepatitis C by conventional testing; 1920 did not and were truly negative. Which one of the following statements is correct with regards to diagnosis of hepatitis C and interpretation of new test results?

A. The prevalence of hepatitis C in the cohort is 10%
B. The sensitivity of the new test is 80%
C. The specificity of the new test is 98%
D. The negative predictive value of the new test is 90%
E. The false-negative rate of the new test is 2%

10. The forest plot below shows the total mortality in patients treated with a beta-blocker versus placebo for hypertension. Which one of the following statements is INCORRECT?

Review: Beta-blockers for hypertension

Comparison: I Beta-blockers vs Placebo or No treatment

Outcome: I Total mortality

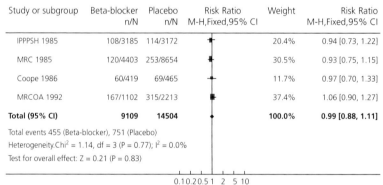

Study or subgroup	Beta-blocker n/N	Placebo n/N	Risk Ratio M-H,Fixed,95% CI	Weight	Risk Ratio M-H,Fixed,95% CI
IPPPSH 1985	108/3185	114/3172		20.4%	0.94 [0.73, 1.22]
MRC 1985	120/4403	253/8654		30.5%	0.93 [0.75, 1.15]
Coope 1986	60/419	69/465		11.7%	0.97 [0.70, 1.33]
MRCOA 1992	167/1102	315/2213		37.4%	1.06 [0.90, 1.27]
Total (95% CI)	**9109**	**14504**		**100.0%**	**0.99 [0.88, 1.11]**

Total events 455 (Beta-blocker), 751 (Placebo)
Heterogeneity.Chi^2 = 1.14, df = 3 (P = 0.77); I^2 = 0.0%
Test for overall effect: Z = 0.21 (P = 0.83)

0.1 0.2 0.5 1   2   5 10
Favours beta-blocker   Favours placebo

Copyright © 2009 The Cochrane Collaboration. Published by John Wiley & Sons, Ltd.

A. The width of the horizontal lines in each study indicates the risk ratio for each study
B. The confidence interval of the test for overall effect crosses 1. This finding suggests there is significant mortality benefit of treating hypertensive patients with beta-blockers compared to placebo
C. To be included in the meta-analysis, studies need to be relatively heterogeneous for meaningful comparison
D. The size of a square in each study indicates the confidence interval of each study in meta-analysis
E. The overall estimated effect of all of the studies in a meta-analysis is represented by a diamond at the bottom of the graph

11. In a city with a population of 10 000, the results of a new diagnostic test for tuberculosis are given below. Which one of the following is the positive predictive value (PPV) of the diagnostic test in this group of patients?

Test result	Tuberculosis	
	Present	Absent
Positive	1800	4000
Negative	200	4000

- A. 50
- B. 31
- C. 90
- D. 18
- E. 45

12. A new laboratory test for a disease has a sensitivity of 90% and a specificity of 80%. Which one of the following is true concerning this new test?
- A. 90% of patients who do not have the disease will have a negative result
- B. If the test is positive, the probability of the disease being present is 90%
- C. 10% of patients who have the disease will have a positive result
- D. If the prevalence of the disease in the population is 1%, in screening this population over 90% will be false positives
- E. Increased laboratory error increases the predictive value of the test

Theme: Statistical test (for Questions 13–15)
- A. Log-rank correlation
- B. Spearman's rank correlation
- C. Wilcoxon signed-rank test
- D. Mann-Whitney U-test
- E. Chi-squared test
- F. Logistic regression analysis
- G. Paired Student's t-test
- H. Unpaired Student's t-test

For each of the studies described below, select the most appropriate statistical test.

13. A study is testing the effects of a new drug A on hypertension. Two groups of hypertensive patients are recruited. One group is treated with drug A for 3 months while the other is not. The study evaluated the reduction of blood pressure after treatment between the two groups. What is the most appropriate statistical test to use for this study?

14. A research fellow is assessing the effectiveness of a new therapy for squamous cell carcinoma (SCC) and recruits newly diagnosed SCC patients to the study. She randomises the total participants to either the existing treatment or the novel treatment arm and performs the standard operation for melanoma excision on the first group (n = 420). She also performs the newly proposed therapy on the second group (n = 390). The treatment arms are double-blinded (both to the researcher and patients); 6 months after the surgery the patients are seen in clinic to assess for recurrence rates. The data shown below are obtained. Which one of the statistical tests would be most suitable for investigating the effect of the novel treatment?

Disease present	Yes	No
Standard treatment	80	340
Novel treatment	60	330

15. The frequency of attendance of 50 basic physician trainees at a weekly educational session was recorded by an observer over a 1-year period. The trainees were assessed at the end of this period with a multiple choice examination with a test score marked out of 100. Which statistical test is the best to evaluate the effectiveness of trainees' attendance on higher examination scores?

Answers

BASIC SCIENCE

1. Answer B
The attributable risk of hyperlipidaemia in patients who had myocardial infarction (MI) in the study group is 23%. The attributable risk is the difference in incidence of MI between those with and without hyperlipidaemia, i.e. 25% − 5% = 20%.

The relative risk is the ratio of those who had a MI in the hyperlipidaemia group to those who had a MI with hyperlipidaemia (0.25/0.05 = 5). A relative risk of greater than 1 implies that hyperlipidaemia is associated with an increased risk of MI, but does not necessarily imply causation.

2. Answer A
Range, standard deviation and variance are common measures of dispersion. The standard deviation is the most widely used measure of the spread of data about their mean. The larger the standard deviation, the more spread out the distribution of the data about the mean.

The range is the measurement of the width of the entire distribution and is found simply by calculating the difference between the highest and lowest values. The range gives no information about the distribution of the values.

In a skewed distribution, the extreme values will affect the mean to a larger degree than they will affect the median. In a normal distribution, 68% of the values should fall between one standard deviation in either direction and over 95% of the values should fall between two standard deviations in either direction.

The variance is the square of the standard deviation and a measurement of the variation among all the subjects in the sample.

3. Answer C
Incidence is the number of newly affected individuals in an at-risk population over a given time (often assumed to be 1 year). Prevalence is the number of cases of a particular disease or condition at a specified time in an at-risk population. Lifetime prevalence is the proportion of a population that at some point in their life (up to the time of assessment) have experienced the condition.

4. Answer D
A type I error occurs when 'the null hypothesis is falsely rejected'. This means that the study claims to find a difference that does not really exist.

A type II error occurs when 'the null hypothesis is falsely accepted'. This means that, although it is suggested that there is no difference between two groups, the study is actually too small to detect a difference.

5. Answer E

In medicine, efficacy indicates the capacity for beneficial change (or therapeutic effect) of a given intervention (e.g. a drug, medical device, surgical procedure or public health intervention). If efficacy is established, an intervention is likely to be at least as good as other available interventions, to which it will have been compared.

When talking in terms of efficacy versus effectiveness, effectiveness relates to how well a treatment works in the practice of medicine, as opposed to efficacy, which measures how well a treatment works in clinical trials or laboratory studies.

CLINICAL

6. Answer E
The analysis of patients dropping out of a study should take into account the adverse effects of a drug (in this case drug Y) causing attrition. Hence, even though patients have dropped out, the 'intention-to-treat' principle requires the patients to be analysed even if they did not receive the treatment. Intention-to-treat analysis is intended to avoid misleading artefacts that can arise in interventional research. For example, if people who have a more serious illness are likely to drop out of a study at a higher rate, even a completely ineffective treatment may appear to be beneficial if the outcome before and after the treatment is compared for just those who complete the study.

7. Answer D
The number needed to treat (NNT) is a helpful way of expressing the potential size of benefit of a therapeutic intervention. It is the reciprocal of the absolute risk reduction (which is the absolute event rate for control – the absolute event rate for treated patients) (Cook and Sackett, 1995).

> NNT = 1/[(Proportion benefiting from experimental intervention)
> – (Proportion benefiting from a control intervention)]

In the example, the absolute risk reduction is 50% – 45% or 0.50 – 0.45 = 0.05. [The relative risk reduction is 10% (5% of 50%).]

Using the information obtained from this trial, the NNT with the new drug treatment to prevent one extra death is 1/absolute risk reduction = 1/0.05 = 20.

Similar calculations can be undertaken to derive the number needed to harm for the adverse effects of treatments. Care needs to be taken when using the NNT to compare trials as the control arm in different trials may vary, as might the study duration, etc. The ideal NNT is 1, where every participant has improved with treatment and no one has with control. The higher the NNT, the less effective is the treatment. However, in preventing death with a simple treatment, such as using aspirin in secondary prevention of stroke, a large NNT, e.g. 25, might still be clinically very useful.

Cook, R.J. and Sackett, D.L. (1995). The number needed to treat: a clinically useful measure of treatment effect. *BMJ* 310, 452–454.
http://www.ncbi.nlm.nih.gov/pmc/articles/PMC2548824/

8. Answer D
The Vioxx Gastrointestinal Outcomes Research (VIGOR) trial in 2000 reported significantly fewer episodes of gastrointestinal bleeding in those taking rofecoxib than those taking naproxen. In the same study, the naproxen users were found

to have one-quarter of the risk of having a myocardial infarction compared to those taking rofecoxib (Avorn, 2012). It was initially speculated that naproxen was cardiac protective due to its anti-platelet effect. In 2004, another randomised clinical trial, APPROVe (Adenomatous Polyp Prevention of Vioxx), was halted 2 months before it was scheduled to end because it was found that rofecoxib had nearly doubled the risk of myocardial infarction and stroke compared to placebo after 18 months. Re-analysis of the original clinical data suggested the gastroprotective advantage was overstated and there was clear evidence of increased risk of cardiovascular death.

Since rofecoxib was withdrawn from the market after it had been approved by the FDA and had been on the market for 5 years, it was withdrawn in phase IV of clinical trials. Clinical trials are conducted in a series of phases:

- Phase I: A new drug or treatment is tested in a small group of people for the first time to evaluate its safety, determine a safe dosage range and identify side effects
- Phase II: The drug or treatment is given to a larger group of patients to assess its effect and safety
- Phase III: The drug or treatment is given to large groups of patients to confirm its effectiveness, monitor side effects, compare it to commonly used treatments, and collect information that will allow the drug or treatment to be used safely
- Phase IV: After the drug or treatment has been marketed, studies are done to gather information on the its effect in various populations and any side effects associated with long-term use

Avorn, J. (2012). 200th Anniversary Article: two centuries of assessing drug risks. *N Engl J Med* 367, 193–197.
http://www.ncbi.nlm.nih.gov/pubmed/22808954

9. Answer C

	Hepatitis C present	Hepatitis C absent	Total
New test positive	36 (a)	40 (b)	76 (a + b)
New test negative	4 (c)	1920 (d)	1924 (c + d)
Total	40 (a + c)	1960 (b + d)	2000 (a + b + c + d)

The prevalence of a disease is the number of people with the disease in the test population at the time of testing. In this instance, the prevalence of the disease in the test population is (a + c)/(a + b + c + d) = 40/2000 = 2%.

Sensitivity and specificity are two statistical test characteristics to describe a population under test. They are often inversely related. Sensitivity is the proportion of subjects with the disease showing a positive test result, while specificity is the proportion of subjects without the disease showing a negative test result. In this instance, the sensitivity is a/(a + c) = 36/40 = 90%.

The false-negative rate can be calculated as the number of false negatives divided by all those who have disease (i.e. the number of true positives + the number of false negatives). The false-negative rate = c/a + c, which is also equal to 1 − Sensitivity = 10%.

The specificity is d/(b + d) = 1920/1960 = 98%.

Positive predictive value is the proportion of those subjects testing positive who actually have the disease, while the negative predictive value is the proportion of those subjects testing negative who do not truly have the disease. In this instance, the positive predictive value of the new test is a/(a + b) = 36/76 = 47%.

There is thus a high false-positive result to the test: b/(a + b) = 40/76 = 53%.

10. Answer E

A forest plot is a graphical representation of multiple randomised controlled studies in a meta-analysis (Lewis and Clarke, 2001). The name refers to the forest of lines produced. Each study is plotted on a horizontal line, represented by a square according to the weight (usually the sample size) that each study contributes to the overall study. The width of the horizontal line represents the confidence interval for each study, which is usually 95%. The overall effect of all of the studies is plotted as a diamond. If the confidence interval of a study crosses the vertical line, which is called 'the line of no effect', then intervention/treatment is neither beneficial nor harmful with respect to the placebo/control.

In the example in this question, the diamond has crossed the line of no effect, which means there is no difference in the mortality in patients treated with a beta-blocker or placebo.

 Lewis, S. and Clarke, M. (2001). Forest plots: trying to see the wood and the trees. *BMJ* 322, 1479–1480.
http://www.ncbi.nlm.nih.gov/pmc/articles/PMC1120528/

 Wiysonge, C.S., Bradley, H., Mayosi, B.M., et al. (2007). Beta-blockers for hypertension. *Cochrane Database Syst Rev*, CD002003.
http://www.ncbi.nlm.nih.gov/pubmed/17253471

11. Answer B

Positive predictive value is the proportion of patients with a positive test result who are correctly diagnosed. In other words, it is the likelihood that an individual with a positive test result truly has the disease in question.

Test result	Disease status		
	Diseased	Not diseased	Total
Positive	a = True positives	b = False positives	a + b
Negative	c = False negatives	d = True negatives	c + d
Total	a + c	b + d	a + b + c + d

Formulae:

Sensitivity = $a/(a + c) \times 100$

Specificity = $d/(b + d) \times 100$

Predictive value of a positive test = $a/(a + b) \times 100$

Predictive value of a negative test = $d/(c + d) \times 100$

Percentage of false positives = $b/(b + d) \times 100$

Percentage of false negatives = $c/(a + c) \times 100$

Using the formula above, the correct answer for this question is $1800/(1800 + 4000) \times 100 = 31$.

The negative predictive value is the proportion of patients with a negative test result who are correctly diagnosed. This is the likelihood that an individual with a negative test result is truly unaffected.

Altman, D.G. and Bland, J.M. (1994). Diagnostic tests 2: predictive values. *BMJ* 309, 102.
http://www.bmj.com/content/309/6947/102.1

12. Answer D

Sensitivity and specificity are indicators of how good a diagnostic test is. The sensitivity is the proportion of people with the disease who test positive. In other words, if the person has the disease, the test result needs to be positive, i.e. 'sensitive' to the presence of disease. Specificity refers to the proportion of people without the disease who test negative. Therefore, if the person does not have the disease, the test result needs to be negative, i.e. 'specific' for the presence of disease.

If a diagnostic test has a sensitivity of 90%, specificity of 80% and the particular disease prevalence is only 1%, the following table can be constructed:

	Disease present	No disease	Total
Test positive	90	1980	2070
Test negative	10	7920	7930
Total	100	9900	10 000

If prevalence is 1%, then 100 of 10 000 will have the disease.

Given that the sensitivity is 90%, then 90 of 100 will test positive.

Given the specificity is 80%, then 7920 out of 9900 will test negative.

The false-positive rate can be calculated to be 95.7% (1980 of 2070).

13. Answer H

In the unpaired (Student's) t-test, two groups can be independent of each other, i.e. individuals randomly assigned into two groups, measured after an intervention and compared with the other group.

In the paired t-test, each member of one sample has a unique relationship with a particular member of the other sample, e.g. the same people measured before and after a new treatment.

The Mann–Whitney U-test is used for non-parametric (not normal distribution) analysis. In this study, it is assumed that both groups have normal distribution of blood pressure values.

Rank correlation co-efficients, such as Spearman's rank correlation co-efficient measure the extent to which, as one variable increases, the other variable tends to increase.

14. Answer E
The chi-square test is a non-parametric statistical technique used to determine if a distribution of observed frequencies differs from the theoretically expected frequencies. Chi-square statistics use nominal (categorical) or ordinal level data, thus instead of using means and variances, this test uses frequencies.

P value generation describes the number generated by calculation of the squared difference between the observed and expected values as a fraction of the expected values. This value is then converted to a P value relative to the degrees of freedom associated with the number of rows and columns involved. P values are useful determinates of whether an observation (or set of observations) generated is likely to be due to chance. For example, a P value of less than 0.05 is often taken to herald significance (i.e. there can be confidence that there is only a 5% risk that the data are due to chance events rather than the ordered effect of a true measurable difference).

15. Answer B
Spearman's rank correlation, named after Charles Spearman, is a non-parametric measure of statistical dependence between two variables. It assesses how well the relationship between two variables can be described using a monotonic function. If there are no repeated data values, a perfect Spearman correlation of +1 or −1 occurs when each of the variables is a perfect monotone function of the other.

18 Intensive care medicine

Questions

BASIC SCIENCE

Answers can be found in the Intensive care medicine Answers section at the end of this chapter.

1. Which one of the following effects is observed with acute metabolic acidosis?
   A. Increased cardiac contractility
   B. Decreased tissue oxygen delivery
   C. Increased adenosine triphosphate (ATP) generation
   D. Increased affinity of haemoglobin for oxygen
   E. Peripheral vasoconstriction

2. Which one of the following physiological changes commonly occurs with non-invasive ventilation in a patient with respiratory failure and chronic obstructive pulmonary disease?
   A. Reduced airway resistance
   B. Alveolar recruitment improving oxygenation
   C. Increased work of breathing
   D. Reduced left ventricular preload
   E. Reduced bronchial secretions

3. Which one of the following correctly describes the effects of norepinephrine (noradrenaline)?
   A. Norepinephrine exerts an agonist effect on $beta_2$-adrenoreceptors
   B. Norepinephrine exerts an antagonist effect on $alpha_1$-adenoreceptors
   C. Adverse effects of norepinephrine are mostly related to $alpha_2$-adrenoreceptor antagonism
   D. Norepinephrine improves blood pressure in the setting of low peripheral vascular tone
   E. Dysrhythmias are common with norepinephrine use

Passing the FRACP Written Examination: Questions and Answers, First Edition. Jonathan Gleadle, Tuck Yong, Jordan Li, Surjit Tarafdar, and Danielle Wu.
© 2013 John Wiley & Sons, Ltd. Published 2013 by John Wiley & Sons, Ltd.

Theme: Pulmonary artery catheterisation findings in states of shock (for Questions 4 and 5)

A. Haemorrhagic shock with low preload
B. Septic shock (warm shock)
C. Septic shock (cold shock)
D. Massive pulmonary embolism
E. Pericardial tamponade
F. Cardiogenic shock caused by left ventricular failure
G. Cardiogenic shock caused by acute ventricular septal defect
H. Anaphylactic shock

For each of the following scenarios, select the most likely diagnosis.

4. A 54-year-old man presents with hypotension, confusion, tachycardia and tachypnoea. Which one of the above conditions is most consistent with the following measurements on pulmonary artery catheterisation?

	Value	Reference range
Cardiac output (L/min)	4.1	5.2–7.4
Central venous pressure (mmHg)	9	2–6
Right atrial pressure (mmHg)	10	1–5
Systolic pulmonary arterial pressure (mmHg)	40	15–25
Pulmonary artery wedge pressure (mmHg)	4	5–12

5. A 70-year-old woman is hypotensive and drowsy 4 days following abdominal surgery. Which one of the above conditions is most consistent with the following measurements on pulmonary artery catheterisation?

	Value	Reference range
Cardiac output (L/min)	9	5.2–7.4
Central venous pressure (mmHg)	4	2–6
Pulmonary artery wedge pressure (mmHg)	14	5–12
Mixed venous saturation (%)*	80	65–75

*Assuming normal arterial oxygen saturation.

CLINICAL

6. Which one of the following has been associated with the best chance of survival with a good neurological outcome after an out-of-hospital cardiac arrest?
  A. Early defibrillation of ventricular fibrillation
  B. Early administration of epinephrine (adrenaline)
  C. Chest compression at a rate of 70/min
  D. Atropine to treat asystolic cardiac arrest
  E. Intravenous calcium chloride during cardiopulmonary resuscitation

7. Which one of the following therapeutic strategies can improve the survival of patients with adult respiratory distress syndrome and acute lung injury?
  A. Early high-dose corticosteroids
  B. Low frequency oscillatory ventilation
  C. Low positive end-expiratory pressure
  D. Low tidal volume ventilation
  E. Supine positioning

8. A 69-year-old woman with stage 3 chronic kidney disease due to perinuclear anti-nuclear cytoplasmic antibody (p-ANCA) associated vasculitis presented with a 24-h history of acute dyspnoea, chest discomfort and watery diarrhoea. She was commenced on azathioprine (75 mg daily) 7 days prior to presentation to replace cyclophosphamide as part of her maintenance immunosuppressive therapy. On examination, she was drowsy, temperature was 35.2 °C. She was found to be hypotensive (blood pressure of 70/40 mmHg), tachycardic (pulse rate 120 beats/min) and the extremities were cold. First and second heart sounds were present without any murmur. She received intensive intravenous fluid therapy but remained hypotensive. A pulmonary artery catheter is placed and the readings are shown below. Which of the following is the most likely diagnosis?

	Value	Reference range
Central venous pressure (mmHg)	13	0–5
Pulmonary artery pressure (mmHg)	40/14	20–25/5–10
Pulmonary capillary wedge pressure (mmHg)	22	6–12
Cardiac output (L/min)	2.2	4–8

  A. Cardiogenic shock
  B. Hypovolaemic shock
  C. Pericardial effusion
  D. Septic shock
  E. Toxic shock syndrome

9. Following acute smoke inhalation, which one of the following treatments is appropriate in the treatment of cyanide intoxication?
   A. Hyperbaric oxygen
   B. Beta-2 agonists
   C. Methylene blue
   D. Glucagon
   E. Hydroxycobalamin

10. Which one of the following treatments can improve gastric motility in critically ill patients in the intensive care unit?
   A. Diltiazem
   B. Fentanyl
   C. Rantidine
   D. Erythromycin
   E. Pantoprazole

11. A 35-year-old man, a victim of a motor vehicle accident, was found to have massive intracranial haemorrhage on computed tomography of his brain. He has been in a coma for the last 3 days in the intensive care unit and is currently on ventilator support. After talking to the family members, a decision was made to determine whether this patient fulfils the brain death criteria. Which one of the following regarding brain death testing is correct?
   A. Sedative drugs should be administered
   B. During apnoea testing, breathing is absent despite an arterial PCO_2 of greater than 60 mmHg (8 kPa) and an arterial pH of less than 7.30
   C. Four-vessel angiography is required to establish intracranial blood flow
   D. Upgoing plantar responses excludes a diagnosis of brain death
   E. There should be a minimum 2-h observation and mechanical ventilation during which the patient has unresponsive coma

12. Which one of the following should be included in the parenteral nutrition for critically ill patients?
   A. Carbohydrate as glucose of 0.5 g/kg ideal body weight/day
   B. Amino acid mixture 0.3–0.5 g/kg ideal body weight/day
   C. Lipid emulsions 1–2 g/kg ideal body weight/day
   D. Weekly multivitamins and trace elements
   E. Separate infusions of lipid from amino acid-containing mixtures

13. Which one of the following is correct concerning patient management after successful resuscitation for ventricular fibrillation cardiac arrest?
   A. Early post-resuscitation electrocardiography accurately identifies acute coronary occlusion
   B. Oxygen supplementation should be administered to achieve oxygen saturation of 85–90%

C. Mechanical ventilation should be adjusted to achieve normocarbia
D. Myocardial dysfunction after arrest is usually irreversible
E. Pyrexia after cardiac arrest is self-limiting and does not require treatment

14. Which one of the following statements is true concerning pulmonary artery catheters?
  A. The pulmonary artery wedge pressure is a measure of left atrial pressure
  B. The use of pulmonary artery catheters is associated with improved intensive care unit survival
  C. There is an increased incidence of ventricular arrhythmias
  D. Left bundle branch block is a common complication
  E. The normal pulmonary artery wedge pressure is 20–25 mmHg

15. In adult comatose patients after cardiac arrest, which one of the following parameters predicts a poor outcome?
  A. Absence of pupillary light and corneal reflexes at 72 h
  B. Absence of vestibulo-ocular reflexes at 12 h
  C. Glasgow coma scale (GCS) of less than 5 at 12 h
  D. Presence of myoclonus
  E. A computed tomography (CT) scan showing cerebral infarction

16. A 65-year-old man presented with a 3-day history of fever and dysuria. His other medical problems included type 2 diabetes, chronic kidney disease (CKD) with serum creatinine of 178 μmol/L due to diabetic nephropathy, hypertension and anaemia with a haemoglobin of 85 g/L. He was transferred to the intensive care unit 2 h after admission because of severe urosepsis (APACHE II score 30) and persistent hypotension (blood pressure 85/50 mmHg) despite intravenous fluid resuscitation. Which one of the following statements concerning treatment options is correct?
  A. Blood should be transfused to maintain a haemoglobin level above 100 g/L
  B. High-dose steroids should be administered
  C. Patients should be placed in the supine position
  D. Blood glucose level should be strictly controlled between 4.5 and 6.0 mmol/L
  E. There is no clear benefit of colloid over crystalloid fluid resuscitation

17. A 60-year-old man presents with sudden onset of palpitations. He is alert and orientated. His blood pressure is 100/70 mmHg. His cardiac rhythm is shown below. Which one of the following medications is contraindicated in this patient to correct the rhythm disturbance?

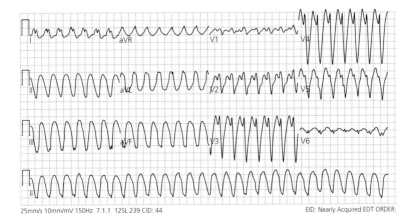

25mm/s 10mm/mV 150Hz 7.1.1 12SL 239 CID: 44   EID: Nearly Acquired EDT ORDER:

    A. Amiodarone
    B. Lignocaine
    C. Verapamil
    D. Magnesium
    E. Procainamide

18. Which one of the following factors is associated with increased chances of a successful spontaneous-breathing trial after prolonged mechanical ventilation?
    A. Pneumonia as cause of respiratory failure
    B. Chronic heart failure
    C. Upper airway stridor at extubation
    D. Partial pressure of arterial carbon dioxide of greater than 45 mmHg after extubation
    E. Daily interruption of sedative infusion

19. A 50-year-old man with cirrhosis due to hepatitis C (from past intravenous drug use) and refractory ascites is being evaluated for liver transplantation. His clinical condition is also complicated by porto-pulmonary hypertension. Which one of the following is an absolute contraindication to orthotopic liver transplantation?
    A. A single hepatocellular carcinoma lesion of 3 cm in diameter
    B. Acute kidney injury due to hepatorenal syndrome
    C. Not responsive to interferon–ribavirin treatment
    D. Pulmonary artery pressure of 55 mmHg
    E. Refractory ascites

Theme: Management of cardiac arrest and arrhythmias
(for Questions 20–23)
   A. Adenosine
   B. Epinephrine (adrenaline)
   C. Amiodarone
   D. Atropine
   E. Calcium chloride (10%)
   F. Flecainide
   G. Lignocaine
   H. Magnesium sulphate

For each of the following scenarios, select the most appropriate treatment to be administered.

20. Which one of the above is administered in the management of pulseless ventricular tachycardia that persists after three shocks?

21. Which one of the above is used in the management of torsades de pointes?

22. Which one of the above should be administered to a patient experiencing palpitations caused by rapid atrial fibrillation (AF) with an accessory pathway?

23. Which one of the above should be administered to a patient who develops ventricular tachycardia at the onset of his regular haemodialysis with pre-dialysis biochemistry showing a potassium level of 7.0 mmol/L (3.4–4.5 mmol/L)?

Answers

BASIC SCIENCE

1. Answer B

Acute metabolic acidosis is common in seriously ill patients and when severe, can be associated with a poor clinical outcome (Kraut and Madias, 2012). Therefore, rapid recognition and provision of effective therapy are essential. The majority of cases of severe metabolic acidosis are caused by lactic acidosis and ketoacidosis. This disorder is associated with the following deleterious effects:

- Decreased cardiac contractility and cardiac output
- Decreased tissue oxygen delivery
- Predisposition to cardiac arrhythmias
- Peripheral vasodilatation
- Resistance to catecholamines
- Pulmonary arterial vasoconstriction; may worsen pulmonary hypertension and induce/worsen right heart failure
- Venoconstriction
- Hypotension
- Decreased adenosine triphosphate (ATP) generation
- Impairment in glucose regulation
- Stimulation of inflammatory mediators
- Impairment of the immune response
- Impaired phagocytosis
- Increased apoptosis.
  The beneficial effects include:
- Decreased affinity of haemoglobin for oxygen. leading to favourable haemoglobin–oxygen dissociation for tissue extraction of oxygen. The reduction in 2, 3-diphosphoglycerate (2, 3-DPG) counteracts this rightward shift. Note that a severe rightward shift also may result in poor haemoglobin saturation when passing through pulmonary capillaries
- Vasodilatation of vessels with increased blood flow to tissues
- Increased ionised calcium with augmented myocardial contractility.

Kraut, J.A. and Madias, N.E. (2012). Treatment of acute metabolic acidosis: a pathophysiologic approach. *Nat Rev Nephrol* 8, 589–601.
http://www.ncbi.nlm.nih.gov/pubmed/22945490

2. Answer B

The aims of managing respiratory failure in acute exacerbation of chronic obstructive pulmonary disease (COPD) are to prevent tissue hypoxia and control acidosis and hypercapnia while medical therapy works to improve lung function and reverse the precipitating cause of the exacerbation. pH is the best marker of severity and reflects acute deterioration in alveolar hypoventilation compared with the chronic stable state.

Non-invasive ventilation (NIV) can involve continuous positive airway pressure (CPAP), whereby the patient breathes spontaneously with positive end-expiratory pressure (PEEP), or biphasic positive airway pressure (BiPAP), whereby the patient breathes spontaneously with pressure support ventilation (PSV) and PEEP. In NIV, the patient receives air or a mixture of air and oxygen from a flow generator through a full facial or nasal mask. NIV augments alveolar ventilation (reverses respiratory acidosis and hypercarbia), leads to alveolar recruitment (reverses hypoxia), decreases the work of breathing (reduces respiratory muscle insufficiency) and reduces left ventricular afterload (improves cardiac output) (Nava and Hill, 2009).

NIV as an adjunct to usual medical care significantly reduces mortality, need for endotracheal intubation, risk of treatment failure and length of hospital stay. There is good evidence for benefit of NIV in patients with moderate respiratory acidosis with a pH of 7.35 or lower and raised partial pressure of arterial carbon dioxide. NIV is contraindicated with respiratory arrest, an unprotected airway, upper airway obstruction, untreated pneumothorax, inability to clear secretions and marked haemodynamic instability.

Nava, S. and Hill, N. (2009). Non-invasive ventilation in acute respiratory failure. *Lancet* 374, 250–259.
http://www.ncbi.nlm.nih.gov/pubmed/19616722

3. Answer D

Norepinephrine (noradrenaline) is a potent sympathomimetic agent produced by postganglionic sympathetic nerve endings, which exerts agonist effects on alpha$_1$ (α_1), alpha$_2$ (α_2) and beta$_1$ (β_1) adrenoreceptors. Its β_1 effect is equipotent to epinephrine (adrenaline). Norepinephrine is used to treat hypotension caused by low peripheral vascular tone, myocardial depression or both. The combination of α_1 and β_1 stimulation increases systemic and pulmonary blood pressure, myocardial contractility and cardiac output. Blood flow may be redistributed away from skeletal muscle, the gastrointestinal tract and kidneys toward the heart and central nervous system. Heart rate can decrease because of intense α_1 stimulation. Compared with epinephrine, norepinephrine lacks β_2-adrenergic effects, which increases the potency of its vasoconstrictive actions. The adverse effects of norepinephrine are related mostly to its potent α_2 agonist effect. Intense peripheral vasoconstriction can cause organ hypoperfusion and ischaemia. Maintaining euvolaemia during norepinephrine infusion improves organ perfusion. Dysrhythmias are rare with norepinephrine use.

4. Answer D

5. Answer G

Commentary for Questions 4 and 5

Shock is a syndrome of hypotension and decreased tissue perfusion. Initially neurohormonal compensatory mechanisms maintain perfusion to vital organs. If appropriate treatment is not promptly instituted, these compensatory mechanisms are overwhelmed, producing ischaemic cellular damage and multiple organ failure and death.

Shock is classified on the basis of its cause and characteristic haemodynamic patterns:

- Hypovolaemic shock is caused by an acute loss of more than 20–25% of the circulating blood volume. An example is haemorrhagic shock from blood loss
- Cardiogenic shock is caused by primary failure of the heart to generate an adequate cardiac output
- Distributive shock is characterised by decreased vascular tone, resulting in arterial vasodilation, venous pooling and redistribution of blood flow. It may be caused by septic shock, anaphylactic shock and neurogenic shock
- Obstructive shock is associated with a mechanical impediment to venous return, arterial outflow of the heart or both. Causes include tension pneumothorax, pulmonary embolism and pericardial tamponade.

The pulmonary artery catheter passes sequentially through the vena cava, right atrium, right ventricle and into the pulmonary artery. It provides useful information, including the central venous pressure (CVP), pulmonary artery (PA) pressure, pulmonary arterial wedge pressure (PAWP), mixed venous blood chemistries and cardiac output (CO). The table below summarises the haemodynamic parameters obtained with pulmonary artery catheterisation (PAC) in different types of shock. Of note in pulmonary embolism, PA pressure is elevated but PAWP can be low. CVP higher than PAWP is a concern as it reflects significant right heart failure not due to left-sided heart failure or valvular heart disease. In ventricular septal defect, there may be a left-to-right shunt giving increased mixed venous oxygen saturation (and PAC may overestimate CO due to increased thermodilution).

	CO	CVP	RA and RV pressures	PAWP	SVR
Hypovolaemic	↓	↓	↓	↓	↑
Cardiogenic					
Left ventricular	↓	↔	↑	↑	↑
Right ventricular	↓	↑	↑	↔/↓	↑
Distributive					
Septic	Variable	↓	↔/↓	↔	↓
Anaphylactic*	↔/↑	↔	↔/↓	↓	↓
Neurogenic	↔	↔	↔/↓	↓	↓
Obstructive					
Pulmonary embolism	↓	↑	↑	↓	↑
Pericardial tamponade	↓	↑	↑	↑	↑

*Anaphylaxis can cause substantial hypovolaemia due to increased permeability and this may result in decreased cardiac output.
CO, cardiac output; CVP, central venous pressure,; PAWP, pulmonary arterial wedge pressure; PE, pulmonary embolism; PT, pericardial tamponade; RA, right atrium; RV, right ventricle; SVR, systemic vascular resistance.

CLINICAL

6. Answer A

Survival from cardiac arrest depends on a sequence of interventions: early recognition and call for help, early cardiopulmonary resuscitation (CPR), early defibrillation for ventricular fibrillation, and post-arrest care in a specialised centre (Nolan et al., 2012). It is important to distinguish between arrhythmias that are responsive to defibrillation and those that are not. High-quality CPR (chest compression depth >5 cm at a rate of >100/min: 'push hard and push fast', allowing recoil and minimising hands-off time) improves survival; feedback devices improve CPR quality but do not increase patient survival.

The use of epinephrine (adrenaline) has not been shown to improve long-term outcome but administration of epinephrine every 3–5 min during CPR is recommended in current guidelines on the basis of expert opinion.

In the past, prior to 2010, atropine was used to treat asystolic cardiac arrest but because of studies showing no benefit, this is no longer recommended during CPR.

Intravenous calcium chloride might have toxic effects on an ischaemic myocardium and might impair neurological recovery, and is therefore given only to patients with hypocalcaemia, hyperkalaemia or an overdose with a calcium antagonist.

Nolan, J.P., Soar, J., Wenzel, V., and Paal, P. (2012). Cardiopulmonary resuscitation and management of cardiac arrest. *Nat Rev Cardiol* 9, 499–511. http://www.ncbi.nlm.nih.gov/pubmed/22665327

7. Answer D

Acute respiratory distress syndrome (ARDS) and its milder form, acute lung injury (ALI), are lung diseases characterised by a severe inflammatory process causing diffuse alveolar damage and resulting in ventilation–perfusion mismatch, severe hypoxaemia and poor lung compliance (Dushianthan et al., 2011). The treatment of ARDS involves general supportive measures (e.g. infection control, early enteral nutrition, stress ulcer prophylaxis and thromboprophylaxis) combined with focused ventilator strategies and treatment of the underlying conditions. There are no effective pharmacological therapies for ARDS.

The main supportive therapy for ARDS is positive pressure mechanical ventilation, which helps to ensure adequate oxygenation. Early ventilation strategies involved volume-controlled ventilation with a tidal volume (Vt) of 10–15 mL/kg to achieve 'normal' arterial blood gases. However, ventilation itself can cause lung injury. Studies demonstrate the importance of using a lower Vt to ventilate the injured lung as opposed to aiming to normalise blood gas variables. The optimal level of positive end-expiratory pressure (PEEP) in ventilated patients with ARDS/ALI remains controversial. PEEP helps to recruit alveolar units and reduces alveoli collapse due to alveolar flooding, and thereby reduces ventilation–perfusion mismatch. Again, the level of PEEP needed to achieve optimal recruitment without causing alveolar over-distension and damage is not established. Of the therapeutic strategies directed specifically at the condition of ARDS and ALI, low-Vt ventilation is the least controversial and widely accepted as standard treatment.

Use of high-dose corticosteroids in patients with early ARDS show equivocal results in decreasing mortality; however, there is some evidence that these drugs may reduce organ dysfunction score, lung injury score, ventilator requirement and intensive care unit stay.

 Dushianthan, A., Grocott, M.P., Postle, A.D., and Cusack, R. (2011). Acute respiratory distress syndrome and acute lung injury. *Postgrad Med J* 87, 612–622.
http://pmj.bmj.com/content/87/1031/612.long

8. Answer A

This patient has cardiogenic shock, manifested by hypotension and evidence of hypoperfusion (decreased mental status and cold extremities). The pulmonary artery catheter results demonstrate volume overload as the central venous and pulmonary capillary wedge pressures are elevated (Summerhill and Baram, 2005). The volume overload and low cardiac output are most consistent with cardiogenic shock.

Septic shock and toxic shock syndrome are types of distributive shock, result from a severe decrease in systemic vascular resistance, and often associated with an increased cardiac output and low pulmonary capillary wedge pressure. Toxic shock syndrome is a rare, life-threatening complication of bacterial infection resulting from toxins produced by *Staphylococcus aureus*, but the condition may also be caused by toxins produced by Group A streptococcus bacteria. Hypovolaemic shock is associated with reduced pulmonary wedge pressure, cardiac output, central venous pressure and pulmonary artery pressure. In significant pericardial effusion leading to tamponade, near equalisation (within 5 mmHg) of the right atrial, right ventricular diastolic, pulmonary arterial diastolic and pulmonary capillary wedge pressures (reflecting left atrial pressure) occurs. The right atrial pressure tracings display a prominent systolic *x* descent and the systolic *y* descent is abolished.

 Summerhill, E.M. and Baram, M. (2005). Principles of pulmonary artery catheterization in the critically ill. *Lung* 183, 209–219.
http://www.ncbi.nlm.nih.gov/pubmed/16078042

9. Answer E

Cyanide intoxication should be considered in patients with smoke inhalation, measured and antidotes, such as hydroxycobalamin, administered if present (Toon et al., 2010). Alternate antidotes such as sodium thiosulphate can be used, but theoretical concerns exist about their potential for the generation of methaemoglobin. Thermal decomposition of nitrogen-containing plastics and polymers can produce smoke containing hydrogen cyanide.

Hyperbaric oxygenation with oxygen delivered at 3 atm is able to reduce the half-life of carbon monoxide from 320 to 20 min. However, data are lacking on the efficacy of this technique. In acute smoke inhalation, pulmonary insults can be delivered by particulates, respiratory irritants and systemic toxins, such as carbon monoxide and cyanide. Smoke inhalation is responsible for the majority of fire-related deaths.

In the management of acute smoke inhalation, high-flow 100% oxygen should be administered immediately via facemask to reduce carboxyhaemoglobin levels as soon as possible (reduces the half-life of carboxyhaemoglobin from 4 h to about 45 min). Securing the airway is vital, which may be compromised by direct thermal injury, oedema or impaired consciousness. Depending on the severity of injury and symptoms, the patient may need to be intubated and ventilated with 100% oxygen. In the case of bronchospasm, nebulised administration of bronchodilators, such as beta$_2$-agonists, improves respiratory mechanics by decreasing airflow resistance and peak airway pressures and have anti-inflammatory properties.

Toon, M.H., Maybauer, M.O., Greenwood, J.E., Maybauer, D.M., and Fraser, J.F. (2010). Management of acute smoke inhalation injury. *Crit Care Resusc* 12, 53–61.
http://www.ncbi.nlm.nih.gov/pubmed/20196715

10. Answer D

The enteral route is the preferred route for delivering nutrition to the critically ill. However, many patients remain intolerant of gastric feeding, with the predominant mechanism being delayed gastric emptying (Deane et al., 2009). This may lead to under-nutrition and increase gastro-oesophageal reflux. Gastric emptying in the critically ill is delayed because of impaired function of the proximal and distal stomach and pylorus, as well as disordered activity in the duodenum. Drug therapy to accelerate gastric emptying can improve the delivery of enteral nutrition: alternatively post-pylorus feeding tubes can be placed.

Currently, combination therapy with intravenous erythromycin and metoclopramide is an effective drug therapy for feed intolerance. This regimen may increase the incidence of diarrhoea. It also has the potential to promote bacterial resistance, but this has not been demonstrated and its clinical importance is unclear. Future therapies may include non-antibiotic motilin agonists, opioid and cholecystokinin antagonists, neostigmine and exogenous ghrelin.

Deane, A.M., Fraser, R.J., and Chapman, M.J. (2009). Prokinetic drugs for feed intolerance in critical illness: current and potential therapies. *Crit Care Resusc 11*, 132–143.
http://www.ncbi.nlm.nih.gov/pubmed/19485878

11. Answer B

The Australian and New Zealand Intensive Care Society (ANZICS) has established clinical guidelines to determine brain death. These should be carried out by two medical practitioners with the requisite knowledge, skills and experience. Some states in Australia require the medical practitioners to have at least 5 years of working experience and at least one person being a specialist not involved in organ retrieval. In Australia and New Zealand, whole brain death is required for the legal determination of death. This contrasts with the United Kingdom, where brain-stem death is the standard. Determination of brain-stem death requires unresponsive coma, the absence of brain-stem reflexes and the absence of respiratory centre function in the clinical setting in which these findings are irreversible. In particular, there must be definite clinical or neuro-imaging evidence of acute brain pathology (e.g. traumatic brain injury, intracranial haemorrhage, hypoxic encephalopathy) consistent with the irreversible loss of neurological function.

Certain preconditions have to be met before brain death testing:
- Absence of hypothermia (temperature is >35°C)
- Adequate blood pressure (e.g. systolic blood pressure >90 mmHg, mean arterial pressure >60 mmHg in an adult)
- Sedative drug effects are excluded
- No severe electrolyte, metabolic or endocrine disturbance
- Intact neuromuscular function
- It is possible to examine the brain-stem reflexes (including at least one ear and one eye)
- It is possible to perform apnoea testing.

For clinical testing there should be a minimum of 4 h observation and mechanical ventilation during which the patient has unresponsive coma (Glasgow coma score of 3), with pupils non-reactive to light, an absent cough/tracheal reflex and no spontaneous breathing efforts.

1. No motor response in the cranial nerve distribution to noxious stimulation of the face, trunk and four limbs, and no response in the trunk or limbs to noxious stimulation within the cranial nerve distribution
2. No pupillary responses to light
3. Absence of corneal reflexes
4. Absence of gag (pharyngeal) reflex
5. Absence of cough (tracheal) reflex
6. No vestibulo-ocular reflexes on ice-cold caloric testing
7. Breathing is absent [despite arterial PCO_2 >60 mmHg (8 kPa) and arterial pH < 7.30]
8. Specify PCO_2 in mmHg or kPa and pH at end of apnoea.

To determine brain death when clinical examination cannot be done, the absence of intracranial blood flow needs to be demonstrated by either intra-arterial angiography or another reliable method, but is not a routine part of testing.

Australian and New Zealand Intensive Care Society. The ANZICS Statement on Death and Organ Donation (Edition 3.1). Melbourne: ANZICS, 2010. http://www.anzics.com.au/death-and-organ-donation

12. Answer C

In the intensive care unit (ICU), patients have increased metabolic needs related to stress, which are likely to accelerate the development of malnutrition, a condition associated with poorer clinical outcomes. Therefore, it is recommended that all patients who are not expected to be on normal nutrition within 3 days should receive parenteral nutrition within 24–48 h if enteral nutrition is contraindicated or if they cannot tolerate enteral nutrition (Singer et al., 2009).

The minimal amount of carbohydrate required is about 2 g/kg of glucose/day. Hyperglycaemia (blood glucose >10 mmol/L) contributes to death in critically ill patients and should be avoided to prevent infectious complications. Studies have shown conflicting outcomes in ICU patients when blood glucose is maintained between 4.5 and 6.1 mmol/L. There is a higher incidence of severe hypoglycaemia in patients treated to the tighter limits, but clear recommendations are lacking. A balanced amino acid mixture of 1.3–1.5 g/kg ideal body weight/day should be administered and should include 0.2–0.4 g/kg/day of L-glutamine. Lipids should be an integral part of parenteral nutrition for energy and to ensure essential fatty acid provision in long-term ICU patients. Essential fatty acids are not synthesised within the human body and must be supplied. All parenteral nutrition prescriptions should include a daily dose of multivitamins and of trace elements. Previously, lipid emulsions were given separately but it is becoming more common for a single solution of glucose, proteins and lipids to be administered.

 Singer, P., Berger, M.M., Van den Berghe, G., et al. (2009). ESPEN Guidelines on Parenteral Nutrition: intensive care. *Clin Nutr* 28, 387–400.
http://www.ncbi.nlm.nih.gov/pubmed/19505748

13. Answer C

Care after cardiac arrest and return of spontaneous circulation (ROSC) substantially influences patient outcomes (Nolan et al., 2012). An 'ABCDE' (airway, breathing, circulation, disability and exposure) approach can be used to identify and treat organ failure. 'Exposure' refers to the need for a comprehensive head-to-toe assessment.

The inspired oxygen concentration immediately after ROSC should be adjusted to achieve normal arterial oxygen saturation (94–98%) when measured by pulse oximetry and arterial blood-gas analysis. Ventilation should be adjusted to achieve normocarbia and monitored using the end-tidal carbon dioxide with waveform capnography and arterial blood gases.

In the setting of cardiac arrest, an early post-resuscitation 12-lead electrocardiogram (ECG) is less reliable for diagnosing acute coronary occlusion than in patients without cardiac arrest. Performing immediate coronary artery angiography in all patients with out-of-hospital cardiac arrest and no obvious non-cardiac cause of arrest, regardless of ECG changes, is becoming increasingly common. Post-cardiac arrest myocardial dysfunction can be severe, but usually resolves after 48–72 h, but this depends on pre-existing dysfunction. In patients with severe cardiogenic shock, an intra-aortic balloon pump should be considered.

Recovery of brain function can be maximised by using targeted temperature management, optimising cerebral perfusion, and controlling seizures and blood glucose levels. Pyrexia associated with systemic inflammatory response is common in the first 48 h after cardiac arrest, and is associated with poor outcome. Therefore, post-cardiac arrest pyrexia should be actively treated and prevented where possible. Mild hypothermia improves outcome after a period of global cerebral hypoxia–ischaemia and it also decreases the cerebral oxygen requirements.

Nolan, J.P., Soar, J., Wenzel, V., and Paal, P. (2012). Cardiopulmonary resuscitation and management of cardiac arrest. *Nat Rev Cardiol* 9, 499–511. http://www.ncbi.nlm.nih.gov/pubmed/22665327

14. Answer A
The following parameters can be measured with a pulmonary arterial catheter: temperature, central venous pressure, right atrial pressure, right ventricular pressures, pulmonary artery pressures, pulmonary artery occlusion pressure, cardiac output and mixed venous sampling.

The pulmonary artery wedge pressure (PAWP) tracing is obtained by inflating the balloon at the distal tip of the catheter, allowing the balloon to obstruct blood flow through a branch of the pulmonary artery. This creates a column of blood between the catheter tip and the left atrium, equilibrating pressure between them so that the pressure at the distal end of the catheter (the PAWP) is equal to that of the left atrium. The PAWP, which is also known as the pulmonary capillary wedge pressure or pulmonary artery occlusion pressure, varies from 6 to 15 mmHg, with a mean of 9 mmHg. The PAWP can estimate the left ventricular end-diastolic pressure (i.e. the left ventricular preload) if there is no obstruction to flow between the left atrium and left ventricle. A variety of haemodynamic and clinical problems can reduce the reliability of this estimate, including mitral valve disease, reduced left ventricular compliance and pulmonary disease.

In intensive care unit patients, heart failure patients and patients undergoing high-risk surgery, the use of pulmonary artery catheters has not been shown to improve survival. Right bundle branch block is a complication of catheter insertion, placing patients with pre-existing left bundle branch block at risk of complete heart block. Ventricular and supraventricular tachycardias are well-recognised complications.

15. Answer A
It is impossible to predict accurately the degree of neurological recovery during or immediately after a cardiac arrest. The neurological examination during cardiac arrest is not helpful in predicting outcome and should not be used. Furthermore, there are no clinical neurological signs that reliably predict poor outcome less than 24 h after cardiac arrest. After cessation of sedation (and/or induced hypothermia), the probability of awakening decreases with each day of coma.

In adult patients who are comatose after cardiac arrest, and who have not been treated with hypothermia and who do not have confounding factors (such as hypotension, sedatives or neuromuscular blockers), the absence of both pupillary light and corneal reflex at 72 h or longer reliably predicts a poor outcome. Absence of vestibulo-ocular reflexes at 24 h or longer and a Glasgow coma motor score of 2 or less at 72 h or longer are less reliable. Other clinical signs, including myoclonus, are not recommended for predicting poor outcome. The presence of myoclonus status in adults was strongly associated with poor outcome, but rare cases of good neurological recovery have been described and accurate diagnosis was problematic. There is insufficient evidence that neuro-imaging or blood tests can accurately predict outcome.

ARC and NZRC Guideline 2010. (2011). Post-resuscitation therapy in adult advanced life support. *Emerg Med Australas* 23, 292–296.
http://onlinelibrary.wiley.com/doi/10.1111/j.1742-6723.2011.01422_15.x/full

16. Answer E

There is good evidence that early resuscitation in patients with severe sepsis or septic shock improves outcome (Annane et al., 2005; Dellinger et al., 2008). Supine body positioning is a risk factor for nosocomial pneumonia in mechanically ventilated patients, a semi-recumbent position reduces the risk. Studies show that transfusion of blood to critically ill patients to maintain a haemoglobin level of greater than 100 g/L does not improve outcome. However, a haemoglobin concentration of less than 70 g/L has become a more widely accepted threshold after the Transfusion Requirements in Critical Care (TRICC) trial. This trial randomised 838 critically ill patients to either a restrictive transfusion strategy (transfusion threshold of <70 g/L) or a liberal transfusion strategy (threshold of <100 g/L) and found that the restrictive strategy decreased in-hospital mortality. Whilst glycaemic control is important, an intensive insulin regimen to keep the level between 4.4 and 6.0 mmol/L has not shown a beneficial effect on mortality. In critically ill patients, a target blood glucose of 4.4–6.1 mmol/L increased the incidence of severe hypoglycaemia, and either increased mortality or had no effect on mortality, when compared to the more permissive blood glucose ranges of 7.8–10 mmol/L. Studies do not support the routine use of steroids in septic shock, but some advocate their use in patients with increasing vasopressor requirements and failure of other therapeutic strategies. There is no clear benefit of colloid over crystalloid fluid resuscitation, but crystalloid redistributes rapidly into the whole extracellular volume, hence larger volumes must be given for intravascular resuscitation.

Annane, D., Bellissant, E., and Cavaillon, J.M. (2005). Septic shock. *Lancet* 365, 63–78.
http://www.ncbi.nlm.nih.gov/pubmed/15639681

Dellinger, R.P., Levy, M.M., Carlet, J.M., et al. (2008). Surviving Sepsis Campaign: international guidelines for management of severe sepsis and septic shock: 2008. *Intensive Care Med 34*, 17–60.
http://www.ncbi.nlm.nih.gov/pmc/articles/PMC2249616/

17. Answer C

All these medications can be useful agents in the treatment of ventricular tachycardia (VT), except for verapamil. Verapamil is contraindicated in this case because it can cause the blood pressure to fall due to negative inotropic action (Roberts-Thomson et al., 2011).

The initial management of a patient with sustained monomorphic VT caused by underlying structural heart disease is determined by the patient's symptoms and haemodynamic state. Direct-current cardioversion is warranted for sustained VT, which produces symptomatic hypotension, pulmonary oedema or myocardial ischemia. Reversible causes of VT, such as electrolyte imbalances, acute ischaemia, hypoxia and drug toxicities, should be corrected.

In patients who are haemodynamically stable, pharmacological reversion of VT can be attempted. Lignocaine can be useful in VT associated with ischaemia or myocardial infarction. However, in patients with slow and stable VT, the efficacy of lignocaine is limited. Intravenous procainamide is an appropriate therapy in these patients, as it rapidly slows and terminates VT. Although procainamide is successful for acute arrhythmia termination in around 75% of patients with sustained monomorphic VT, its use can be limited by hypotension, which occurs in approximately 20% of these individuals. Amiodarone is also useful, but its onset of action is slower than that of lignocaine or procainamide, and the results of acute termination studies have been variable. Transvenous catheter pace termination, by application of ventricular pacing at a faster rate than the VT ('overdrive'), can also be performed to treat sustained VT. The most common form of idiopathic VT is focal VT arising from the right ventricular outflow tract, which accounts for approximately 60–70% of idiopathic VTs. These focal VTs can manifest as recurrent premature ventricular contractions or paroxysmal monomorphic VT, usually with left bundle branch block morphology and a marked inferior axis. Patients, who are typically aged 30–50 years, often present with palpitations and, occasionally, presyncope. The treatment of patients with focal VT depends on the frequency and severity of symptoms, as this condition has a benign course in the vast majority, with a low incidence of sudden cardiac death. Patients with minimal symptoms do not necessarily need treatment. For those with severe symptoms or those who have developed a tachycardia-mediated cardiomyopathy, the options include pharmacological therapy or radiofrequency catheter ablation. Acute termination of focal VT can be achieved by vagal manoeuvres, such as carotid sinus massage.

Roberts-Thomson, K.C., Lau, D.H., and Sanders, P. (2011). The diagnosis and management of ventricular arrhythmias. *Nat Rev Cardiol* 8, 311–321.
http://www.ncbi.nlm.nih.gov/pubmed/21343901

18. Answer E

Approximately 15% of patients in whom mechanical ventilation is discontinued require re-intubation within 48 h (McConville and Kress, 2012). Rates of extubation failure vary considerably among intensive care units (ICUs). For example, the average rate of failed extubation in surgical ICUs ranges from 5% to 8%, whereas it is often as high as 17% in medical or neurological ICUs. Patients who require re-intubation have an increased risk of death, a prolonged hospital stay and a decreased likelihood of returning home, as compared with patients in whom discontinuation of mechanical ventilation is successful.

Risk factors for unsuccessful discontinuation of mechanical ventilation include:
- Failure of two or more consecutive spontaneous-breathing trials
- Chronic heart failure
- Partial pressure of arterial carbon dioxide of greater than 45 mmHg after extubation
- More than one co-existing condition other than heart failure
- Weak cough
- Upper airway stridor at extubation
- Age 65 years or older
- Acute Physiology and Chronic Health Evaluation (APACHE) II score of greater than 12 on the day of extubation
- Pneumonia as the cause of respiratory failure.

Treatment approaches include a progressive reduction of ventilator assistance. Increasingly, tracheostomy is performed in patients who require prolonged weaning. However, the timing of tracheostomy remains controversial. Potential advantages of tracheostomy include easier airway suctioning and improvements in the patient's comfort and ability to communicate. Although some studies have suggested that early tracheostomy might reduce short-term mortality, the length of stay in the ICU and the incidence of pneumonia, others have not shown such benefits. A recent meta-analysis led to the conclusion that there is insufficient evidence to warrant a recommendation for early tracheostomy.

Daily interruption of sedative infusion has been associated with reduction of the duration of mechanical ventilation.

Trials of spontaneous breathing assess a patient's ability to breathe while receiving minimal respiratory support. To accomplish this, ventilators are switched from full respiratory support modes, such as volume-assist control or pressure control, to ventilatory modes, such as pressure support, continuous positive airway pressure (CPAP) or ventilation with a T-piece (in which there is no positive end-expiratory pressure). Ideally, a trial of spontaneous breathing is initiated while the patient is awake and not receiving sedative infusions.

For a spontaneous-breathing trial to be successful, a patient must breathe spontaneously with little or no ventilator support for at least 30 min without any of the following:
- Respiratory rate of more than 35 breaths/min for more than 5 min
- Oxygen saturation of less than 90%
- Heart rate of more than 140 beats/min

- Sustained change in the heart rate of 20%
- Systolic blood pressure of more than 180 mmHg or less than 90 mmHg
- Increased anxiety or diaphoresis.

McConville, J.F. and Kress, J.P. (2012). Weaning patients from the ventilator. *N Engl J Med* 367, 2233–2239.
http://www.ncbi.nlm.nih.gov/pubmed/23215559

19. Answer D

The ultimate treatment for cirrhosis and end-stage liver disease is liver transplantation (Schuppan and Afdhal, 2008). Once decompensation has occurred in all types of liver disease, mortality without transplantation is as high as 85% over 5 years. Porto-pulmonary hypertension (defined by the co-existence of portal and pulmonary hypertension) is rare, but occurs in up to 16–20% of patients with refractory ascites. The development of porto-pulmonary hypertension seems to be independent of the cause of portal hypertension. Although most patients with porto-pulmonary hypertension have cirrhosis as the underlying disease, the syndrome has been described in patients with portal hypertension due to non-hepatic causes, such as portal venous thrombosis in the absence of chronic hepatic disease. Thus, portal hypertension seems to be the required driving force of pulmonary hypertension. The mechanisms by which portal hypertension causes pulmonary hypertension remain incompletely understood. The development of severe pulmonary hypertension in patients who have cirrhosis is an ominous prognostic sign. The condition is deemed irreversible and a pulmonary artery pressure of more than 40 mmHg precludes liver transplantation.

Other absolute contraindications include:
- Extrahepatic malignant disease
- AIDS responding poorly to highly active anti-retroviral therapy
- Cholangiocarcinoma
- Severe uncontrolled systemic infection
- Multiorgan failure
- Active substance abuse.

The Milan criteria suggest that the mortality and recurrence of hepatocellular carcinoma is acceptable if liver transplantation is done for either a single tumour of less than 5 cm in diameter, or no more than three tumours with the largest being less than 3 cm in diameter. Recurrence of infection with hepatitis C virus is universal following liver transplantation, with an accelerated natural history compared with hepatitis C infection in immunocompetent patients.

Schuppan, D. and Afdhal, N.H. (2008). Liver cirrhosis. *Lancet* 371, 838–851.
http://www.ncbi.nlm.nih.gov/pmc/articles/PMC2271178/

20. Answer C
Amiodarone is an anti-arrhythmic drug with complex pharmacokinetics and pharmacodynamics. It has effects on sodium, potassium and calcium channels, as well as alpha- and beta-adrenergic blocking properties. Two randomised trials demonstrated the benefit of amiodarone over conventional care, which included lignocaine in 80% of cases, or routine use of lignocaine for shock refractory, recurrent ventricular tachycardia (VT) or ventricular fibrillation (VF), for the endpoint of survival to hospital admission, but not to survival to hospital discharge (Nolan et al., 2012).

Additional studies have reported improvement in defibrillation response when amiodarone is given to patients with VF or haemodynamically unstable VT. In view of the short-term benefits, amiodarone should be considered for refractory VF or VT. There is little evidence to suggest a survival-to-discharge advantage with any anti-arrhythmic drug used during resuscitation from out-of-hospital or in-hospital cardiac arrest. Amiodarone is given intravenously with an initial dose of 300 mg. An additional dose of 150 mg could be considered. This may be followed by an infusion at a rate of 15 mg/kg over 24 h.

Amiodarone is recommended following the third shock; however, in situations where two or three stacked shocks are given in the first 'round', amiodarone is not given until two further shocks, with 2 min of cardiopulmonary resuscitation in between each round, have been given.

Nolan, J.P., Soar, J., Wenzel, V., and Paal, P. (2012). Cardiopulmonary resuscitation and management of cardiac arrest. *Nat Rev Cardiol* 9, 499–511. http://www.ncbi.nlm.nih.gov/pubmed/22665327

21. Answer H
Magnesium is an electrolyte that is essential for membrane stability. Hypomagnesaemia causes myocardial hyperexcitability, particularly in the presence of hypokalaemia and digoxin. Compared with placebo, magnesium has not been shown to increase return of spontaneous circulation (ROSC) or survival for patients in VF in the pre-hospital, intensive care and emergency department settings. Magnesium should be given for hypomagnesaemia and torsades de pointes, but there is insufficient data for or against its routine use in cardiac arrest.

22. Answer F
The goals of acute drug therapy for rapid atrial fibrillation (AF) with an accessory pathway are prompt control of the ventricular response and stabilisation of the haemodynamic state (Link, 2012). Treatment of AF with an accessory pathway requires a parenteral drug with rapid onset of action that lengthens antegrade refractoriness and slows conduction in both the AV node/His–Purkinje system and the accessory pathway. Treatment is not to differentially block the AV node as this may increase antegrade conduction down the accessory pathway and accelerate the ventricular rate. Flecainide is effective at slowing conduction through both

normal pathways as well as accessory pathways, and is therefore less prone to diverting conduction toward the accessory path. It also has greater effect at higher atrial rates. It is a potent inhibitor of sodium channels and therefore slows conduction. The effect of flecainide can be seen as lengthening of the PR interval and widening of the QRS complex on the electrocardiogram. Flecainide is also known to be negatively inotropic and may result in bradycardia and hypotension. Other side effects include visual blurring and oral paraesthesiae. Cardioversion is required for haemodynamically unstable patients.

 Link, M.S. (2012). Clinical practice. Evaluation and initial treatment of supraventricular tachycardia. *N Engl J Med* 367, 1438–1448.
http://www.ncbi.nlm.nih.gov/pubmed/23050527

23. Answer E
Calcium is essential for normal muscle and nerve activity. It transiently increases peripheral resistance, myocardial excitability and contractility. Calcium may have toxic effects on an ischaemic myocardium. Therefore, it is to be given only to patients with hypocalcaemia, hyperkalaemia or who have overdosed on a calcium antagonist. Randomised controlled trials and observational studies have demonstrated no survival benefit when calcium was given to in-hospital or out-of-hospital cardiac arrest patients. In ventricular fibrillation, calcium did not restore spontaneous circulation.

Hyperkalaemia raises the resting membrane potential, causing a narrowing between resting membrane potential and threshold potential for action potential (AP) generation. Calcium restores this initial narrowing back towards 15 mV by raising the threshold potential to being 'less negative'. APs generated from less negative voltages are slower since sodium channels in phase 0 are voltage dependent for velocity (Vmax). Calcium restores Vmax, resulting in improvement in ECG changes within minutes of administration.

Index

Note: Page numbers in normal type refer to questions, Page numbers in **bold** refer to answers. Alphabetical order is letter-by-letter so that spaces are ignored. For example, 'J wave' comes after 'Jod-Basedow effect'.

Passing the FRACP Written Examination: Questions and Answers, First Edition. Jonathan Gleadle, Tuck Yong, Jordan Li, Surjit Tarafdar, and Danielle Wu.
© 2013 John Wiley & Sons, Ltd. Published 2013 by John Wiley & Sons, Ltd.